Goodbye DIABETES

preventing and reversing diabetes the natural way

DR. WES YOUNGBERG
with ELISE HARBOLDT, RN

Hart Books

PO Box 2377, Fallbrook, CA 92088 · (800) 487-4278

The author assumes full responsibility for the accuracy of all facts and quotations as cited in this book.

Editors: Conna L. Bond and Nicole M. Batten
Design: Mark A. Bond
Typeset: 11/15 Dante

PRINTED IN U.S.A.

1 2 3 4 5 6 7 8 9 10

Youngberg, Wes
Goodbye Diabetes: preventing and reversing diabetes the natural way / Wes Youngberg with Elise Harboldt—2nd ed.
Includes bibliographical references and index.
ISBN: 978-1-878046-42-0
1. Health—Health Concerns. 2. Health—Diabetes

To order additional copies of *Goodbye Diabetes* by Dr. Wes Youngberg, call 1-800-487-4278 or visit www.goodbyediabetes.com.

CONTENTS

—Praise for Goodbye Diabetes—

"Diabesity, like a huge earthquake at the bottom of the sea, is causing an enormous and dangerous tsunami that is already beginning to wash up on nations worldwide. This silent, devastating epidemic is forecast to not only overwhelm the world's healthcare resources, but also its economies in lost productivity and additional medical costs. But, unlike the tsunami caused by an earthquake on the sea floor, this epidemic can be turned around. Yes! The vast majority of diabetes is reversible. The devastating effects of the diabesity tsunami are not inevitable.

"I believe *Goodbye Diabetes* is destined to help reverse this dangerous epidemic. It is well-written and easy to read. It is well-documented and evidence-based. It is clinically savvy and based on years of clinical success using lifestyle change to treat diabetes and related chronic diseases.

"I recommend this book for all who want to help turn back the tsunami of diabesity and diabetes crashing upon the world. Read it, follow its solid advice, and share it with others. We will all be glad you did. It is no exaggeration to say our future just may depend upon it."

John Kelly, MD, MPH
Founding President, American College of Lifestyle Medicine
Co-Investigator, Diabetes Wellness Research for the Marshall Islands

---

"Type 2 diabetes is much more than just a sugar problem. In this book, Dr. Youngberg lays out the scientific evidence in a simple yet practical way, showing the many causes and effects of this disease. His practical treatment experience is presented in real-life stories from his own lifestyle medicine practice. These stories demonstrate that effective lifestyle treatment of type 2 diabetes is doable and beneficial. *Goodbye Diabetes* is a great resource for educating my patients about what needs to be done to really treat type 2 diabetes."

George Guthrie, MD, MPH, CDE, CNS
Department of Family Medicine, Florida Hospital

"A delightfully hopeful look at what could be a devastating diagnosis. Dr. Youngberg outlines solid scientific evidence for the benefits of a healthy lifestyle and gives practical suggestions for change. Be fascinated by the content, persistently practice it, and enjoy your life to the fullest."

Betty Jo Vercio, RN, MS, CDE
Diabetes Educator, Adventist Health Medical Group
Walla Walla, Washington

—Foreword—

by Richard Hart, MD, DrPH

America is slowly and unwittingly committing suicide. Type 2 diabetes, heart disease, and other preventable conditions are increasing at alarming rates. For the first time in centuries, American children may have shorter lifespans than their parents. This epidemic of lifestyle disease is cause for serious concern. It calls for deliberate and aggressive action.

In this clearly written plan for optimal health, Dr. Youngberg has outlined the powerful tools needed to prevent or reverse these debilitating lifestyle diseases. Sprinkled liberally with patient case histories and practical suggestions, this book outlines a pathway that is easy to understand. The author has also provided numerous references to document his recommendations.

Through the years, I have watched Wes's career and admired his ability to distill complex information into a user-friendly format. *Goodbye Diabetes* is the result of years working with patients who needed both information and courage to make fundamental lifestyle changes. Through the pages of this book, you can sense both Wes' enthusiasm and his patients' gratitude for the dramatic health improvements they have experienced.

The beauty of *Goodbye Diabetes* is its emphasis on simple changes that can make a profound difference. These strategies are available to all, regardless of income or accessibility to healthcare. From defining diabetes through debunking, detecting, and finally defeating diabetes, these improvements are simple, practical, and possible.

The lifestyle changes outlined in this book are supported by ample scientific evidence. They are the most effective treatments for diabetes and prediabetes. Dr. Youngberg has successfully packaged this information in a clear and engaging way. His important contribution will be a valuable tool in the battle against lifestyle disease.

In discussing the potential benefits of nutritional supplements, Dr. Youngberg emphasizes that supplements may have a secondary role in diabetes management but should not be used as substitutes for the far more effective strategies of diet, exercise, and other lifestyle interventions. Using a supplement as an excuse for a poor diet will not bring the results hoped for. Fortunately, moving toward a plant-based diet will fulfill the majority of nutrient requirements.

For over 100 years, Loma Linda University has been at the forefront in research and promotion of healthy living. As a former professor of Dr. Youngberg's, I am very pleased with his important contribution to health promotion.

An old Afghan proverb says, "Drop by drop, we make a river." America desperately needs a river of social support, public-health education, commercial initiative, media attention, and community enthusiasm to save us from our current lifestyle. This takes teamwork. Our faith-based communities can be involved. Our school systems need to catch the message and change the way that children eat and play as they grow. Our restaurants need to cater to health, not just to sales, tastes, and appetites. Our medical community needs to slow down and take the time to help individuals address the source of their problems, instead of just masking hypertension or diabetes symptoms with more pills. We must move beyond the latest popular prescriptions and their billion dollar markets to a realistic understanding of the cause, prevention, and reversal of disease.

Can it be done? Absolutely. We have tackled similar challenges before. Our successes in tobacco cessation point the way to a combined approach that engages all sectors of society in this battle. Perhaps healthcare reform and "bundled payments" will motivate the medical community to devote more time and energy to wellness and prevention. Even more likely, patients and the public at large will demand more for the protection of their health.

I truly hope *Goodbye Diabetes* becomes a must-read for all those who are committed to a healthy and productive life, for themselves and those they love.

Richard Hart, MD, DrPH
President, Loma Linda University

—Introduction—

Don't deny the diagnosis. Defy the verdict.
—Norman Cousins

"Don't get your hopes up about this island, Dr. Youngberg. People won't follow your advice. Diabetes is just part of the culture."

I had just moved my family across the Pacific Ocean to the beautiful island of Guam. My goal was to teach the Guamanian and Micronesian people how to better care for their health. At the time, the island was facing a staggering health crisis. Diabetes death rates were nearly five times higher than in the U.S. mainland. Obesity and heart disease were skyrocketing. Thousands of people were suffering and dying from diseases that I knew were preventable and reversible. I wanted to be part of the solution.

Two days after my arrival, I was told it couldn't be done. This well-meaning physician explained to me that the only thing the medical community could offer the islanders was to support them through the inevitable complications of type 2 diabetes.

Dialysis could help. Insulin could help. Coronary angioplasty and vascular stenting could help. But preventing or reversing the disease process? Impossible!

I took this physician's comment as a challenge to prove him wrong. I worked with a fantastic team to develop an outpatient diabetes-reversal program, collaborated with government officials to improve diabetes screening guidelines, and promoted health education in the community.

But more importantly, I worked with people. People whose lives had been devastated by the nightmare of diabetes. People who had been taught to believe that disease was their destiny. People who deserved to know the truth about how disease was caused and how it could be prevented or reversed.

I watched these people experience the miracle of transformation. I saw the light come back into their eyes as they realized they could take control of their health, one choice at a time. I saw blood sugars stabilize, pounds melt away, cholesterol and blood fats normalize. I saw the joy that people experience when the burden of disease is lifted and life becomes full of new possibilities.

Did every person on the island change? No. But many did. The legend is told of a young man who frequently walked the beach after the tide came in, picking up washed up starfish, then throwing them back to the sea. When asked what he was doing, the young man replied: "The sun is up, and the tide is going out. If I don't throw them in, they'll die." The questioner responded: "Don't you realize there are miles and miles of beach, with starfish along every mile? You can't possibly make a difference!" At this, the young man bent down, picked up another starfish, cast it into the ocean, and replied: "I made a difference for that one."

The book you hold in your hands has the potential to make a difference for you. It is an expression of what I have learned over the past twenty-three years as I have dedicated my career to the prevention and reversal of lifestyle disease. The passion I had for the people of Guam is the same passion I take to work every day as I continue to help people reverse diabetes. It is this same passion that motivated me to share *Goodbye Diabetes* with you.

The same valuable strategies that helped my patients on Guam can also help you to take control of your health and change the course of your future. Whether you're diabetic, prediabetic, or just curious about how to optimize your health, you will find hope-filled, life-saving instruction in the pages ahead.

Congratulations for taking the first step to improve your health. I hope and pray this book will make a difference for you.

Sincerely,

Wes Youngberg, DrPH, MPH, CNS, FACLM

—Acknowledgments—

It takes a great team to make the many elements of a book come together. I would like to extend my sincere appreciation to the key individuals who contributed to this process. It has been a privilege to work with each of you:

Elise Harboldt — You have shown an amazing ability to effectively communicate my life work into book form. I can't imagine accomplishing what we did without your untiring tenacity and commitment to excellence. Thanks for being you.

Dan Houghton — Without your vision and enthusiasm, this project would never have materialized. Thank you for challenging and encouraging me to get the job done. I couldn't ask for a better publisher.

Mark and Conna Bond — Mark, you know how to make things look good! Thank you for the creative genius you poured into the design and layout. Conna, thank you for your tireless editorial work. Your eye for verbal detail and precision is very much appreciated.

Nicole Batten — Many thanks for your editorial contributions.

Brenda Davis — You have a contagious passion for health and nutrition. Thank you for sharing your valuable insights.

And Many Others — Thank you for taking the time to review, advise, critique, and improve this book: Evelyn Kissinger, Kaya Chong, Richard Hart, John McDougall, Betty Jo Vercio, Wayne Dysinger, Eric Ngo, George Guthrie, Ernie Medina, John Kelly, Susan Harboldt, Hans Deihl, Charles and Meredith Brinegar, Scott Krenrich, David Katz, and others.

My Family — Betsy, Dakota, Madison, and Katie. You know me best and love me most. Thank you for believing in me and supporting me in this project.

And Finally, My Parents — John and Millie Youngberg. I couldn't ask for better role models. I am motivated and inspired by your passion to help others experience optimal health.

PLEASE NOTE: This book contains stories and case studies involving patients the author has worked with in the past. Their names and identities have been changed to protect their privacy and in the interest of confidentiality. The information in this book is for educational purposes only. It is designed to help you make informed decisions about your health, but is not intended to be a substitute for professional medical advice. Always consult your healthcare provider to determine the appropriateness of the information for your own situation. If you need specific advice, seek help from a medical professional who is knowledgeable in that area. The author and publisher specifically disclaim all responsibility for any liability, loss, or risk, personal or otherwise, which is incurred as a consequence, directly or indirectly, of the use and application of any of the contents of this book.

SECTION 1

Defining Diabetes

—ONE—

The Diabedemic

(THE DIABETES EPIDEMIC)

I FIRST MET JOHN ON A SUNNY SATURDAY AFTERNOON on the island of Guam. At the time, I was the director of a wellness clinic on the island. It was a rewarding job at a dream location, with a tropical climate, beautiful beaches, and warm, friendly people.

This particular day, I was enjoying a restful time with my family when the phone rang. A local colleague and friend requested that I come to the hospital immediately to see one of his patients.

I found John alone in his hospital room, shaken from the events of his day. A 45-year-old firefighter, John should have been in prime health, enjoying the beautiful weekend with his family. Instead, he was lying in a bed at the Guam Memorial Hospital after a nearly fatal brush with acute kidney failure caused by uncontrolled type 2 diabetes.

Until that weekend, John hadn't realized that anything was wrong. He knew he was diabetic but wasn't too concerned—lots of people were diabetic, and they seemed to be okay. Not realizing the severity of his situation, he hadn't taken the initiative to aggressively address the problem until it was almost too late. For John, this was a wake-up call.

As I glanced through the many lab reports and notes in his chart, I recognized how serious John's condition was. Sky-high blood sugar levels.

Hypertension. High cholesterol. Kidney failure. This was possibly John's last chance to make major changes in his lifestyle, reverse his diabetes, and avoid serious and even deadly complications.

I told John that, regardless of his current health status, it wasn't too late to reverse his condition and reduce his risks. Realizing the urgency of the situation, John became highly motivated to do whatever it took to improve his health. I then told him about the six-month wellness program we were just starting at our clinic. The day after being discharged from the hospital, John was in my office, ready to begin the program.

John was just one of many millions of people who suffer from diabetes or prediabetes. Fortunately, his story gets better—much better. In fact, I'll share the rest later in this chapter. You will be surprised and encouraged at the positive results he experienced. But first, let's examine the problem of diabetes a little more closely.

THE GOOD NEWS AND THE BAD NEWS

When it comes to diabetes, there's good news and bad news. The bad news is that diabetes is a worldwide epidemic affecting hundreds of millions of people. Since you're reading this book, I'm assuming that you or someone you care about is in this group.

The good news is that you don't have to stay there. In the vast majority of cases, diabetes can be prevented or reversed. This book is about the good news—for you and for the millions of others who want to say goodbye to diabetes.

In order to understand the good news, however, you must first understand the bad news. Before looking at solutions, you need to identify the problem. In this first chapter we will look at the "bad news." Don't get discouraged as you read through what may seem like alarming information. There is hope for all who are affected by diabetes.

THE DIABETES EPIDEMIC

Do you know someone who has diabetes? Statistics from the Centers for Disease Control and Prevention (CDC) show that diabetes has been increasing at an alarming rate.[1] In 1980, only 2.5 percent of the U.S. population had diabetes.[2] Today, 8.3 percent of the U.S. population is diabetic. That's 25.8 million Americans!

Americans aren't the only ones who should be concerned. The World Health Organization now estimates that 346 million people worldwide have diabetes.[3]

The numbers don't end there. Catherine Cowie, PhD, who directs the diabetes epidemiology program for the National Institutes of Health, spearheaded a comprehensive study to determine the prevalence of diabetes in American adults. More than 7,000 Americans were tested, using two different methods. The study showed that, as of 2006, more than 40 percent of Americans 20 or older had diabetes or prediabetes. Almost one-third of individuals 60 and older had full-blown diabetes, and an astounding three-fourths of those 75 and older had diabetes or prediabetes.[4]

Prediabetes, a condition characterized by higher than normal blood glucose levels not yet elevated enough to be diagnosed as diabetes, puts people at a high risk for cardiovascular disease, even if it never progresses to full-blown diabetes.[5] As it progresses, more complications occur.

Researchers estimate that, for every person with diabetes in the United States, there are *at least* three more people with prediabetes.[6, 7] If this ratio is consistent worldwide, you can conservatively estimate that more than 1 billion people suffer from prediabetes or diabetes—roughly 15 percent of the world's population!

If the current trend continues, the question will no longer be "Do you know someone who has diabetes?" but rather "Do you know anyone who *doesn't* have diabetes?"

THE SILENT KILLER

While it's alarming to discover the enormity of the diabetes problem, it's even more disturbing to consider that at least a third of diabetics in the United States don't even *know* they have the disease.[8, 9] With so many cases of diabetes remaining undiagnosed in the United States—the most medically advanced society in the world—you can only imagine the extent of undiagnosed diabetes worldwide.

Diabetes progresses slowly and silently. It often doesn't manifest noticeable symptoms until the condition is well advanced. People who aren't aware of their risk often remain unscreened and undiagnosed. Because symptoms are not an adequate guide, it is critical to know how to evaluate your risk for diabetes and associated complications. We will talk more about testing later in this book.

THE COST OF DIABETES

Diabetes is a costly disease, both financially and otherwise. In 2007, the CDC estimated that approximately $174 billion was spent on diabetes in the United States. Diabetics spend more than twice as much on healthcare as nondiabetics.[10] But the real cost of diabetes isn't measured in dollars, but rather by the enormous toll it takes on a person's quality and quantity of life.

It is inconvenient to live with diabetes. Diabetics struggle with the burden of constantly regulating their blood sugar levels, taking medications, and trying to avoid complications. Many are fighting an uphill battle.

Diabetes and prediabetes are major contributors to heart attack, stroke, hypertension, and other vascular problems. Diabetes is also considered *the* leading cause of blindness, kidney failure, and non-traumatic lower-limb amputations, as well as numerous other complications.[11]

Not only does diabetes impair a person's quality of life, but it also shortens one's lifespan. Diabetics are twice as likely to die prematurely as people without diabetes. Diabetes is currently ranked as the seventh-leading cause of death in the United States.[12]

This is a conservative number, however, as it only takes into account death certificates that list diabetes as the *primary* cause of death. Keep in mind that, while cardiovascular disease, cancer, and stroke are listed as the first, second, and fourth causes of death, all three of these conditions are often related to or worsened by the presence of prediabetes and diabetes.

The numbers aren't expected to get any better. In fact, the World Health Organization projects that by 2030, diabetes deaths will double.[13]

THE DANGER OF DIABETES

With such a marked increase in diabetes in the United States and worldwide, some have concluded that it's simply a normal, unavoidable progression of aging. Patients diagnosed with type 2 diabetes are often told that their condition is chronic: "Once a diabetic, always a diabetic," or, "You will have this condition for the rest of your life."

In order to understand the mainstream thinking regarding diabetes, let's take a look at some definitions found in these popular sources:

WIKIPEDIA (DIABETES MELLITUS):

"All forms of diabetes have been treatable since insulin became available in 1921, and type 2 diabetes may be controlled with medications. Both type 1 and 2 are chronic conditions that usually cannot be cured."

THE AMERICAN DIABETES ASSOCIATION:

"There is no cure for diabetes, however, it is very treatable. The treatments available help control blood glucose levels, which can result in fewer complications and slower disease progression."

THE MAYO CLINIC:

"There's no cure for type 2 diabetes, but you can manage—or even prevent—the condition."

People are led to believe that if they have type 2 diabetes, they can "manage" or "control" the situation with insulin and other medications. If they're lucky, they can avoid serious complications and "slow" the progression of the disease, but an actual cure is impossible. They're told that lifestyle interventions such as diet and exercise can help manage the condition, but the disease will still be chronic.

What you believe about diabetes will play a crucial role in whether you take appropriate action to prevent or reverse the disease. It is crucial to know the facts:

1) DIABETES IS DANGEROUS. Regardless of how many people suffer from the disease, diabetes is a serious health threat. We shouldn't allow it to become "normal" in our thinking.

Both prediabetes and diabetes exponentially increase the risk for cardiovascular disease and many other complications. Although diabetes progresses over time, even the early stages of development (before diagnosis) are dangerous.

In future years, we will see the effects of this disease multiply. Many diabetics will increasingly develop life-threatening complications, and many prediabetics will continue down the same path.

2) DIABETES IS PREVENTABLE. At least 90 percent of diabetes cases need never exist.[14] Type 2 diabetes accounts for the overwhelming majority of cases, and is caused by lifestyle and environmentally-related factors.[15] The best way to say "goodbye" to diabetes is to never say "hello." With the right education and proper preventive choices, diabetes can be stopped before it starts.

3) DIABETES IS REVERSIBLE. For those who have already been diagnosed with the disease, there is hope! The same habits that help healthy people *avoid* diabetes can help the majority of type 2 diabetics to *reverse* the disease and avoid its complications, and can help type 1 diabetics improve their health. If you're struggling with prediabetes or type 2 diabetes, don't settle for "managing" your condition when you can greatly improve and possibly even reverse it! The strategies in this book can help you to have the same kind of success as my patient John.

BACK TO JOHN'S STORY

Remember, John had almost died of acute kidney failure. Let me tell you the rest of the story. John was ready to do whatever it took to improve his health, so he signed up for our six-month wellness program.

For the first two weeks of the program, we monitored participants very closely. We met as a group five days each week for four hours each day. We monitored everyone's blood sugar, blood pressure, and weight. Participants did aerobic exercise for forty-five minutes each morning and took short walks after their meals. Healthy, plant-based meals were provided on site, and specially prepared meals were sent home. We provided interactive classes and lectures to teach the basics of living a healthy lifestyle. John stayed focused and did his best.

After the first two weeks, John was able to stop taking his usual 100 units of insulin. His blood sugars, which had been in the 400s, were now consistently under 110 before meals, and under 140 two hours after meals.

John's blood pressure lowered significantly, and he was able to discontinue all his antihypertensive medications.

As the months passed, John's situation continued to improve. He lost 30 pounds, felt better, looked better, and noticed major improvements in his overall performance. His kidney function improved. He started enjoying life again and was able to move forward—in control of his health and confident about his future success.

John's situation is not unusual. He is one of many people who have overcome significant health complications caused by uncontrolled diabetes. His story should provide hope to anyone suffering from this disease. Diabetes shouldn't be a death sentence or a forecast for chronic disease. Instead, it should be a wake-up call. The same blueprint John followed can prove effective for anyone who wants to say "Goodbye diabetes!"

CHAPTER SUMMARY

- Diabetes and prediabetes have reached epidemic proportions and continue to rise.
- Diabetes causes complications that devastate health and quality of life.
- Both prediabetes and diabetes greatly increase the risk of cardiovascular disease.
- Diabetes is a leading cause of death in the United States.
- People with diabetes spend twice as much money on healthcare as those without diabetes.
- Diabetes is a dangerous disease and must not be considered the "new normal."
- At least 90 percent of diabetes cases are preventable.
- The majority of type 2 diabetes cases are reversible if corrective action is taken quickly.

— TWO —

Diabetes for Dummies

Know your enemy and know yourself and
you can fight a thousand battles without disaster.
—Sun Tzu

THESE WORDS ARE FOUND IN *THE ART OF WAR*, AN ANCIENT military treatise written by Chinese general Sun Tzu. Dated to 500 BC, this classic work has played a significant role in shaping both ancient and modern military strategy. It also has implications with regard to strategies for battling diabetes.

In any battle, you need to understand both your enemy and yourself. It's just common sense. The goal of this chapter is to help you do just that, especially if you're new to diabetes.

WHAT EXACTLY IS DIABETES?

Diabetes is simply *having blood sugar levels so high, and for so long, that they eventually cause significant health complications, if not corrected.* Various criteria are used to diagnose diabetes. If you meet even one of them, you are diabetic.

The criteria are as follows:

- A fasting blood glucose of 126 mg/dL or higher.
- A blood glucose of 200 or higher, two hours after an oral glucose tolerance test.
- A random blood glucose of 200 or higher taken at any time and accompanied by classic diabetic symptoms.
- A Hemoglobin A1c level of 6.5 percent or higher.

More information about testing is included in Chapters 7 and 8.

Numerous complications are associated with diabetes, but the single most important (and most devastating) complication is heart disease. At least 65 percent of people who have diabetes eventually end up suffering a premature heart attack or stroke.[1] There are other significant complications as well, but *one of the primary goals* in addressing diabetes is to reduce the risk of the nation's number one killer—heart disease.

But let's back up. How does diabetes happen? What causes blood sugar levels to get so high? What is happening inside the body? In order to best explain what diabetes is, I will first explain what it is not. I will help you understand how a healthy body functions so you can better appreciate how diabetes counteracts that process.

HEALTHY HAL

Hal is the perfect picture of health. He is in excellent shape. He sleeps eight hours every night, exercises daily, eats the most nutritious food possible, and follows every other health principle he knows about. Hal has optimal blood sugars, and no trace of diabetes or even prediabetes. Let's take a look at what happens inside Hal's body right after he eats.

Hal has just finished his favorite Italian meal and has gone outside to do some yard work. Although from his perspective the meal is over, from his body's perspective it's just beginning.

The food that Hal has eaten begins the digestion process and is broken down into several different nutrients. One of the most important of these nutrients is glucose. Glucose is a simple sugar that is critical for survival. It is the primary source of energy for Hal's cells.

The glucose enters Hal's bloodstream from his digestive tract and begins to circulate, causing his blood glucose (blood sugar) levels to rise. The glucose needs to enter Hal's cells to give them energy, but there's one problem. The cells are "locked." Circulating glucose can't cross through a cell membrane by itself. It needs a "key" to let it in. This key comes in the form of insulin, which is a hormone secreted by the pancreas.

Thankfully, Hal's pancreas detects the need. Responding to the natural rise in blood sugar, it secretes insulin. The insulin travels to Hal's cells—which are eager to accept it—and then connects to insulin receptors on the outside of the cell membrane, unlocking the doors to the cell and allowing glucose to enter.

As the glucose enters Hal's cells, his blood sugar levels naturally decrease and stabilize, and his cells are provided with energy. Four to five hours later, Hal's cells need glucose again. He eats dinner, and the process repeats itself. Hal's story illustrates how a healthy body absorbs glucose for energy use.

Although Hal is an outstanding example of health, he does not represent the 35 to 40 percent of Americans who are prediabetic or diabetic.[2] What is happening inside their bodies? How do their stories differ from Hal's?

THE IDEAL: A person who does not have diabetes or prediabetes is able to metabolize glucose normally. The pancreas responds to rising blood sugar levels by secreting insulin. This insulin attaches to receptors on cell membranes, unlocking the cells and allowing glucose to enter. Blood sugar levels stabilize, cells receive energy, and the cycle continues.

TYPE 1 TINA

Like Hal, Tina is health-conscious and tries to make good choices. However, she has disadvantages that Hal doesn't have. Tina has type 1 diabetes. This means that her pancreas has been damaged and does not produce any significant amount of insulin.

When Tina eats her favorite Chinese meal, her digestion process starts out just like Hal's. Her food is broken down into nutrients, including glucose. The glucose leaves her digestive tract and is absorbed into her bloodstream. Her blood sugar levels rise. The glucose needs to be able to enter her cells, but it requires insulin to do this.

Tina's pancreas doesn't produce insulin like Hal's does. How is the glucose supposed to enter her cells? Without insulin, more and more glucose builds up in her bloodstream, causing her blood sugar levels to rise. This can be very dangerous.

Tina was 15 years old when she first developed this problem. She noticed that she was urinating more frequently than usual and was extremely thirsty. She also started eating everything in sight, but nothing seemed to satisfy her hunger. Tina was losing weight, even though she was eating more than usual. She also felt fatigued. Tina's parents were concerned and took her to the doctor.

After multiple tests, Tina was diagnosed with type 1 diabetes. Her doctor explained that, because her pancreas was no longer producing insulin, she would have to take insulin injections. Tina would have to monitor her blood sugar levels very closely and tailor her insulin doses to keep those levels stable. If Tina stopped taking insulin, she could have serious and even deadly complications within days, or even hours.

Tina also learned that controlling her blood sugars would decrease her risk for serious chronic complications associated with diabetes, including heart disease, high blood pressure, kidney failure, severe nerve damage, and blindness.

Thankfully, Tina is reducing those risks by managing her blood sugars with insulin injections. However, Tina does more than just take insulin. She uses lifestyle strategies to help make her body *more receptive* to insulin. The more receptive her body is to insulin, the less she has to take, and the less likely she is to experience the negative effects of insulin resistance and high insulin doses. We'll discuss this more in the next chapter.

TYPE 1 DIABETES is characterized by the inability of the pancreas to produce insulin, and is treated with insulin injections. It generally results from damage done to the pancreatic cells by toxins, infections, viruses, or physical factors. Only 5 to 10 percent of people with diabetes have this type.[3] It is usually diagnosed in children and young adults, but can occur at any age. This condition is chronic, but it can be well managed. Blood sugar levels must be carefully monitored to prevent complications. Lifestyle interventions such as diet and exercise also play a key role in reducing risks associated with this type of diabetes.

TYPE 2 TOM

Tina is a rare case, representing only 5 to 10 percent of diabetics. Tom, on the other hand, is mainstream, representing at least 90 percent of all cases of diabetes.[4] Tom is a 53-year-old, type 2 diabetic. He has a hectic schedule full of responsibilities and deadlines. With so many priorities to juggle, his lifestyle takes a toll on his health. Tom is about 30 pounds overweight. He wants to exercise but has an early work commute each morning and is exhausted by the time he gets home. Several years ago, Tom was alarmed to discover that he had type 2 diabetes.

Just like Hal and Tina, when Tom eats, glucose enters his bloodstream, and his blood sugar level begins to rise. In response, his pancreas attempts to secrete enough insulin.

For several years prior to his diagnosis, Tom's pancreas had been overworked. It was forced to produce enormous amounts of insulin in an attempt to stabilize his blood sugars. Unlike Tina, who couldn't produce any insulin, Tom was producing extra. But his blood sugar levels were still high. Why wasn't the insulin working?

Tom's cells had become *resistant* to insulin. His receptors weren't as eager to allow insulin to unlock the cells and allow glucose to enter. Because of this resistance, it started to take increasing amounts of insulin to control Tom's blood sugar, causing his pancreas to work harder.

After years and years of producing so much insulin, Tom's pancreas is burned out and no longer able to produce the large amounts it used to. To rectify the problem, Tom's doctor prescribes insulin injections and oral medications to help force the glucose into Tom's cells. Tom doesn't realize that this, in and of itself, isn't a good long-term solution. There are many simple strategies Tom can implement to help improve his health and possibly even *reverse* his condition.

TYPE 2 DIABETES is the most common form. Millions of Americans have been diagnosed with this disease. In type 2 diabetes, the body becomes resistant to insulin, requiring more insulin than normal to control blood sugars. The pancreas has to work extra hard to produce the extra insulin. Over time, the pancreas loses its ability to keep up with the increased insulin demand. This leads to pancreatic fatigue, a decrease in insulin production, and high blood sugar levels.

PREDIABETIC PAM

Meet Pam. Pam hasn't yet been diagnosed with type 2 diabetes, but she has been heading in that direction for several years. Pam represents the millions of Americans who are unaware that they are at risk—about 35 percent of the U.S. adult population.[5]

Pam is active in her community and with her family. She loves to cook dinner for her husband and two teenagers. Pam recently had lab work done and discovered that her triglyceride and cholesterol levels are a little high. She also had a fasting blood glucose test, with results on the high end of normal.

What Pam doesn't realize is that she is already at greatly increased risk for heart disease. She is already experiencing insulin resistance and other metabolic problems. The sooner Pam acknowledges that her condition is serious, the sooner she can implement simple lifestyle strategies to reduce her risk factors and halt the progression of the disease.

PREDIABETES is an early form of diabetes marked by blood glucose levels that are significantly higher than normal, but not yet high enough to be diagnosed as diabetes. Prediabetes is considered a significant risk factor for developing full-blown diabetes. It is also a strong indicator of early and progressive heart disease.[6] Prediabetes is diagnosed when there is a fasting blood glucose level of 100 to 125 mg/dL, or a two-hour glucose tolerance level of 140 to 199 mg/dL. More information about testing is included in chapters 7 and 8.

GESTATIONAL GINA

Gina is thrilled to be eight months pregnant! She has been getting regular prenatal checkups, preparing the nursery room for her baby, and reading every baby book she can get her hands on. About six months into her pregnancy, Gina was tested for gestational diabetes as part of her typical prenatal care. She had never had diabetes before and was surprised when she tested positive. Gina realized that both she and her baby were at risk.

Gina quickly learned how to monitor and control her blood sugars. She made adjustments to her diet and started walking for 20 minutes after each meal (in addition to her regular exercise program). Gina is doing her best to keep herself and her baby as healthy as possible.

GESTATIONAL DIABETES occurs in women who didn't have diabetes prior to becoming pregnant, but whose blood sugar levels rise during pregnancy. It threatens the health of both mother and baby, and puts the baby at a much higher risk for developing diabetes in the future. Prediabetes is a major risk factor for developing gestational diabetes. (Prediabetes also increases risk to mother and baby, whether or not gestational diabetes develops.) Pregnant women are typically tested for gestational diabetes at 24 to 28 weeks. Gestational diabetes affects an estimated 18 percent of all pregnancies.[7] Ideally, women wishing to become pregnant should get tested and address any underlying blood sugar problems—prior to conception, or very early in the pregnancy.

FOCUS ON PREDIABETES AND TYPE 2

Tina, Tom, Pam, and Gina help us to understand the different types of diabetes: type 1, type 2, prediabetes, and gestational diabetes. Although their stories may differ slightly from others with the same conditions, they provide typical examples of the four types of diabetes.

Prediabetes and type 2 diabetes represent the overwhelming majority of diabetic cases. In this book, we will primarily focus on these two types. We will generally use the term *diabetes* to refer to type 2 diabetes, recognizing that prediabetes is type 2 diabetes in its early stages. However, it's important to recognize that the same mechanisms that drive prediabetes and type 2 diabetes also drive (or at least contribute to) all other forms of the disease.

The wellness strategies in this book apply to all forms of diabetes, and are relevant and beneficial for everyone. Regardless of which type of diabetes you may be suffering from or wanting to prevent, this book provides you with valuable tools to improve your health.

In the next chapter, we'll take a closer, behind-the-scenes look at what drives diabetes and its associated complications.

CHAPTER SUMMARY

- Diabetes commonly comes in three forms: type 1, type 2, and gestational diabetes.
- In type 1 diabetes, the pancreas does not produce insulin. This type of diabetes accounts for 5 to 10 percent of all diabetic cases.
- In type 2 diabetes, body cells become more resistant and less sensitive to the insulin that is produced, requiring more insulin to control blood sugars.
- Prediabetes is type 2 diabetes in its early stages.
- Prediabetes greatly increases the risk of developing type 2 or gestational diabetes.
- Prediabetes increases the risk of heart disease.
- At least 79 million Americans are prediabetic. Most are unaware of their risk.
- Gestational diabetes affects 18 percent of all pregnancies.

—THREE—

A Metabolic Mess

Diabetes is kind of like a messy room.

My youngest daughter, Katie, is a spunky, creative kid. She has bright red glasses, a rambunctious personality, and more energy than her parents know what to do with.

But Katie is selective about where she invests her energy—it doesn't usually get channeled into cleaning her room. It's amazing how quickly Katie's room seems to explode after a required cleaning. Legos®, stuffed animals, clothes, missing homework assignments, and art projects litter the floor and the shelves. Drawers stay pulled open, the bed remains unmade, and underneath the bed is a jumbled assortment of, well... just about everything. Katie's room is a mess.

My oldest daughter Madie is an organization expert. Madie can enter a messy room or chaotic situation, survey the scene, and within moments know exactly how to turn things around. Madie helps Katie (as well as the rest of the family) to stay organized.

With some encouragement from Madie, Katie has discovered that, little by little, with each toy returned to its proper place, dirty laundry put in the laundry basket, bed made, drawers closed, and trash thrown away, her room can be transformed into a clean and orderly living space.

Diabetes and prediabetes are similar to a messy room. Just like Katie has multiple toys, clothes, and other items that combine to make her room a mess, diabetes is driven by multiple factors, creating an overall metabolic mess in the body.

The dictionary defines *metabolism* as: "The sum of the physical and chemical processes in an organism."[1] A metabolic mess simply means that multiple physical and chemical processes in the body are malfunctioning and causing damage.

The good news is that, just as Katie can clean her room one item at a time, diabetes and prediabetes can be greatly improved, and possibly even reversed, by cleaning up the metabolic mess, one good choice at a time. Just like Madie provides help and encouragement for Katie to clean up her messes, this book provides you with the tools you need to clean up your own metabolic mess.

In this chapter, you will learn about the "messy" internal environment that contributes to diabetes and prediabetes. Once you understand this metabolic mess, you can take steps to change that environment into one in which diabetes cannot progress, or maybe even exist.

A metabolic mess simply means that multiple physical and chemical processes in the body are malfunctioning and causing damage.

THE CIRCULATION SECRET

If I had to explain in just one sentence what the most important strategy is for overall health and wellness, this is what I would say:

Perfect health depends on perfect circulation.

The circulatory system (which includes the heart, the blood vessels, and the blood) is constantly in motion, transporting nutrients, oxygen, and water to every system, organ, and cell in the body. In order to have a healthy circulatory system, the heart and blood vessels need to be clear and unobstructed, the blood needs to be pure and filled with the right nutrients, and the heart needs to work efficiently and effectively to pump this blood throughout the body.

The number one leading cause of death in the United States is heart disease, and the fourth leading cause is stroke.[2] Both of these conditions are caused by problems in circulation.

But what about diabetes? Does poor circulation impact the progression of diabetes? Does diabetes damage the circulatory system? What's the connection?

Most people think of diabetes in a compartmentalized way. They believe that diabetes is a disease that causes blood sugar problems, and that for some reason, it leads to a variety of complications. For this reason, they often attempt to control their blood sugars primarily through medications, hoping that this will reduce their risk for complications.

But *why* does diabetes cause the complications that it does? Do the complications have anything in common? Will focusing only on blood sugar management *really* solve the underlying problem?

When I lecture on diabetes, I frequently ask the audience: "What are the complications associated with diabetes?" They respond with the typical answers: kidney failure, blindness, amputations, and nerve damage. "But what's the *number one* complication associated with diabetes?" I ask. They usually look puzzled and guess one of the other complications already mentioned.

But the number one complication associated with diabetes—and therefore the number one thing we should be concerned about—is cardiovascular disease. Studies show that people with diabetes who have never had a heart attack are just as likely to have one as those without diabetes who have already had a heart attack.[3] At least 65 percent of diabetics will die prematurely from complications associated with cardiovascular disease, caused by damage to the circulatory system.[4] This same circulatory damage is also what causes other complications associated with diabetes.

With this in mind, a more accurate way to explain the complications associated with diabetes would be to say: "The multiple factors that cause diabetes also cause *circulatory damage*, which leads to complications such as heart disease, stroke, amputations, kidney damage, nerve damage, and blindness." Yes, these complications are caused by diabetes, but they are primarily caused by the fact that *diabetes damages the circulatory system.*

The next logical question is: "What's the best way to combat diabetes and the circulatory damage that it causes?" Is it to focus on blood sugar management? While blood sugar management is very important and can help prevent circulatory damage, this is only one piece of the puzzle. A more comprehensive and effective approach is to understand and address all the factors that contribute to diabetes and that affect circulatory health. Let's examine these factors now.

INSULIN RESISTANCE

In the last chapter, we discussed how a healthy body regulates blood sugar. In a prediabetic or diabetic person, this process is impaired.

Glucose is the primary energy source for cells. The carbohydrates we eat break down into glucose, and that glucose enters the bloodstream. Ideally, the glucose will then enter the body's cells to provide the energy needed for optimal function. The majority of glucose is stored in muscle and liver cells.

Insulin is a hormone secreted by the beta cells of the pancreas. It acts like a key to unlock the cells, allowing the glucose molecules to enter. Without insulin, glucose is not able to enter the cells, and the blood sugar rises. This is what happens in type 1 diabetes, where the pancreas isn't producing insulin.

But people with prediabetes and type 2 diabetes initially have a very different problem. They *are* producing insulin. Surprisingly, many of them are producing exponentially more insulin than they were before developing problems. What's happening? If insulin is present, why is the blood sugar still high? It doesn't make sense until we understand the concept of insulin resistance.

Insulin resistance is the main driver of diabetes and prediabetes. It simply means that the cells (especially the muscle and liver cells) won't allow insulin to unlock them for sugar storage. The cells have become "fat and sassy." These muscle cells are full of energy with no expectation of using that energy anytime soon. Most likely, they have not regularly been subjected to physical activity. The muscles essentially say: "We already have all the sugar we need. Why would we want to store more?"

Unable to enter the cells, glucose builds up in the bloodstream—causing high blood sugar. The pancreas detects the rising glucose level and responds by secreting more insulin in an attempt to force glucose into the cells. The more resistant the muscles are to insulin, the higher the amount of insulin the pancreas must produce in an attempt to control blood sugars. Hyperinsulinemia occurs when the pancreas is making a heroic effort to lower glucose levels by producing more insulin than it would under normal circumstances.

This creates an unhealthy roller coaster ride of blood sugars. While insulin resistance raises blood sugars too high, hyperinsulinemia can drop them too low. This leads to hypoglycemia, headaches, cravings for unhealthy foods, and severe emotional reactions including mood swings, anger, and irritability.

In many cases, prediabetics and diabetics have these high insulin levels for years, or even decades, before they realize that there is a problem. Blood sugar problems are present but can go undetected by conventional screening techniques, because the pancreas is overworking to keep sugar levels down.

Expecting the pancreas to produce large amounts of insulin on a daily basis for years and years on end is like expecting yourself to run a 10K every day and a marathon every weekend.

Unfortunately, even the pancreas has limitations. Expecting the pancreas to produce large amounts of insulin on a daily basis for years and years on end is like expecting yourself to run a 10K every day and a marathon every weekend. It's impossible to keep up this pace for long without damaging your body. Eventually, pancreatic fatigue sets in and insulin production dramatically decreases. Without the extra insulin production, blood sugar levels shoot up.

Often, this is the point at which people first realize that they have a problem. This is unfortunate, because by this time the body has been under stress for years, the pancreas has been damaged, and blood sugar levels are out of control.

HIGH BLOOD SUGAR—A STICKY SITUATION

Now that we understand what causes high blood sugar, let's take a look at how this impacts the body. When glucose is unable to enter the muscle or liver cells, it builds up in the bloodstream. Glucose is sticky. As it circulates through the body, it attaches to proteins on the membranes of all different kinds of cells. Over time, this leads to a glazy, sticky buildup on cells, tissues, and organs. This is called glycosylation.

Have you ever spilled honey? Honey tastes good, but it can be a gooey, sticky mess. It's hard to clean it off your hands, dishes, or to wipe it off of the counter. Imagine spilling honey in your bloodstream. Picture the honey sticking to everything it touches, causing those surfaces to become sticky. This is how glycosylation works. Glycosylation occurs everywhere that blood flows and causes damage to the kidneys, eyes, nerves, arteries, heart, and every other organ and system you can think of.

As this sticky sugar attaches to proteins on cell membranes, it morphs the structure of those proteins. By changing the structure of cellular proteins, glycosylation changes the function of cells. Proteins in cells are like the software in a computer. When computer software is infected with a virus, the computer doesn't work the way it is supposed to. In the same way, whenever the structure of a protein is altered, the cell becomes dysfunctional.

Glycosylation also causes cholesterol to become more sticky, increasing the tendency for plaque buildup in the arteries.[5] This impairs circulation and increases the risk for cardiovascular disease.

The Hemoglobin A1c, or glycated hemoglobin test, reveals how much glycosylation is occurring in the body. It tests the amount of sugar build-up on the hemoglobin proteins of red blood cells. For every percentage point the Hemoglobin A1c level increases, representing a 30 point increase in the average daily blood sugar level,[6] the risk for heart attack increases by 14 percent, the risk for amputation or death from peripheral vascular disease increases by 43 percent, and the risk for kidney disease, vision loss, and nerve damage increases by 37 percent. This demonstrates a very significant correlation between the amount of glycosylation caused by high blood sugars and the risk for diabetes-associated complications.[7] See page 85 for a chart showing this correlation.

Glycosylation also causes damage by activating the body's inflammatory response, contributing to a state of chronic, low-grade inflammation.[8] Let's take a closer look at inflammation and how it relates to diabetes.

INFLAMMATION

Inflammation is arguably the most overlooked factor in the development of diabetes and cardiovascular complications. Inflammation is the immune system's natural response to protect itself against injury or invasion. It helps the body get rid of whatever shouldn't be there. For example, let's pretend you accidentally step on a nail covered with cow manure. Unfamiliar and dangerous bacteria have now been introduced into your bloodstream. The inflammatory response calls immune cells to the scene to clean up the area, destroy the bacteria, and get rid of the infection. Temporary acute inflammation can help your body protect itself against infection, trauma, and allergy. The normal inflammatory response helps the body to heal properly.

Chronic inflammation is a different story. Chronic inflammation occurs when the immune system *perpetually* produces an inflammatory response to hidden toxins, infections, foreign substances, or damaged tissues and cells. In an attempt to destroy substances that don't belong in the body, chronic inflammation actually damages the body itself.

In an attempt to destroy substances that don't belong in the body, chronic inflammation actually damages the body itself.

While conducting a diabetes reversal workshop for the president of Palau, I had the opportunity to go scuba diving at Blue Corner, the island's most famous dive site. Led by a guide, our group was to dive and drift to about 60 feet underwater, hooking in to the Blue Corner reef. We would stay there during the tide change, which is when sea creatures are most visible and the view of the reef is spectacular.

As our small diving group entered the water, I was alarmed to see the fins and bodies of about ten sharks ahead. I looked down, only to realize that there were 10 to15 sharks below me. To my right were at least 20 more sharks. It was the same to my left. Our guide had told us that we would see sharks, but I hadn't expected to be surrounded by them! I did my best to stay in the middle of the group, hoping that if a shark attacked, it would prefer someone on the outside! The closer we drifted toward the reef, the closer the sharks swam to us until they were only a few feet away.

Thankfully, the dive provided a breathtaking view, and the sharks left us alone. With such a high concentration of marine life at the reef, the sharks always have their fill of fish, so they aren't usually interested in consuming humans—unless someone throws chum in the water.

Chum is a bait mixture of fish parts and blood. It is used to lure fish, especially sharks. At the smell of blood, sharks go crazy, and a *Jaws*-like frenzy ensues. The same sharks that swim serenely by scuba divers will instantaneously transform into ferocious predators, attacking anyone and everyone in sight.

A shark attack caused by chum is very similar to an inflammatory response gone bad. Normally, there are thousands of white blood cells circulating in the blood, occasionally engulfing bacteria or toxins. These immune cells are much like the sharks that swim close to the reef, occasionally engulfing fish. However, when a chronic infection or irritation is present, these same cells become aggressive and hostile. While attempting to target the invader, they end up damaging everything in sight, causing inflammation throughout the body.

Inflammation is a primary cause of plaque buildup in the arteries.[9] White blood cells attempt to get rid of toxic cholesterol by engulfing it. These white blood cells become engorged with the cholesterol and die, becoming sticky, pus-filled cholesterol carriers. As thousands of these sticky cells combine, plaque is formed.

Chronic inflammation is associated with a major increase in risk for many degenerative diseases.[10] The Cardiac CRP blood test measures the level of inflammation in the body. The higher the average Cardiac CRP level, the higher the risk for developing cancer, heart disease, stroke, Alzheimer's, and diabetes.[11] (You'll learn more about the Cardiac CRP test later in this book.)

Chronic inflammation can be caused by multiple factors, including environmental toxins, unhealthy chemicals in junk food, and any type of infection.[12] One of the biggest causes of chronic inflammation, however, is glycosylation, caused by high blood sugar.[13] You will recall that glycosylation changes the structure and function of cells. The immune system considers these altered cells to be diseased and damaged, so it activates an inflammatory response against them. The problem is that since glycosylation occurs everywhere in the body, inflammation also occurs everywhere. The sugary, sticky, glycosylated mess is too big for the immune system to clean up fast enough. This mess overwhelms the body's ability to heal. The inflammation remains, causing constant chemical stress everywhere in the body.

The good news is that inflammation can be reversed. But the cause of the inflammation must be discovered and addressed. Dr. Sidney Baker, MD, professor emeritus at Yale Medical School, has a good way of describing this: "If you're sitting on a tack, it takes a lot of aspirin to make you feel good. If you're sitting on two tacks, removing just one does not result in a 50 percent improvement."[14] This is a humorous way of explaining that chronic inflammation cannot be cured simply by taking anti-inflammatory medications, or by addressing only some of the factors contributing to the problem. In the following chapters, you will discover comprehensive strategies for identifying and addressing inflammation.

HIGH BLOOD PRESSURE

The CDC estimates that one third of U.S. adults (18 and older) suffer from high blood pressure, also known as hypertension.[15] Blood pressure measures the force of the blood circulating in the body. High blood pressure indicates that the heart has to work harder than it normally would to keep blood flowing.

HYPERTENSION technically exists if you have a blood pressure of 140/90 or higher. However, as it relates to diabetes, even prehypertension (120/80 to 139/89) can signal a problem. When I see a patient with prehypertension or hypertension, I automatically suspect that they have prediabetes or diabetes, unless testing proves otherwise. If your blood pressure is in this range, it is important that you be thoroughly evaluated for prediabetes and diabetes.

The prevalence of hypertension increases with age. Over 50 percent of American adults age 55-64 have high blood pressure. This jumps to 64 percent of men and 70 percent of women age 65-74, and 65 percent of men and 80 percent of women age 75 and older.[16]

These statistics are even higher among diabetics. Diabetics are at least twice as likely to suffer from high blood pressure as nondiabetics.[17] What's the correlation between diabetes and hypertension?

Dr. Gerald Reaven, renowned endocrinologist and professor emeritus at the Stanford University School of Medicine, reports that up to half of hypertension cases are caused by insulin resistance.[18] Hypertension is one of the earliest warning signs that insulin resistance may be present in the body.[19]

You've learned that one of the purposes of insulin is glucose storage, but insulin also functions in other ways as well. Insulin acts as a vasoconstrictor to tighten and squeeze the arteries. As insulin levels go up, small muscles inside the artery walls begin constricting. Because the heart meets more resistance, it has to work harder to pump and circulate blood throughout the body. This causes blood pressure to rise. High insulin levels also contribute to hypertension by causing the kidneys to filter out magnesium and other minerals that naturally reduce blood pressure.

Hypertension damages the integrity of blood vessels, compromising circulation throughout the entire body. It greatly increases the risk for heart disease, strokes, and all other diabetic complications.

Hypertension is one of the earliest warning signs that insulin resistance may be present in the body.

ATHEROSCLEROSIS

Atherosclerosis, or hardening and narrowing of the arteries, occurs when cholesterol, fat, and other substances infiltrate the artery walls, causing plaque buildup. This plaque impairs circulation, and over time can obstruct the arteries. Atherosclerosis is the leading cause of heart attack, stroke, and peripheral vascular disease. Diabetes is a leading cause of atherosclerosis.[20]

The same metabolic mess that causes diabetes also causes atherosclerosis. All of the factors discussed in this chapter damage the arteries and compromise circulation.

WHY IT MATTERS

Insulin resistance, high blood sugar, glycosylation, inflammation, high blood pressure, atherosclerosis—these are processes that create the metabolic mess. Each process contributes to, and is affected by, the others. These processes work in tandem to damage the circulatory system, driving diabetes, cardiovascular disease, and a host of related complications.

This information may sound alarming. You're probably thinking, *Is it really that complicated? I thought all I had to do was manage my blood sugars. Do I really have to worry about all this other stuff?*

The good news is that, by having a thorough understanding of the problem, we can better understand how to address it. It's also encouraging to realize that, when it comes to cleaning up the metabolic mess, the same, simple strategies that help to improve blood sugar levels and reduce insulin resistance also help to reduce inflammation, blood pressure, and atherosclerosis. Although the problem may sound complex, the solutions are simple.

No matter how "messy" your health may be right now, there is hope. Just as Katie's messy room can be transformed into an organized, livable place, you can clean up your metabolic mess and experience optimal health. Every single risk factor described in this chapter can be improved—and possibly even reversed—by applying the comprehensive lifestyle strategies outlined in this book.

CHAPTER SUMMARY

- Diabetes is a "metabolic mess" caused by multiple factors.
- The number one complication associated with diabetes is heart disease.
- Perfect health depends on perfect circulation.
- Diabetes is dangerous because it damages the circulatory system.
- Almost all diabetic complications are the result of circulatory damage.
- Effective treatment of diabetes must address everything that impacts circulation, not just blood sugar management.
- Insulin resistance occurs when the cells become resistant to allowing insulin to unlock them so glucose can enter.

- High blood sugar sticks to cells, causing glycosylation. This damages cells throughout the body.
- Chronic inflammation causes the body to damage itself.
- High blood pressure causes strain on the heart and damage to the arterial walls.
- Atherosclerosis is narrowing and hardening of the arteries and is made worse by diabetes.
- There is hope! It's possible to clean up the metabolic mess.

SECTION 2

Debunking Diabetes

—FOUR—

The Diabetic's Genetics

DO YOU REMEMBER WHERE YOU WERE ON DECEMBER 31, 1999? As the clock turned toward midnight, the world seemed to hold its breath—waiting, hoping, and praying that the infamous "Y2K" bug was just a millennial myth. The weeks and months leading up to New Year's Day were filled with media buzz, frantic speculation, and fear of the unknown. While skeptics minimized the concern, many apprehensive businesses and individuals anticipated the worst. The long awaited hour finally came and went. To our relief, there was no life-altering, world-shaking crisis.

Several months later, however, a life-altering event *did* occur. Although it didn't get as much mainstream publicity as the Y2K scare, the discovery and mapping of the entire human genome marked the beginning of a new frontier in medicine.[1] This discovery promised to revolutionize our understanding of genetics and to transform individual healthcare into a more personalized, effective approach.

THE HUMAN GENOME

The human genome is the collection of all the genetic information in humans. Inside the nuclei of almost every cell in your body are 46 chromosomes. Half of these are from your mother, and half are from your father. Your genetic blueprint is stored on these chromosomes inside your genes.

Genes contain a code of instructions for making everything the body needs, especially proteins. These proteins are essential to life. They help carry out almost all functions of the human body.

Humans have approximately 20,000 genes.[2] In the spring of 2000, The Human Genome Project successfully finished decoding and mapping these genes. The code, and therefore the structure, of each human gene was determined. The information was stored in databases and made available to researchers everywhere. This opened up a whole new world of genomic research—exploring patterns of gene expression, identifying which genes contribute to which diseases, and developing new therapies to target genetic flaws. Over a decade later, the research continues. This wealth of information helps us to better understand our risk for developing diseases like diabetes.

DID I INHERIT DIABETES?

In the first few chapters of this book, we've examined the problem of diabetes and the multiple metabolic factors that drive the condition. This may have left you with questions: *Isn't diabetes a genetic condition? I thought I inherited it from my parents. How can I prevent or reverse something that was passed down to me genetically?*

Diabetes does have a genetic component. In fact, all diseases have a genetic component, or else they wouldn't exist. But does a genetic predisposition to a certain disease always mean that developing the disease is inevitable? No!

For example, consider the case of identical twins. Identical twins have identical genes. From birth, they share the same exact genetic blueprint. So why is it that one identical twin can be diagnosed with terminal cancer, while the other twin remains cancer free? One twin can be lean and fit, while the other is obese. One twin can be diabetic, the other diabetes-free. These questions can be answered, at least in part, by epigenetics.

EPIGENETICS

You were probably taught in your middle-school biology class that the genes a person inherits determine their destiny. This long-held theory teaches that, at the beginning of life, every person is "dealt a hand" of genes. These genes largely determine whether or not you will contract certain diseases. Some people inherit "good genes," while others inherit "bad genes." Since we don't have a choice as to which genes we inherit, we must simply hope for the best.

For decades, this has been the mainstream teaching regarding genetics. However, in recent years a wealth of new research has proven that this theory isn't true. Research in the field of epigenetics has challenged traditional viewpoints.

Epigenetics comes from two words. The first is the Greek word *epi* meaning "on top of" or "in addition to," and the second word is *genetics*. Epigenetics refers to the factors that affect the way genes work, independent of the genes themselves.

Regardless of what genes we have, there are thousands of factors that influence the way those genes are expressed. The environment that we live in, the choices that we make, and the habits that we form all have profound effects on how our genes function. The role these factors play in the epigenetic phenomenon is best illustrated in the following story about a startling scientific discovery made ten years ago at Duke University.[3, 4, 5]

Epigenetics refers to the factors that affect the way genes work, independent of the genes themselves.

Randy Jirtle, PhD, directs a large genomics research laboratory at Duke. Several years ago, he began researching Agouti mice. These fat mice are genetically bred to become obese. They are born with a yellow coat instead of a brown coat. Under normal laboratory conditions, the agouti mice rapidly gain weight and then develop diabetes and heart disease. The majority of the mice die prematurely of cancer. The poor Agouti mice inherit a triple-whammy of significant health risks.

Dr. Jirtle and his fellow researchers were curious to learn if they could change the Agouti gene in these mice. They were astonished to discover that, by feeding the fat yellow mice a special nutritional supplement along with their regular Purina mouse chow, the mice began giving birth to lean, brown-coated mice within a short time period. The brown-coated mice did not develop obesity, diabetes, heart disease, or cancer.

SAME GENES, DIFFERENT OUTCOMES

Although a traditional view of genetics would assume that the Agouti gene had been eradicated from the offspring and that the brown-coated mice were genetically different, that isn't what the researchers found. When they compared the genetic codes, they discovered that the brown mice still had the Agouti gene. Although they looked completely different and were much healthier, the lean, brown-coated mice were genetically identical to the fat, sick, yellow-coated mice.

Although the special diet fed to the Agouti mice did not change their actual genes, it completely changed the way their genes worked. The additional nutrients had such a powerful effect that they actually deactivated the Agouti gene.

The good news is that gene expression changes don't just occur in mice. They also occur in people! Every lifestyle choice you make has the potential to turn your good genes on and your bad genes off. Epigenetics teaches that you are not a helpless victim when it comes to your genetics. Instead, you play an active role in the way your genes are expressed.

Every lifestyle choice has the potential to help turn your good genes on and your bad genes off.

After the Agouti mouse experiment, Dr. Jirtle concluded: "Epigenetics is proving we have some responsibility for the integrity of our genome. Before, genes predetermined outcomes; now, everything we do—everything we eat or smoke—can affect our gene expression and that of future generations. Epigenetics introduces the concept of free will into our idea of genetics."[6]

GOOD GENES ON, BAD GENES OFF

Dean Ornish, MD, is one of the most well-known and highly-respected advocates of lifestyle and nutritional medicine. In 1990, he published groundbreaking research that proved for the first time to the scientific community that heart disease could be reversed through changes in diet, exercise, and stress management.[7]

In 2008, Dr. Ornish undertook another fascinating research project in the field of epigenetics.[8] This study followed 30 men who had been diagnosed with low-grade prostate cancer, but who had opted out of conventional treatment methods such as surgery, radiation, and hormone therapy. These men were placed on a three-month lifestyle program that included a healthy plant-based diet, moderate exercise, stress management, and weekly support group meetings.

The goal of the study was to see whether these lifestyle changes would change the way that the men's cancer genes were expressed. Each participant underwent genetic testing prior to the beginning of the study and again after three months of implementing the lifestyle program.

The results were remarkable. Not only did the men experience significant health improvements such as weight loss, lower blood pressure, and lower cholesterol, but they also showed evidence of major epigenetic changes. At the beginning of the study, 453 genes known to promote disease had been specifically tested and found to be active. Just three months later, follow-up testing revealed that all 453 disease-promoting genes had been deactivated. Additionally, the 48 disease-preventing genes that had been inactive at the beginning of the study were now all active after the lifestyle changes. To put it simply, lifestyle changes turned on all the good genes, and turned off all the bad genes!

Dr. Ornish believes this study provides hope for anyone battling genetic predispositions. He says, "It's an exciting finding because so often people say, 'Oh, it's all in my genes, what can I do?' Well, it turns out you may be able to do a lot. In just three months, I can change hundreds of my genes simply by changing what I eat and how I live. That's pretty exciting! The implications of our study are not limited to men with prostate cancer."[9]

THE BEST APPROACH

According to the National Cancer Institute, 1 in 8 American women will develop breast cancer.[10] Sadly, an estimated 40,000 American women die of breast cancer each year.[11] In the 1990s, researchers discovered two specific genes, BRCA-1 and BRCA-2, that play a role in the prevention of breast and ovarian cancer.[12] When these genes function properly, breast cancer is not likely to occur. However, when a mutation is present in either of these genes, a woman is at much higher risk for developing breast and ovarian cancer.

This new knowledge led many women to undergo genetic testing to determine their risk. Those who tested positive for mutations in the genes knew that they had a much higher chance of developing breast and ovarian cancer. Many of these women chose to undergo prophylactic mastectomies and oophorectomies, as a pre-emptive strike against cancer. Even women in their 20s and 30s were undergoing these procedures!

It may be that these surgeries have saved the lives of some women who would have otherwise developed cancer. But what if there were a better approach? What if, instead of undergoing radical procedures, these women had followed the same lifestyle approach as the men in Dr. Ornish's study? Such an approach would be noninvasive and would avoid the emotional consequences of lifelong disfiguration. It would also be comprehensive, reducing health risks not only for breast and ovarian cancer, but for many other diseases as well. Ongoing research in this area suggests that the best and most simple approach to avoid disease is to take full advantage of your epigenetic potential.

THE DIABETIC'S GENETICS

What about diabetes? What is the genetic connection? Researchers have discovered that multiple genes are associated with the development of type 2 diabetes. But does that mean that people with those genes will automatically inherit the disease? No. It simply means that they have inherited a genetic predisposition and are at an increased risk for developing diabetes if those genes are expressed. The disease will not develop unless triggered by lifestyle or environmental factors that allow the diabetes genes to become active.

Francis Collins, MD, current director of the National Institutes of Health and former director of the Human Genome Project, describes it this way: "Genetics loads the gun and environment pulls the trigger."

In between college classes and work, my son Dakota enjoys going to the shooting range for target practice. One of his favorite sayings is: "Guns don't kill people. People kill people." This principle applies to health as well. I tell my patients who are concerned about their family history and genetic risk: *Genes don't kill people; unhealthy choices kill people.*

THERE IS HOPE

Understanding how genes function provides hope for all of us. Each of us inherited a unique collection of genes—some helpful and some harmful. However, we're not helpless victims when it comes to genetics. We have the ability to re-engineer our genetic risk and enhance our genetic potential—one choice at a time.

Does this mean that we have found the solution to all genetic diseases? No. We are just now scratching the surface of our epigenetic potential. There are certain diseases we still don't understand well. However, our current understanding of epigenetics suggests that all diseases can be positively influenced through lifestyle medicine.

The things we do, the things we eat or drink, the activities that we're involved in, our thoughts and attitudes—all have a significant influence on how our genes are expressed. The daily choices we make, however small they may seem, have a profound influence on our health, as well as on the health of future generations.

As you follow the principles outlined in this book, you will see noticeable changes in your health and performance. These changes may be measured by improved blood sugar and cholesterol levels, weight loss, and reduced blood pressure. While these changes are rewarding, it's also exciting to realize that, for every change that you see, multiple changes are occurring behind the scenes that you don't see. The same lifestyle choices that help you say goodbye to diabetes will also help you say goodbye to many other genetic risks.

CHAPTER SUMMARY

- Genes contain information that influences how the body functions.
- The way your genes are expressed has a profound impact on your health.
- Epigenetics refers to changes that occur in gene expression, while the actual genetic code remains the same.
- A genetic predisposition to a certain disease does not necessarily mean that the disease must exist.
- Genes associated with diabetes can be activated or deactivated by lifestyle and environmental factors.
- There is hope for all who have genetic predispositions for diabetes, and many other diseases.
- You can turn good genes on and bad genes off one choice at a time.

—FIVE—

There's a Cure For Sure!

IN THE TIME IT TAKES YOU TO READ THIS SENTENCE, approximately 200,000 people will perform a Google search.[1] In the past decade, Google and other Internet search engines have revolutionized the way millions of people seek information.

When I did a Google search for the word "diabetes," I found 304,000,000 results. I was especially interested to know what the top search results would say about whether or not diabetes could be cured. Here are the top six hits:

1. **U.S. National Library of Medicine:**
   "Diabetes is a lifelong (chronic) disease.... There is no cure for diabetes."

2. **American Diabetes Association:**
   "There is no cure for diabetes."

3. **Wikipedia:**
   "Type 1 and 2 [diabetes] are chronic conditions that usually cannot be cured."

4. ***New York Times:***
   "There is no cure for diabetes."

5. **WebMD:**
   "Avoid products that promise a cure for diabetes. There is no cure."

6. **The Mayo Clinic:**
   "There is no cure for type 2 diabetes."

What? The top six search results all claim that there's no cure? Then why is this book called "Goodbye Diabetes?" you may wonder. As a clinician who has worked with diabetics for more than 20 years, I chose the title *Goodbye Diabetes* because I strongly believe there *is* a cure. I am not alone in that belief. Many other researchers and clinicians have also concluded that *there is a cure for type 2 diabetes!*

WHY THE CONTRADICTION?

As you have seen, this is a controversial issue. How can we know for sure what to believe? Before we continue the discussion, we need to make sure we understand *exactly* what it means to be "cured of diabetes." Take a look at these definitions of the word "cure."

cure:

To restore to health.

To effect a recovery from: *cure a cold.*

To remove or remedy (something harmful or disturbing): *cure an evil* [2]

TYPE 2 DIABETES

We learned in Chapter 2 that diabetes is simply *having blood sugar levels so high, and for so long, that they eventually cause significant health complications, if not corrected.* But there is more to it than that. The American Diabetes Association has issued four specific diagnostic criteria that can independently determine the presence of diabetes:[3]

- A fasting blood glucose of 126 mg/dL or higher.
- A blood glucose of 200 or higher, two hours after an oral glucose tolerance test.
- A random blood glucose of 200 or higher, taken at any time and accompanied by classic diabetic symptoms.
- A Hemoglobin A1c level of 6.5 percent or higher.

With these definitions in mind, when we ask the question, *Is there a cure for diabetes?* we are really asking, *Can someone who once met the criteria for type 2 diabetes improve their condition so significantly that they no longer meet the criteria? Can someone with diabetes be restored to health?* And if a person who used to meet the criteria for diabetes no longer does (without the aid of medication), wouldn't it be safe to say that that person has been cured of diabetes? The answer is... absolutely yes!

IS THERE A CURE FOR OBESITY?

Claiming that there is no cure for diabetes is similar to claiming that there is no cure for obesity. "Once a diabetic, always a diabetic" is as illogical as "Once obese, always obese."

When Lisa first came to my office, she weighed 248 pounds. Lisa was active and fit throughout college, but gained quite a bit of weight during her pregnancies. After a difficult divorce, Lisa turned to food for emotional comfort. Her weight spiraled out of control. She came to me depressed, disappointed in herself, and desperately wanting to change.

Obesity is defined as having a Body Mass Index (BMI) of 30 or higher.[4] The BMI is calculated based on a person's height and weight. At 5 feet 6 inches tall, Lisa's BMI was 40, placing her at a much higher risk for heart disease, diabetes, cancer, and many other diseases.

Now, suppose I had said to her: "Lisa, you weigh 248 pounds. Your BMI is 40. You are obese. In fact, you will always be obese. Even if you lose 120 pounds and lower your BMI to an optimal level of 21, you will still be obese. It doesn't matter how skinny you get, you will always be obese, and there's nothing you can do about it. However, you can try to "control your obesity" by losing weight. That way you won't be as likely to have complications resulting from your obesity." If I'd said those things to Lisa, she would think I was crazy—and she would be right!

Specific criteria define what it means to be overweight and obese. (A BMI over 25 is considered overweight, and a BMI over 30 is considered obese[5]). If Lisa were to drop from a BMI of 40 to a BMI of 21, she would drop from obesity to a normal, healthy weight. She would no longer be considered obese, because she would no longer fit the criteria.

In the same way, hundreds of patients have come to me with type 2 diabetes. Their blood sugars and/or Hemoglobin A1c levels have fit the criteria for a diabetes diagnosis. When I sit down with these patients, I don't tell them, "You have type 2 diabetes. Unfortunately, you will always be diabetic. There is no cure. However, you should try to manage your condition to prevent complications." No! I say, "You have type 2 diabetes. This is a wake-up call. You can do something about it! The good news is that the majority of people with type 2 diabetes can reverse the disease, and I want to help you do just that."

I have seen hundreds of patients reverse their diabetes by following comprehensive lifestyle programs. Patients who once fit the criteria for diabetes no longer have blood sugar or Hemoglobin A1c levels that fit those criteria. And if, without pharmaceutical intervention, they no longer fit the criteria for diabetes, *it's safe to say that they are no longer diabetic!*

Of course, there's always the risk of relapse. A person who has lost weight and reversed their obesity can fall into old, unhealthy patterns and become obese again. But that doesn't mean that there is no cure for obesity. In the same way, if a person who has reversed—or cured—type 2 diabetes abandons positive lifestyle changes and reverts to former choices that contributed to the disease, diabetes can develop again. But this does not mean that they weren't really cured, or that a cure doesn't exist. It simply means that the human body must be treated the way it was designed to be treated for the cure to be permanent.

A diabetic relapse can also be triggered by acute illness, trauma, or major stress. For example, anyone who has had diabetes for an extended period of time knows that catching a cold or flu causes their blood sugars to shoot way up. However, former diabetics who continue to address these problems head-on will find that they can once again stabilize their blood sugars.

MY INTEREST IN DIABETES

The year was 1985. I was studying at Loma Linda University in Loma Linda, California. Because I had minimal financial aid in my first year of professional training, I was taking a light class load. Eager to learn, I took advantage of my spare time by attending numerous conferences and lectures around campus.

Loma Linda is a mecca of health and healing. It includes a state-of-the-art medical center and children's hospital, as well as a health science institution comprised of eight different schools and more than 55 programs. In 2005

Loma Linda was featured in the November issue of *National Geographic* in an article entitled "The Secrets of Living Longer." It was listed as one of the top three places in the world where people live the longest—together known as "Blue Zones."[6] Because of its strong emphasis in health and health research, Loma Linda University offers a wide variety of lectures and seminars on nearly every health topic you can think of. These lectures provided me with invaluable information that expanded on what I was learning in class.

I was fortunate enough to attend a lecture by James Anderson, MD, a world-renowned endocrinologist and researcher, and professor emeritus of medicine and clinical nutrition at the University of Kentucky. Dr. Anderson was lecturing on his work in diabetes reversal. He shared multiple examples where he took hospitalized type 2 diabetic patients who were following the standard American diet and placed them on a high fiber, primarily plant-based diet.[7] The amount of medications normally needed by these patients dropped drastically. The need for insulin and oral medications dropped anywhere from 75 to 90 percent in just a few weeks.

Dr. Anderson claimed that type 2 diabetes was reversible. This was the first time I had ever heard this claim. The prevailing teaching was that there was no cure for diabetes, but Dr. Anderson was clearly showing that his patients had been successful in reversing their conditions.

His lecture piqued my interest in diabetes and, in many ways, set the stage for my future career. It provided me with a scientific, evidence-based foundation to apply in my own clinical practice. As I began working with diabetic patients, I found that the same strategies that helped Dr. Anderson's patients to reverse diabetes also helped my patients to reverse diabetes.

THE DIABETES DEBATE

In 2004—19 years after I attended Dr. Anderson's lecture—the president of the Guam Medical Society called and invited me to give a lecture at an upcoming regional medical conference. I agreed and asked him what he would like me to speak about. "I'd love for you to talk about reversing diabetes with nutrition," he said. Wanting to be sure that he knew what to expect, I asked, "Are you *sure* you want me to talk about reversing diabetes? It's a pretty controversial topic." "Yes," he replied, "I'm sure they will love it."

The weekend of the conference arrived. More than 500 physicians and health professionals were gathered from all over the Pacific. As I stood up to address them, I started with this disclaimer, "I just want to go on record as saying that I didn't choose the title of this lecture, 'Reversing Diabetes.' It was actually the president of the medical society who chose it." Not knowing how people would react to the information, I grinned and hoped I was off the hook.

I went on to present the latest research and rationale as to how diabetes can be reversed through nutritional strategies. I told the stories of several patients who had come to me suffering with type 2 diabetes. After following specialized lifestyle medicine plans, they no longer fit the criteria for diabetes. I also showed a clip of the recently released film, *Supersize Me.* In this entertaining documentary, Morgan Spurlock eats nothing but McDonald's food for 30 days. Over the course of just one month, Spurlock gains twenty-five pounds and his cholesterol increases from 165 to 230. He also begins experiencing mood swings, depression, sexual dysfunction, and fat accumulation in his liver.

Throughout the film, Spurlock interviews different health professionals. The clip I showed was of Spurlock interviewing Adam Naaman, MD, and Carl Geisler, MD—two well-known bariatric surgeons. They made an interesting claim about the effect of bariatric surgery on diabetes: "We have established now that the only procedure that really cures diabetes is obesity [gastric bypass] surgery."[8]

I clarified that I was not recommending bariatric surgery for diabetes treatment, but simply sharing this information to make them aware of studies showing that diabetes is indeed curable. While I believe that lifestyle strategies like nutrition and exercise are the optimal way to reverse diabetes, research helps demonstrate that a cure is possible.

I finished my 90-minute lecture, feeling that it had gone well. As I was preparing to take questions from the audience, a physician and leader of the conference stood up to speak. "As the chairman of the scientific committee, I want to go on record that I completely disagree with Dr. Youngberg's assertion that diabetes is reversible."

The physician went on to explain that, as a nephrologist (kidney doctor) who sees many patients with diabetes, he believed he would be giving people false hope to tell them that their diabetes could be reversed.

The speaker who preceded me was a geneticist who lectured about a future cure for diabetes using genetic re-engineering. As the nephrologist continued to critique my lecture, he challenged, "Perhaps someday in the future when we learn more about genetic engineering—we may reverse diabetes—but not now." With that, he sat down, waiting for my response. As you can imagine, the audience had grown very quiet, waiting to see what would happen next.

"First of all, most of us were trained to believe that diabetes is not reversible," I said. "It's our natural bias to believe what we learn in school. But evidence is showing that this belief simply isn't true. I'm glad that you mentioned genetic engineering, because that's exactly the way that nutritional medicine operates. We don't have to wait until researchers discover gene therapies to stop diabetes. We have the power to turn good genes on and bad genes off by the lifestyle choices we make today."

Two days later, I was listening to the news as I drove to work. The radio host announced a groundbreaking health study that had just been published in *The Journal of the American Medical Association* (JAMA). That large study with thousands of participants showed that 77 percent of diabetic individuals who had undergone gastric bypass surgery were able to reverse or "completely resolve" their diabetes within one year.[9]

I was excited about the new research, but wished that I had been able to reference it in my lecture the previous Sunday. I parked my car, headed into the office building, and got on the elevator. Who was there to meet me but the nephrologist who had challenged my lecture? His kidney dialysis center was right across from my lifestyle medicine clinic. We were the only two people in the elevator! My initial impression was to say: "Hey, did you hear the news this morning about the new JAMA study and diabetes reversal?" Thankfully, I resisted the urge, greeted him, and then kept my mouth shut. I knew that he would find out soon enough.

I'm glad that I chose not to rub it in, because within months this same nephrologist asked me to collaborate with him on several research projects involving diabetes in the Pacific region. Once he saw the evidence for himself, he began to recognize the value of the information I had presented.

I can understand why this nephrologist initially believed that diabetes was incurable. He was dealing with patients in the very final stages of diabetes. He was treating renal dialysis patients whose kidneys couldn't function without being hooked up to a dialysis unit. Even though he was a good doctor, he thought it was impossible because he had never seen diabetes reversal happen. From my perspective, I knew a cure was possible, because I had seen it happen time and time again.

When physicians say that diabetes is not curable, they are expressing conclusions based on their own understanding and experience. This does not mean that they are not excellent, well-trained doctors. It just means that they may not have had the opportunity to see diabetes reversal for themselves.

THE PREVAILING DOGMA

It is estimated that clinical knowledge doubles every year-and-a-half. With an increase in technology and communication, researchers are conducting thousands of clinical trials and studies each month. We live in an exciting era. We're constantly discovering new information about science and health.

But there's a difference between information and application. Clinicians, healthcare organizations, and educators all face the difficult challenge of updating medical care, policies, and procedures based on current information. Often, there is a significant lag time between information and application.

Although scientific evidence and common sense both strongly suggest that there is a cure for type 2 diabetes, the prevailing medical dogma still says, "Once a diabetic. Always a diabetic."

The good news is that, in response to the growing awareness that type 2 diabetes is reversible, the American Diabetes Association has commissioned a task force to explore this issue. Their goal is to develop official criteria that will determine when diabetes has been cured.[10]

A DIFFERENT PERSPECTIVE

I'm thankful that a growing number of clinicians, researchers, and former diabetics are ignoring the prevailing medical dogma and telling the world that *there is a cure for type 2 diabetes!* But don't just take my word for it. Here's what they have to say:

Dean Ornish, MD

"Got diabetes? Get rid of it."

As mentioned in the previous chapter, Dr. Ornish is a highly respected pioneer of lifestyle medicine. A Harvard-trained internal medicine specialist, Dr. Ornish has spent the past 33 years researching and implementing lifestyle strategies to help people reverse disease. Dr. Ornish is a sought-after speaker, best-selling author, and effective practitioner.

When President Bill Clinton wanted to lose weight and shape up for his daughter Chelsea's wedding, he sought the help of several physicians, including Dr. Ornish. Clinton had a history of heart disease, and had undergone a quadruple bypass surgery in 2004. Knowing that he still had blockage in his arteries, Clinton hoped that lifestyle changes would not only improve his weight, but also his heart.[11] He carefully followed the plant-based diet and moderate exercise program prescribed to him, and quickly began seeing results. After losing 24 pounds, lowering his cholesterol, and essentially reversing his heart disease, Clinton was convinced that Ornish was on to something big.

Not only does Dr. Ornish help people reverse heart disease, lose weight, and lower cholesterol, but he also helps people to reverse diabetes: "Although heart disease and diabetes kill more people worldwide than all other diseases combined, these are completely preventable and often reversible for at least 95 percent of people today by changing our diet and lifestyle." [12]

John McDougall, MD

"A simple cure is possible for essentially everyone with type 2 diabetes."

For the past thirty years, Dr. John McDougall has cared for thousands of patients suffering from a variety of degenerative diseases, including diabetes. He is the medical director of the McDougall Program, a ten-day residential lifestyle program in Santa Rosa, California. That program is designed to optimize health and jumpstart the reversal of diabetes and other diseases. Like Dr. Ornish, Dr. McDougall is a best-selling author and sought-after speaker.

He is considered an authority in his field. Dr. McDougall has seen first-hand that there is a cure for type 2 diabetes. Thousands of people have reversed their type 2 diabetes by following Dr. McDougall's plan. One of these people is Jason Wyrick.

Jason Wyrick

In his late twenties, Jason should have been the picture of perfect health. Instead, he found himself in a hospital bed in Austin, Texas. He was more than 100 pounds overweight, had a dangerous infection, and had just been diagnosed with type 2 diabetes. Jason was told that he would need to take insulin for the rest of his life.[13]

Jason believes he was diabetic for at least two years before the diagnosis. He had been fatigued and moody, and had experienced problems with his eyesight, which had dramatically deteriorated.

Hospitalization was a wake-up call for Jason. Fortunately, he found a friend who had been through a similar experience. After researching her options, she had started a low-fat, plant-based diet, which she read about in Dr. McDougall's books. Within a few months, her symptoms were gone, and soon after that, she no longer fit the criteria for diabetes.

Jason decided to give it a shot. He switched to a plant-based diet, avoiding meat, dairy products, and refined foods, as well as increasing his intake of fruits, vegetables, legumes, and whole grains.

How is Jason doing now? Here's his report: "I have lost over one hundred pounds, cured my diabetes, regained my eyesight, achieved the ability to think quickly again, and I'm in better shape than when I was an athlete in high school... My [fasting] blood sugar is now 89 mg/dl..." Jason's new lifestyle impacted every aspect of his life: "After I made that change, I could go out, I could take classes, I could go to the gym, I could go see a movie, I could do work, and... *I could do it all in the same day*!"[14] Jason's story provides hope for anyone suffering from type 2 diabetes.

Neal Barnard, MD

Dr. Neal Barnard is a physician and clinical researcher with the George Washington School of Medicine and the president of the Physician's

Committee for Responsible Medicine. Dr. Barnard has authored 14 books on nutrition, collectively selling over two million copies. One of these books is *Dr. Neal Barnard's Program for Reversing Diabetes.*[15] In 2003, the National Institutes of Health gave Dr. Barnard a $350,000 research grant to study the effects of a low-fat, plant-based diet for diabetes treatment. The results were published in the American Diabetes Association's *Diabetes Care* magazine.[16] Several years ago, I met with Dr. Barnard for lunch to discuss the impact of his study. He was enthusiastic about the results. Let's look at the story of one of the participants in Dr. Barnard's study.

Nancy Boughn

Nancy Boughn was diagnosed with type 2 diabetes in 1996. Through the years, she tried to control her condition, but wasn't very successful. In 2003, two of her friends who also had diabetes started experiencing serious complications. One friend lost her eyesight. The other friend had to begin dialysis because her kidney function had deteriated so drastically. Nancy was very concerned for her own health. "I thought it was time to take another step in the right direction, making sure that this didn't happen to me," she said. She saw an ad in the *Washington Post*, looking for diabetics who were interested in being part of Dr. Barnard's study for the National Institutes of Health. Knowing that something drastic needed to change, Nancy joined the study.[17]

At the beginning of the study, Nancy weighed 196 pounds, and her Hemoglobin A1c was 8.3 percent. This means that she was at a high risk for cardiovascular disease, stroke, kidney disease, nerve damage, and blindness.

Nancy began following a plant-based diet—avoiding all animal products and eating a variety of vegetables, fruits, whole grains, and legumes (beans, peas, and lentils). Here's what Nancy reported in a video interview at the conclusion of the study:

"Almost immediately upon starting this diet, I noticed that I felt better generally, and I could tell that my blood glucose numbers were dropping, because of course I checked them a number of times a day. In a period of five months, my A1c number went from 8.3 to 6.4, and I also lost all my joint pain. So I consider that an added bonus. And then immediately the weight started falling off. We were in the study for 18 months and I lost 48 pounds.... The study is over and we've had the final results, and everything about my numbers look great across the board."[18]

Joel Fuhrman, MD

"If you're a type 2 [diabetic], we won't be *controlling* your diabetes, we'll be having you become *undiabetic.*"

Dr. Joel Fuhrman is one of the nation's leading experts in nutritional medicine. He has appeared on *Today, Good Morning America, The Dr. Oz Show,* CNN, ABC, CBS, NBC, FOX, Discovery Channel, and many other TV and radio programs and networks. Dr. Fuhrman is the research director of the Nutritional Research Project, an initiative of the National Health Association.

Dr. Fuhrman directs a clinic in New Jersey. There, he has treated thousands of patients with diabetes and helped them to completely reverse the disease. He has authored numerous articles and books, including the *New York Times* bestseller *Eat to Live.* Dr. Fuhrman is a strong believer in the power of lifestyle and nutritional medicine to cure diabetes. "The cure for type 2 diabetes is already known—removing the cause can reverse the disease. Don't *live* with your diabetes and don't simply *control* your diabetes...*get rid of it*!"[19]

Tony Bennett

Fifty-six-year-old Tony had been feeling lousy for several months. His sister, who had been diabetic for the past 25 years, used her glucose meter to test his blood sugar. It was 491. After a trip to the ER, Tony was prescribed metformin and aspirin, referred to an endocrinologist, and sent home. He was not given any advice regarding his diet.

A few weeks later, the endocrinologist prescribed several additional medications for Tony. He began taking them but soon experienced serious side effects. Because he did not have medical insurance, Tony's options were limited. He couldn't afford to continue doctor visits or medications. While researching diabetes on the Internet, he found Dr. Fuhrman's website and ordered the books *Eat to Live* and *Eat for Health.* He was skeptical at first, but decided to give the program a chance. Dr. Fuhrman's program focuses on a nutrient-dense, low-fat, plant-based diet. Tony began that diet and stopped taking all of his medications. *(Please consult your doctor before changing your medications.)*

After just three months on the new diet, Tony's weight dropped from 220 to 195 pounds, and his Hemoglobin A1c dropped from 8.9 to 6.0 percent. This reduced his risk of a heart attack by over 50 percent. Tony no longer fit into the diagnosable criteria for diabetes. In other words, Tony's diabetes had been cured![20]

WHAT IT ALL MEANS

Drs. Dean Ornish, John McDougall, Neal Barnard, Joel Fuhrman, and researchers and clinicians like them have helped to revolutionize our understanding of the connection between diet and disease. People like Jason, Nancy, and Tony provide evidence that lifestyle and nutritional changes really work. Their stories help to validate what I have seen first-hand in my own clinical practice.

After spending more than 20 years treating people with type 2 diabetes, I have seen evidence in the lives of my patients that there is a cure! The cure is not found in a magic pill or potion. It is found in nourishing and treating our bodies according to their design. The growing body of evidence shows that the lifestyle interventions outlined in this book provide a powerful cure for diabetes.

CAN EVERYONE BE CURED?

Although it is possible for most type 2 diabetes cases to be reversed through the vigorous application of lifestyle medicine, some patients try very hard but still do not get their lab values and blood sugars into the target ranges. Try as they might, they still need medication to control their blood sugar levels.

Diabetes is a progressive disease. The earlier it is detected and treated, the better the prognosis. While the majority of type 2 diabetics can become non-diabetic, some people may still fit the criteria for diabetes even after following a comprehensive lifestyle program.

For example, some type 2 diabetics have sustained so much damage to the pancreatic tissue that they may always need some insulin. This is because their type 2 diabetes has progressed for so long that it has actually become more like type 1 diabetes.

Is there hope for this group of people? Are the lifestyle strategies still worth following? Absolutely! The good news is that this group will still benefit tremendously from following the same diabetes reversal plan. They will increase their sensitivity to insulin, cut down on the amount of medication needed, and dramatically reverse their risk for heart disease and other complications.

Remember that health is not solely defined by blood sugar levels. Although blood sugar levels are important, lifestyle strategies improve health in many other ways. Since the ultimate goal is *to be healthy*—not to *just* control blood sugars—there is hope for 100 percent of diabetics (both type 1 and type 2) to improve their overall wellness by following this plan.

THE POWER OF HOPE

I love the statement by the apostle Paul that says we are "saved by hope."[21] This concept applies to all aspects of our lives. In order to accomplish any goal, we must first have hope that the goal is possible and that it is within our reach. It is my hope that the information in this chapter has inspired *you* with hope that it is possible to improve your health and reverse—or greatly improve—your diabetes.

Another favorite quote of mine is by Seneca, the ancient Roman orator: "It is part of the cure to wish to be cured." Knowing that a cure exists gives us hope. The more we wish for the cure, the more motivated we will be to do everything in our power to obtain it and to say, "Goodbye diabetes."

CHAPTER SUMMARY

- Overwhelming evidence shows that there is a cure for type 2 diabetes.
- Most type 2 diabetes cases are reversible.
- A person who no longer fits the criteria for diabetes (without taking medications) should no longer be considered diabetic.
- Thousands of people have reversed type 2 diabetes by following simple lifestyle strategies, including a high-nutrient, plant-based diet.
- There is hope for all who struggle with diabetes!

SECTION 3

Detecting Diabetes

— SIX —

Warning Signs

ON APRIL 15, 1912, THE RMS TITANIC SANK TO ITS watery grave at the bottom of the Atlantic Ocean. Just four days before, 2,208 passengers and crew members had boarded the vessel—the largest and most luxurious passenger ship of its time. They were confident that the *Titanic* would carry them safely and comfortably from Southampton, England, to New York City in just eight days.

Touted as the "safest ship ever built," the *Titanic* was thought to be unsinkable. But, after striking an iceberg, it took only three hours for the *Titanic* to sink. When Phillip Franklin, vice president of the company that built the *Titanic,* received the report that the ship had struck an iceberg and sunk, he did not believe it. "There is no danger that *Titanic* will sink. The boat is unsinkable and nothing but inconvenience will be suffered by the passengers." Later that day, Franklin sobbed as he informed reporters of the "horrible loss of life" accompanied by the sinking of the ship. Of the 2,208 passengers and crew who boarded the ship, only 705 survived.

One hundred years later, the story of the *Titanic* still captivates the hearts of those who hear it. What really happened? Why did so many people have to die? Could the collision have been prevented? Once it occurred, could it have been dealt with more effectively? There are answers to these questions, and some of these answers are rather unsettling.

LESSONS FROM THE TITANIC

The *Titanic* tragedy claimed the lives of more than 1,500 people. Although this disaster took the ship and the entire world by surprise, it didn't come without prior warning. Warnings were ignored and unheeded, adequate safety precautions were overlooked, and rescue measures fell short of their potential. I share this story because I believe that the *Titanic* can teach us powerful lessons about diabetes.

TITANIC LESSON #1: BEWARE OF COMPLACENCY

The story of the *Titanic* illustrates all too well that complacency can kill. The *Titanic* struck an iceberg at 11:40 p.m. on Sunday, April 14. Earlier that day, the ship had received at least six telegraphs from neighboring ships—warning of approaching ice. But the telegraph operators were overwhelmed with sending and receiving personal correspondence telegraphs between passengers and their loved ones. They delivered a few—but not all—of the warning messages to the bridge (the commanding center of the ship). But even the messages that were delivered went unheeded. The *Titanic* sailed on at almost maximum speed.

The captain and crew had full confidence in their ship. They were distracted by their various duties and social engagements—caught up in the excitement of the voyage. They didn't take the warning signs seriously. They reasoned that, if an iceberg was present, they would see it in plenty of time to change their course and avoid collision. "If we can't see it, it must not be a problem."

All too often, we are tempted to have the same complacent attitude toward our health. Unless something feels drastically wrong, we assume that everything is OK. "If I can't see it or feel it, it must not be a problem."

Unfortunately, by the time the people on the *Titanic* saw, felt, and heard the iceberg it was too late. In the same way, if we complacently wait for major disease symptoms to appear before evaluating or addressing our health, we place ourselves in danger.

Diabetes is called the silent killer. Often the disease process is underway for ten or fifteen years before symptoms are felt. You can't feel diabetes until the disease is well advanced.

Dangerously high blood sugars can damage the body for years, yet go completely undetected. The first sign of a problem can be a heart attack, stroke, kidney damage, or vision problems. By the time these events occur, the body has already been seriously damaged. The good news is that we don't have to be complacent. We can choose to plan ahead and pay attention to the warning signs that are available to us.

TITANIC LESSON #2: PAY ATTENTION TO WARNING SIGNS

Just like the *Titanic* received multiple warnings indicating that danger was ahead, multiple signs and symptoms signal the approach of prediabetes and diabetes. Here are some of the official warning signs that increase risk for diabetes:

RISK FACTORS FOR DIABETES[1]

- You're 45 years or older.
- You're overweight or obese.
- You do not exercise regularly.
- You have elevated blood pressure.
- Your cholesterol and/or triglyceride blood fat levels are not normal.
- You have a family history of diabetes.
- You are Black, Hispanic, Native American, Asian, or Pacific Islander.
- You've had gestational diabetes or have given birth to a baby weighing more than nine pounds.

Although the above list isn't exhaustive, it is the official standard published by the American Diabetes Association in an attempt to warn people about major risk factors for diabetes. Let's take a closer look at these risk factors.

AGE

Risk of type 2 diabetes increases with age—especially after age 45. In 2008, Catherine Cowie, PhD, director of the diabetes epidemiology program for the National Institutes of Health, documented the correlation between diabetes and age:[2]

Age	Diabetes Risk	Prediabetes Risk	Total Risk (Diabetes and Prediabetes)
12-19 yrs.	0.3%	16.0%	16.3%
20-39 yrs.	3.1%	17.9%	21.1%
40-59 yrs.	12.4%	34.6%	47.0%
60-74 yrs.	30.0%	36.8%	66.7%
75+ yrs.	29.1%	46.7%	75.7%

As you can see, the risk for both prediabetes and diabetes dramatically increases with age. However, it's important to remember that, in and of itself, age does not determine the incidence of diabetes. Diabetes can happen at almost any age. I've treated patients as young as seven and eight years old with advanced prediabetes.

Historically, type 1 diabetes was called "childhood onset diabetes" and type 2 diabetes was called "adult onset diabetes." Children rarely develop type 2 adult onset diabetes. However, with increasingly unhealthy diets, sedentary lifestyles, and obesity among school-age children, this trend has changed. Because more and more children are developing the adult form of diabetes, diabetes is now defined simply as "type 1" or "type 2."

That is why it's important not to wait until someone is 45 to determine whether they are at risk. It's also important to remember that although most elderly people have diabetes or prediabetes, the disease does not automatically occur with age. Other risk factors must be present for the disease to develop. The good news is that, just as diabetes can occur at almost any age—diabetes can be prevented or reversed at almost any age.

WEIGHT

Being obese or overweight is one of the most significant risk factors for developing type 2 diabetes. Results from the Nurses' Health Study (an ongoing research initiative affiliated with Harvard University) suggest that 50 to 70 percent of all new cases of diabetes could be prevented by maintaining a normal weight or losing weight if necessary.[3]

Losing even 10 pounds can go a long way toward helping to prevent or reverse prediabetes or diabetes.[4] The at-risk weight chart in this chapter will help you determine whether or not your weight is putting you at risk.

Weight isn't the only number to consider, however. Body fat percentage should also be taken into account.[5] People who weigh more than average, but are lean and carry a lot of muscle weight, are much less likely to develop diabetes than those who have a high body fat percentage. A six-foot-tall man weighing 180 pounds may be fit, lean, and healthy, while his friend—also six feet tall and 180 pounds—may be out of shape with a high body fat percentage and numerous associated risks. The same is true for women. A 5-foot-3-inch-tall woman weighing 125 pounds may have a high body fat percentage and increased risk, while another woman of the same height and weight may be lean, fit, and healthy.

Because the issues of weight and fat are so important, we have dedicated an entire chapter to discuss them in more detail. In Chapter 16 you will find valuable information on how to evaluate and manage your weight and body fat percentage.

FAT DISTRIBUTION

Although any amount of excess fat can increase diabetes risk, fat in the midsection (belly fat) is the most dangerous.[6, 7] People who are "pear shaped" tend to carry more weight in the lower body; particularly the hips and thighs. People who are "apple shaped" carry more weight in their abdominal region. This contributes to more visceral fat (fat surrounding the organs) and increases the risk for heart disease, diabetes, several forms of cancer, and numerous other diseases.[8] To determine whether your fat distribution puts you at increased risk for disease, you can calculate your waist-to-hip ratio according to the directions in Chapter 16.

WHAT IF I'M NOT OVERWEIGHT?

Although excess weight and abdominal fat contribute significantly to the risk of developing type 2 diabetes, people who are not overweight or over-fat can still develop the disease. While weight may not put them at risk, other risk factors may be involved. That's why it's important for everyone to be properly screened and evaluated, regardless of weight.

INACTIVITY

Despite the growing awareness of the health benefits of exercise, 7 out of 10 Americans do not exercise regularly.[9] It is estimated that inactivity contributes to approximately 300,000 deaths annually in the United States, including deaths caused by heart disease, stroke, and diabetes.[10] Data from the Harvard Nurses' Health Study reveals that engaging in regular, moderate exercise can reduce the risk of diabetes by 30 to 50 percent.[11]

Exercise plays a powerful role in reducing insulin resistance.[12] As muscles are used, they burn their sugar stores, and then require more fuel in the form of glucose. In fact, muscles require up to 20 times more glucose during exercise than during rest.[13] When muscles are exercised regularly, they begin to accept more sugar for storage because they know that it will be used up. Starting a regular exercise program is one of the most important strategies for reducing insulin resistance.

The three most important types of exercise for preventing or reversing diabetes are:

- Regular aerobic exercise (5 to 7 days per week for a minimum of 30 minutes or more each day).
- After-meal exercise (light to moderate exercise for 10 to 15 minutes immediately following each meal to help prevent after-meal blood sugar spikes).
- Strength training (20 to 40 minutes, 1 to 3 times per week).

We will discuss these types of exercise in more detail in Chapter 15 and will address how to incorporate them into your wellness plan.

As with other risk factors, it is important to note that not everyone who has diabetes is inactive. Even athletes sometimes develop diabetes. When this occurs, we must determine whether their exercise plan is adequate. Does it combine all three of the important exercise types? People sometimes get regular aerobic activity but do not exercise after meals or participate in strength training. It's important that any exercise program is comprehensive.

We must also remember that multiple factors combine to create diabetes. Inactivity is a significant piece in the puzzle, but it's not the only contributing factor. Consequently, exercise is an extremely important tool to prevent or reverse diabetes, but it should be accompanied by all the other strategies outlined in this book.

HIGH BLOOD PRESSURE

High blood pressure, also known as hypertension, is a warning sign that prediabetes or diabetes may be brewing. Although one third of all American adults suffer from high blood pressure,[14] diabetics are twice as likely to have hypertension as nondiabetics.[15] As mentioned in Chapter 3, insulin resistance is a leading causes of hypertension.

If you have high blood pressure, it's important to be evaluated for prediabetes and diabetes. Too often, doctors prescribe medications to lower blood pressure yet fail to determine or address the underlying cause of the problem. If you have elevated blood pressure or take medication to control your blood pressure, you are probably resistant to insulin and may have prediabetes or diabetes.

Addressing high blood pressure with lifestyle strategies can help to prevent or reverse heart disease and diabetes, as well as to decrease or eliminate the need for blood pressure medication.

HYPERTENSION technically exists if you have a blood pressure of 140/90 or higher. However, as it relates to diabetes, even prehypertension (120/80 to 139/89) can signal a problem. When I see a patient with prehypertension or hypertension, I automatically suspect that they have prediabetes or diabetes, unless testing proves otherwise. If your blood pressure is in this range, it is important that you be thoroughly evaluated for prediabetes and diabetes.

HIGH CHOLESTEROL

Cholesterol is a fatty steroid that provides structure for cells and helps to synthesize hormones. Everyone needs some cholesterol to survive. However, every cell in the body is able to produce this cholesterol. Our bodies naturally produce all the cholesterol we need. It is not necessary to ingest any additional cholesterol from food.[16]

Animal products such as meat, cheese, milk, fish, and eggs all contain cholesterol. These foods can raise cholesterol to unhealthy levels. This contributes to plaque build-up in the arteries and increases the risk for heart attack or stroke.

When foods with cholesterol are exposed to air, the cholesterol combines with oxygen and becomes oxidized. Oxidized cholesterol is very sticky and highly accelerates plaque build-up.[17] Foods high in oxidized cholesterol include custards and puddings, pancake and cake mixes, Parmesan cheese, lard, and ice cream.[18]

While it is very important to avoid high cholesterol foods, it's surprising to discover that saturated and trans fat actually raise cholesterol levels far more than dietary cholesterol does.[19, 20] Saturated and trans fats stimulate the liver and cells to produce more cholesterol than the body needs.

Even among people with high cholesterol, 75 percent of this cholesterol is produced inside the body, while only 25 percent can be attributed to dietary cholesterol.[21] People with high cholesterol aren't just *eating* more of it—they're *producing* more of it.

A high nutrient diet that is low in saturated fat, trans fat, and cholesterol will lower both the production and the accumulation of excess cholesterol.

Elevated cholesterol is one of the major risk factors for cardiovascular disease. If your cholesterol is high, it's important to lower it and to identify other risk factors.

CHOLESTEROL TARGET LEVELS[22]

- » Your total cholesterol should *at least* be under 200, optimally under 180, and ideally under 160.
- » Your HDL ("good") cholesterol should be higher than 40 for men, and higher than 50 for women.
- » Your LDL cholesterol should *at least* be under 130, optimally under 100, and ideally under 70.

HIGH TRIGLYCERIDES

Triglycerides are fats that circulate in the blood or are stored in fat tissue. When you eat more calories than your body needs, these calories are converted to triglycerides. The body needs some of these stores to be used between meals or in the event of a food shortage. However, many people have triglyceride levels that are dangerously high.[23]

Even people at healthy weights can have high triglycerides. Why is this? Not only can *too much* food raise triglyceride levels, but the *wrong types* can raise them as well. Sugary foods and refined grains, alcohol, saturated fat from animal products, junk food, and excess calories all contribute to heightened triglycerides.[24]

High triglyceride levels are closely correlated with insulin resistance.[25] High triglycerides levels should be taken as a warning sign that diabetes or prediabetes may be present.[26]

If your fasting triglyceride levels are over 150 mg/dL, this is a serious red-flag indicating that you may be heading in the direction of diabetes.[27] Optimal levels are less than 100, but levels over 150 show a significant increase in risk.

FAMILY HISTORY

A family history of diabetes—particularly a parent or sibling—increases your risk of developing the disease as well. However, it is encouraging to remember that, although you may inherit a genetic predisposition to diabetes, the disease will not develop unless triggered by lifestyle or environmental factors. As we discussed in Chapter 4, "The Diabetic's Genetics," genes do not determine our destiny. Healthy choices have the power to turn disease-preventing genes on and disease-promoting genes off.

RACE

Diabetes knows no racial or ethnic boundaries. In recent years, as the Western diet and sedentary lifestyle have spread throughout the world, we have seen diabetes develop among people groups who used to be essentially diabetes-free. For example, while 30 years ago diabetes was virtually non-existent in China, today over 92 million Chinese adults have full blown-diabetes, and roughly 150 million have prediabetes.[28] No race is immune to diabetes. There are some races, however, that are at a higher risk for developing diabetes:[29]

AT-RISK PEOPLE GROUPS

- Blacks
- Hispanics
- Native Americans
- Asians
- Native Hawaiians and other Pacific Islanders

These ethnic groups are more likely than whites to develop type 2 diabetes. However, diabetes can occur in people of any race. Although certain groups may have a stronger genetic predisposition toward diabetes, the disease will not occur apart from other factors. A good example of this is the island of Nauru.

THE FAT LITTLE ISLAND

Nauru is a tiny island country located in Micronesia, in the South Pacific. With a population of 9,378, Nauru is the world's smallest republic.[30] Although the island of Nauru is small—the people are not. In fact, Nauru holds the record for having the most obese population in the world. Ninety-seven percent of men and 93 percent of women are overweight or obese.[31] Not surprisingly, Nauru also has the highest rates of diabetes of any country in the world. Nearly half of Nauruans have full-blown diabetes, and many have prediabetes.[32] The average life expectancy on the island is just 56 years for males and 65 years for females.[33]

Being born into the Nauruan culture significantly increases the risk for developing type 2 diabetes. Why? Is it simply a genetic phenomenon? Has it always been this way? The answer is no.[34]

NAURUANS IN 1914

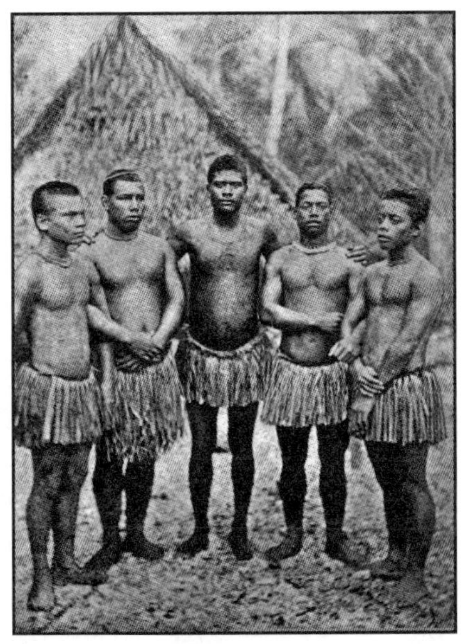

The picture on the right, taken in 1914, shows a group of young, athletic-looking Nauruan men.[35]At that time, Nauruan's were hunter-gatherers, living off the land.[36] They survived on raw or boiled fish, pandunas plants, bananas, and coconut fruit.

Around the same time, the Pacific Phosphate Company began strip-mining in Nauru.[37] Nauru had rich phosphate deposits close to the surface. The country quickly became a major phosphate exporter, which led to an economic boom which lasted for several decades. For a brief period in the late 1960s and early 1970s, Nauru had the highest per-capita income of any country in the world.[38]

But the economic prosperity took a toll on the health of the islanders. With increased wealth, they became less active. Their diet changed as well. They began importing processed, fatty food from Australia and New Zealand.

Eventually, the phosphate deposits on Nauru ran out. Phosphate mining had destroyed much of the soil and vegetation on the island, making agricultural development difficult. The once-wealthy country spiraled into economic collapse.

Today, the Nauruans continue to survive on processed, imported foods. It is virtually impossible for the average Nauruan to purchase healthy food. Only 3 percent of the population has the luxury of regularly eating fruits and vegetables.[39]

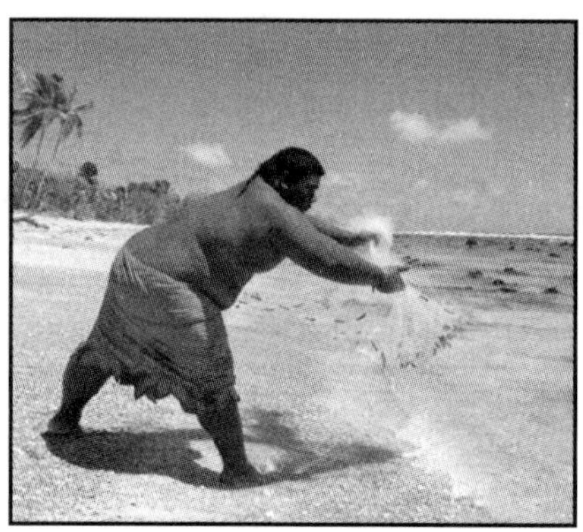

This unfortunate chain of events explains why so many Nauruans suffer from obesity and diabetes today. Although the islanders do have a genetic predisposition to diabetes, the disease did not develop until they moved away from a natural diet and active lifestyle.

Nauru teaches a valuable lesson regarding diabetes and racial risk. People born into ethnic groups with higher rates of diabetes are not destined to develop the disease unless they follow lifestyle habits that contribute to the disease. Unfortunately, because of economic limitations, many Nauruans do not have adequate healthful options available to them. But the majority of us do have healthful options. As we make an effort to take full advantage of these options, we can eliminate genetic risk.

GOOD NEWS ABOUT RISK FACTORS

Regardless of how many risk factors you have for diabetes, you can take action to reduce your risk. Are you 45 years or older? Regardless of your age, you can improve your health. Are you overweight or obese? The nutritional strategies outlined in this book will help you lose weight and decrease your risk. Are you inactive? You can begin a moderate exercise program. Do you have high blood pressure, high cholesterol, or high triglycerides? You can follow natural strategies to significantly reduce those levels. Do you have a family history of diabetes? You can overcome that risk and give hope to future generations. Are you from a racial or ethnic group that has high rates of diabetes? You can outsmart the disease regardless of the statistics.

TITANIC LESSON #3: TAKE SYMPTOMS SERIOUSLY

Even after the *Titanic* struck the iceberg, there didn't seem to be any cause for alarm. Although a deadly wound had been dealt to the bottom of the ship, everything on the upper levels still appeared normal. But disturbing reports soon began to emerge. The mail room was flooding, the cargo room was flooding, and it was impossible to stop the water from coming in. After an inspection of the damage, the ship's designer delivered the grim news to the captain—the damage was fatal. Within hours, the ship would sink.

The crew began boarding passengers into lifeboats. The *Titanic* was equipped with 20 lifeboats, enough to hold approximately half of the passengers on board. It was difficult, however, to convince passengers to board the boats. Oblivious to what was happening, the passengers believed it was more dangerous to board the lifeboats than to stay on the warm, cozy ship. Many lifeboats left the ship only half-full. Lifeboat number one, which could have held at least 65 people, left with only 12. Crew members began knocking on doors, waking people up and telling them to get on deck. Because of the confusion and lack of information, many passengers delayed.

As news spread around the ship and distress rockets were launched, more and more passengers started to realize what was happening. The mood grew frantic. People who had refused to board the lifeboats before now scrambled toward them. By this time, the last few lifeboats had been launched, and were filled to capacity.

Many people died that night because they were waiting for stronger warnings—for more evidence showing that it was necessary to get off of the ship. They ignored the subtle signs that there was a problem, waiting for more obvious signs to appear. But by the time those signs appeared, it was too late.

People with diabetes and prediabetes are in danger of making the same mistake. When early warning signs are ignored, the condition progresses and symptoms begin to show. Sometimes they are subtle at first, and sometimes they are severe. But early symptoms—or complications—must be taken very seriously and addressed as quickly as possible.

COMPLICATIONS OF DIABETES INCLUDE[40]

- Heart attack or stroke.
- Peripheral vascular disease (damage to blood vessels outside the heart).
- Vision impairment or blindness.
- Tingling or loss of sensation in arms, hands, legs, or feet.
- Kidney disease or failure.
- Sores or wounds on feet or legs.
- Gum or periodontal disease.

By the time these symptoms occur, the disease most likely has been progressing for decades. Corrective action must immediately be taken to halt further progression before it's too late.

THE CINNABON® STORY

I recently received an email from a former colleague on Guam, informing me that my friend and former patient, Jasmine, had passed away. Jasmine had type 2 diabetes and had developed enormous sores on her legs and feet. She needed to have both legs amputated, but died before the procedure could be done. She was only 53 years old.

Five years earlier, Jasmine had attended our diabetes reversal program for several weeks. She was a warm, friendly woman who seemed eager to learn. However, as the weeks progressed I realized that, although she was interested in learning about diabetes, she was not motivated to put into practice what she learned. Busy with her career and family, Jasmine stopped attending the lectures and canceled her consultations with me.

A few months later, I stopped by the office where Jasmine worked. As I climbed the stairs to the office complex, I noticed the sweet, warm smell of cinnamon buns. The man climbing the stairs behind me was carrying a big box full of Cinnabons to share with the office staff.

After conducting my business, I went to Jasmine's desk to greet her. She was embarrassed to have me see her eating a Cinnabon. "Oh! Dr. Youngberg! I can't believe you're here—right when I'm eating this!" she said. I always tell my patients that I am not the food police and that I want them to be comfortable around me. So I just greeted her and encouraged her to set up another appointment so we could continue addressing her diabetes.

Knowing that Jasmine's blood sugar levels were frequently in the 300s and 400s, I was concerned for her health and hoped she would recognize her risk and take action. She was already experiencing multiple diabetic complications, and I knew her condition would get worse unless she made drastic changes.

Unfortunately, Jasmine never set up another appointment. She ignored her symptoms, allowing herself to minimize the risk in her own mind. Eventually, the disease progressed until it was too late. Like the passengers on the *Titanic* who did not take advantage of their chance to escape, Jasmine did not take advantage of her chance to reverse her diabetes. Sadly, she missed out on years—possibly even decades—she could have enjoyed with her friends and family.

TITANIC LESSON #4: ACT QUICKLY AND THOROUGHLY

Although the sinking of the *Titanic* was an event too tragic to even imagine, there were 705 people who were fortunate enough to survive.

LIFEBOAT #6

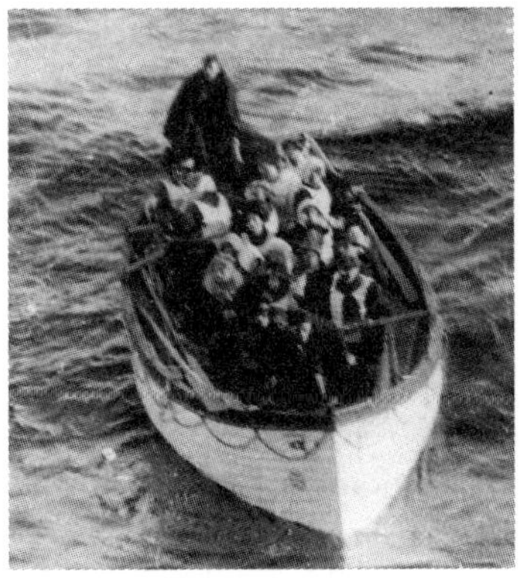

Pictured at right are eleven women and six men who occupied *Titanic* lifeboat number six. Many passengers were still hesitant to leave the apparent safety of the *Titanic*. But these people acted quickly and escaped. They were willing to accept the discomfort of floating in a rowboat on the cold Atlantic Ocean because they believed it could possibly save their lives. Because they quickly took aggressive action, their lives were spared. Although it wasn't *comfortable* for them to get in the lifeboat, in the end it was much more comfortable than *not* getting in.

When it comes to preventing or reversing diabetes or prediabetes, the sooner you take aggressive action, the more likely you are to save your health—and your life. Don't wait for stronger warnings or symptoms to occur. *Now* is the time to take charge of your health.

WHAT NEXT?

Because diabetes and prediabetes are silent killers and often go undetected until their advanced stages, it's essential that you get tested and screened early on to determine whether you are at risk. The first step in transforming your health is to have a proper understanding of your current health condition. This can only happen when you test! In the next few chapters, we will look closely at tests that can help you identify your risk for prediabetes and diabetes.

CHAPTER SUMMARY

- You can't afford to be complacent about your health.
- You can take action to prevent disease before it ever starts.
- There are multiple risk factors for developing diabetes, including age, excess weight or obesity, inactivity, high blood pressure, high cholesterol, high triglycerides, family history of diabetes, and race.
- You can overcome these risk factors by making healthy lifestyle choices.
- Diabetes is a silent killer. Don't wait for signs and symptoms to appear. Evaluate and address your health now!
- There are multiple symptoms that appear in the advanced stages of diabetes. These include heart attack or stroke; peripheral vascular disease; vision impairment or blindness; tingling or loss of sensation in arms, hands, legs, or feet; kidney disease or failure; sores or wounds on feet or legs; and gum or periodontal disease.
- By the time these symptoms appear, diabetes has been developing for years. Corrective action must be taken immediately to halt further progression and possibly reverse the disease.
- Lifestyle change seems difficult at first, but if you take aggressive action to improve your health, the results will be well worth the effort.
- Testing is essential to evaluating and addressing your health. We'll examine this in the coming chapters.

—SEVEN—

How Are Your Sugars?

Have you ever wondered how long diabetes has existed or how it was first diagnosed? Although our understanding of the disease has increased dramatically in the past 150 years, records of diabetes have existed for much longer.[1] The ancient *Egyptian Ebers Papyrus,* dated to 1550 BC, describes a condition characterized by "abundant urine," (a symptom of diabetes) and details treatments for improving the problem. This description is thought to be the first known record of the disease.

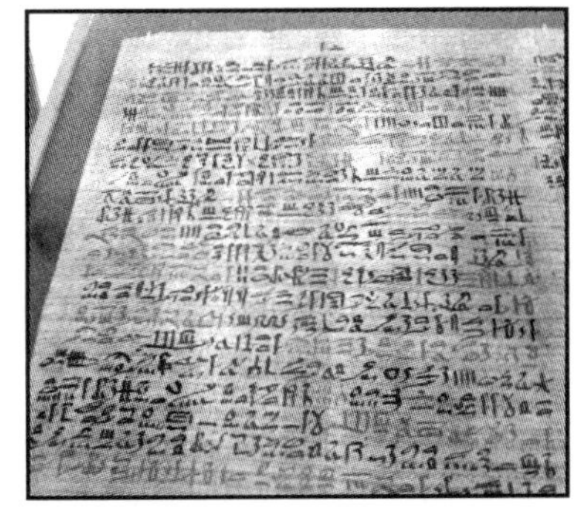

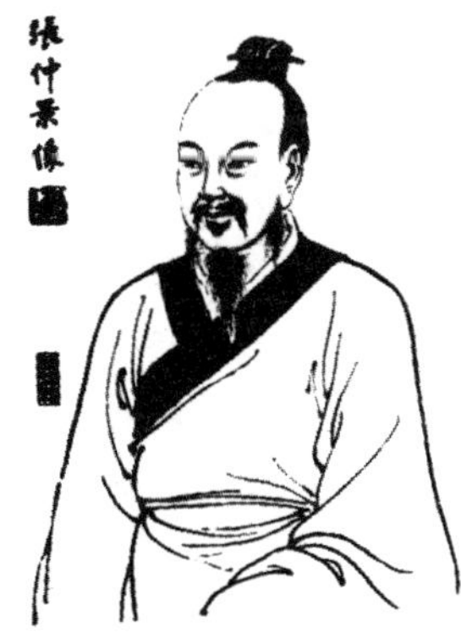

Almost 2,000 years ago, Chinese physician, Chang Chung-Ching, reported that diabetic urine was so sweet that dogs were attracted to it. Thus, the first test for the disease was the urine taste test. There is record that early Greeks, Egyptians, and Indians tested for diabetes by either tasting urine or setting it out to see whether it attracted insects and animals.

Although crude, this method of testing is scientifically logical. When blood sugars reach diabetic levels after meals, the kidneys release some of the excess sugar into the urine, causing it to be sweet. The ancient researchers didn't make a connection between sugar in the urine and sugar in the blood, but they did know that sweet urine meant there was a problem.

Thankfully, medical testing has progressed since that time. We now have multiple tests available that determine the presence and extent of prediabetes or diabetes—no urine tasting required! It is extremely important to take full advantage of this testing.

Because diabetes is a "silent killer" and often doesn't cause noticeable symptoms until the advanced stages, it is very important to screen people for the disease as early as possible. Not only does testing for prediabetes and diabetes provide a basis for diagnosis, but it also helps in the development of individualized treatment plans and in the measurement of improvements as these plans are followed.

WHO SHOULD BE SCREENED?

How can you know whether you need to be screened or tested for prediabetes or diabetes? Let's look at the screening criteria suggested by the American Diabetes Association:

"Screening should be considered by healthcare providers at three-year intervals beginning at age 45. Testing should be considered at a younger age or be carried out more frequently in individuals who are overweight and have one or more of the other risk factors."[2] These "other risk factors" are the same risk factors discussed in the previous chapter.

RISK FACTORS FOR DIABETES[3]

- You're 45 years or older.
- Excessive weight or obesity.
- You do not exercise regularly.
- You have elevated blood pressure.
- Your cholesterol and/or triglyceride blood fat levels are elevated.

- You have a family history of diabetes.
- You are Black, Hispanic, Native American, Asian, or Pacific Islander.
- You've had gestational diabetes or have given birth to a baby weighing more than nine pounds.

In addition to people with these risk factors, those who have previously identified blood sugar problems, a history of heart disease, or polycystic ovary syndrome should also be screened earlier and more frequently.[4]

I think it's important to reiterate the American Diabetes Association's statement that: "Testing should be considered at a younger age or be carried out more frequently in individuals who are overweight and have one or more of the other risk factors."

You may recall from the age chart in Chapter 6 that an estimated 16 percent of American adolescents, ages 12 to 19, are prediabetic or diabetic. Twenty-one percent of Americans ages 20 to 39 are diabetic or prediabetic.[5] This means that 1 in 5 American adults (and many American adolescents) under age 40 already fit the criteria for diabetes or prediabetes. These people cannot afford to wait until age 45 to be screened!

But how early and how often should they be screened? The American Diabetes Association isn't very specific about that. The organization states: "The decision to test for diabetes should ultimately be based on clinical judgment and patient preference."[6]

BETTER SAFE THAN SORRY

After more than 20 years of screening people for diabetes, my clinical judgment leads me to believe that, when it comes to testing, *it's better to be safe than sorry.*

A mother recently came to my clinic with her two daughters—Emily, age 14, and Megan, age 12. She wanted me to evaluate her health and the health of her girls. Emily was thin and lean. She didn't have any noticeable risk factors. Her mother was more interested in addressing her acne problem. Because I like to look at the big picture when evaluating my patients, I also asked Emily about other aspects of her health. She mentioned that sometimes she felt fatigued. I did not suspect that she would have a problem with diabetes or prediabetes. She didn't have any risk factors, except that her grandmother was diabetic. Wondering if she might be hypoglycemic (have low blood sugar), I decided to order a four-hour glucose tolerance test (discussed later in this chapter).

When the results came back, I was surprised to discover that Emily was in the advanced stages of prediabetes. Her younger sister, Megan, was also prediabetic.

I applaud their mother for her willingness to have her family's health thoroughly evaluated. Their story is a reminder that diabetes and prediabetes can show up much earlier than age 45. People with a family history of diabetes—or with any of the other risk factors listed above—need to be intentional about early and regular screening. The earlier diabetes is caught, the better the chance of stopping it in its tracks.

It's important for patients and clinicians to realize that broad and thorough testing can identify conditions that would normally go unnoticed. If you're willing to look at the big picture and test comprehensively, you're more likely to be able to detect and fix what's wrong. This chapter will provide you with practical information on how to evaluate your blood sugar levels to determine your risk for diabetes or prediabetes.

THE FASTING BLOOD GLUCOSE TEST

The fasting blood glucose (or fasting blood sugar) test is the most common test used to diagnose diabetes. It measures the level of glucose in the blood after a person has not eaten for 12 or more hours. This usually means that no food or drink (except for water) is to be taken after 8 p.m. the night before the test which is taken the following morning. Sometimes the test is ordered by itself, other times it's part of a more comprehensive metabolic profile.

FASTING BLOOD GLUCOSE CRITERIA[7]

Normal = 70–99 mg/dL
Prediabetes = 100–125 mg/dL
Diabetes = 126+ mg/dL

If the fasting blood sugar is 126 or higher, the test should be repeated on a different day. If the results are verified, a diagnosis of diabetes will be confirmed.

Until recently, the majority of physicians have screened patients only for diabetes—not prediabetes. However, because of the growing awareness that prediabetes exponentially increases the risk of heart disease and stroke, in 1997 new guidelines were introduced for physicians to evaluate and diagnose prediabetes as well.[8]

A fasting blood glucose level between 100 and 125 indicates that prediabetes is present. Because some physicians are still unaware of these updated national guidelines, it's important to ask your doctor to tell you the specific values of your blood sugar and to address your risk for prediabetes. You can also use "The Five Stages of Blood Sugar," discussed in the next chapter, to determine whether your blood sugar levels are compromised.

TESTING AT HOME

While I do suggest that you find a clinician who can properly guide you in testing, evaluation, and management, I also encourage you to test your blood sugar at home.

People are sometimes hesitant to be screened by a physician, but once they test at home and realize they have a problem, they are more motivated to go in for additional testing. Also, if you have blood sugar problems, you will need to test regularly; so if you haven't already, it will be necessary to learn how to do this yourself.

You can purchase an inexpensive blood sugar monitoring kit at your local pharmacy without a prescription. The kit will include instructions on how to use it. Typically, you prick your finger with a small lancet, which produces a small droplet of blood. You place a drop of this blood on a test strip that has been inserted into the blood glucose meter. Within seconds, the meter determines your blood sugar level and displays the results. You can use a home kit to determine your fasting blood glucose as well as other important glucose levels throughout the day.

IS THE FASTING BLOOD GLUCOSE TEST ENOUGH?

There's no doubt that a fasting blood glucose test can provide you with valuable information about your health. However, it's also beneficial—and in my opinion even more important—to evaluate how your blood sugar levels respond to meals. After all, you eat on a regular basis. The way your body responds to rising blood sugars after eating or drinking is typically a *better indicator* of diabetes or prediabetes than a fasting glucose test. One way this can be determined is by taking a glucose tolerance test.

THE GLUCOSE TOLERANCE TEST

In my opinion, the glucose tolerance test is the *most* accurate and comprehensive test available for determining a predisposition for prediabetes or diabetes.[9] The glucose tolerance test shows how the body metabolizes and uses sugar (glucose) after it is ingested. It's not uncommon for people to have a fasting blood glucose level in the optimal range, but to be diagnosed as diabetic after an oral glucose tolerance test.

This test involves taking a fasting blood sugar level just before drinking a glucola drink—a concentrated, sweet drink that contains 75 grams of glucose. This is a metabolic stress test, designed to determine how your body responds to glucose.[10] Blood sugars are tested again at certain times after the drink is consumed. The results reveal the body's ability to control blood sugars effectively over time.

TWO HOURS

The two-hour glucose tolerance test can be officially used to diagnose diabetes.[11] A clinician will test the fasting blood sugar before a glucola drink is given, give the glucola drink, and then test the blood sugar again two hours after the drink is finished. A blood sugar level of 200 or higher after two hours is a definitive diagnosis of diabetes. A blood sugar level of 140 to 199 is prediabetes.[12]

The story of Emily, the 14-year-old patient mentioned previously, illustrates the value of the two-hour glucose test. Although I didn't suspect that Emily had a problem with prediabetes or diabetes, I ordered a glucose tolerance test to check for hypoglycemia. Emily's fasting blood glucose was 73—a perfect level. However, I was surprised to discover that her two-hour glucose tolerance level was 195—just five points away from an official diagnosis of diabetes. Emily had advanced prediabetes. This condition would have gone undetected for years, and possibly even decades, if I had only considered her fasting glucose level. The two-hour test revealed that Emily had a problem and gave her the opportunity to begin addressing her condition at an early age, before the condition had time to progress.

Because an official diagnosis for prediabetes or diabetes can be determined by either the fasting blood glucose test or the two-hour glucose tolerance test, these are the two most common tests that clinicians use.[13] But when I perform a two-hour glucose tolerance test, I also like to check the blood sugar at one hour.

ONE HOUR

Although the one-hour glucose tolerance test is not part of the official criteria used to diagnose diabetes, it also provides valuable information. This test is more sensitive in detecting early tendencies toward blood sugar problems than the fasting and two-hour tests are. For this reason, I recommend that any time a glucose tolerance test is done, it should include a one-hour reading.

Researchers have determined that a blood sugar level of 155 or higher one hour after consuming 75 grams of glucose is an independent risk factor for cardiovascular disease.[14] Since the primary focus of diagnosing diabetes and prediabetes is to help prevent and lower the risk of cardiovascular disease, it is important to pay attention to this test.

Emily's younger sister, Megan, is a good example of someone who benefited from the one-hour glucose tolerance test. Because Emily and Megan's mom wanted me to thoroughly evaluate both of her daughters, I ordered a glucose tolerance test for Megan as well. Megan's fasting blood sugar was 79—an optimal level. Her two-hour level was 100—also a normal level. If that were all the information we had, it would have appeared that Megan had optimal blood sugars. However, I also ordered a one-hour level to be drawn. When the results came back, I realized that Megan did in fact have a blood sugar problem. Her one-hour level was 200.

Because the one-hour test is not diagnostic, Megan could not be officially diagnosed as "prediabetic." However, this test showed me that she was experiencing blood sugar spikes after meals, which, if left untreated, would cause serious damage to her body over time. Thankfully, the one-hour test caught the problem, and Megan is learning how to manage her blood sugars after meals. Megan is very fortunate to have learned about her risk at such a young age. This gives her the opportunity to take control now and to avoid serious complications in the future.

PEPSI®-JELLY BEAN CHALLENGE

Just as there is a way to test your fasting blood sugar at home, there is also a do-it-yourself way to perform a modified glucose tolerance test at home. I call this the Pepsi-Jelly Bean Challenge.

Several years ago, I was reading an article in a medical journal that described an alternate method of doing the glucose tolerance test.[15] Typically, all pregnant women are given a glucose tolerance test at 28 weeks to screen for gestational diabetes. Many pregnant women dislike the sugary sweet drink and have trouble getting or keeping it down. To make it easier on them, some clinics began allowing them to eat jelly beans instead of drinking the glucola drink.

This idea appealed to me for several reasons. I realized that people would be more eager to do the test if they were able to eat jelly beans or other sugary snacks. This would also give them the flexibility of testing at home using their own glucose meter and food or drinks. In addition, it would wake them up to the fact that their favorite snacks and drinks could seriously impact their blood sugars.

I have had multiple patients take the glucose tolerance test with the glucola drink and test positive for diabetes or prediabetes. These patients tend to minimize their risk, saying, "Well of *course* my blood sugar went up after drinking that drink. But I would never drink something *that* sweet on a regular basis!" For this reason, I developed the Pepsi-Jelly Bean Challenge.

I named it after Pepsi's popular marketing campaign, the "Pepsi Challenge." But the goal of the Pepsi-Jelly Bean Challenge isn't to determine whether Pepsi or Coke® tastes better. It's to show people how either of these drinks—along with any other sugary drinks or snacks—affect their blood sugars.

To take the Pepsi-Jelly Bean Challenge, get your favorite soda or drink and your favorite starchy snacks (cookies, candy, crackers, etc.). After checking and recording your fasting blood glucose level, eat your snacks and drink your drink. One hour later, and two hours later, check and record your blood glucose levels again. Then use "The Five Stages of High Blood Sugar" chart in Chapter 8 to determine whether you have prediabetes or diabetes. The success of the Pepsi-Jelly Bean Challenge is illustrated by the story of Chris.

Several years ago, I was teaching a university wellness class. Knowing that more than 20 percent of these students probably had prediabetes or diabetes,[16] I wanted to make them aware of the importance of blood sugar management. I asked everyone to bring their favorite sugary and starchy snacks to our next class period—sodas, juice, cookies, candy, crackers, etc. Each person was to bring 75 to 100 grams of sugar or starch, which is 300 to 400 calories.

When the next class period came, the students were prepared. At the beginning of class, the students ate and drank their sugary snacks. About an hour later, I had the staff from my clinic test the students' blood sugar levels. Quite a few students were surprised to discover that their blood sugars were running high. However, one young man was deeply concerned.

Chris approached me at the end of class looking utterly defeated. "I don't know what I'm going to do," he said. "My blood sugar was 350. I didn't even know that I had a problem." Working his way through college, 25-year-old Chris was under a lot of stress. He was about 50 pounds overweight, and smoked two packs of cigarettes a day. "Let's check it again once it's been two hours since your snack," I told him. We did, and it was well above 200.

Although Chris had a family history of diabetes, he was young and didn't think that it could happen to him. Thankfully, he had enrolled in this required wellness class and discovered that he had a problem. Chris became highly motivated to address his condition. He remembered his Uncle Joe, who had his leg amputated from out-of-control diabetes, and his grandfather who had gone blind before passing away. He wanted to overcome his genetic risk and outsmart the disease.

Throughout the rest of the class, I worked with Chris to address his diabetes. He started exercising every day. He started eating well. His energy returned. By the end of 10 weeks, Chris had lost 30 pounds, stopped smoking, and dramatically improved his blood sugar levels. In fact, he no longer fit the criteria for diabetes. Because of a simple Pepsi-Jelly Bean Challenge and Chris' motivation to change—his health had been transformed.

DIRECTIONS FOR THE PEPSI-JELLY BEAN CHALLENGE

Necessary Supplies

- Blood glucose monitoring kit and supplies
- Sugary, starchy snacks equaling 75-100 grams of starch or sugar total (i.e. 300-400 calories from sugar).
- These snacks can include:
- Sodas (not diet)
- Juice
- Jelly Beans
- Candy
- Crackers
- Sugar cookies

Note: Avoid eating any significant amount of fat or protein.

Performing the Test

1. Take and record your fasting blood glucose level. (Although technically a fasting glucose level is obtained after twelve hours of not eating or drinking anything except water, for the sake of this test you only need to wait three or more hours. By this time, blood sugar levels will be very close to fasting levels.
2. Eat and drink your sugary snacks and beverages.
3. After one hour, take and record your blood glucose level.
4. After two hours, take and record your blood glucose level.
5. Evaluate your fasting, one-hour, and two-hour blood glucose levels according to the criteria outlined in Chapter 8 to determine whether your blood sugars are compromised.

Note: If you don't want to drink soda or candy, you can eat a starchy meal such as spaghetti or pancakes. Just be sure that the majority of the calories are coming from carbohydrates, not protein or fat. (For example, if you're eating spaghetti, avoid eating alfredo sauce or meatballs. Just stick with the spaghetti. If you're eating pancakes, avoid adding butter or eggs or any other protein at the same time.)

Sometimes when I suggest the Pepsi-Jelly Bean Challenge to patients, they don't think it will apply to them. They assume that because they don't regularly eat sugary snacks or drink soda, they don't have a blood sugar problem. It's important to note that many starchy foods eaten on a regular basis can cause blood sugar spikes. I tell these patients that they can pick their favorite 100 percent juice and whole wheat crackers. The test results will still reveal any tendency toward high blood sugar. The Pepsi-Jelly Bean Challenge evaluates more than just the effect of junk food on blood sugars; it provides information on how the body processes glucose in general.

RANDOM BLOOD GLUCOSE

The Random Blood Glucose test is another way of determining the presence of diabetes. If a blood sugar level taken at any random time throughout the day is 200 or higher and is accompanied by diabetic symptoms, this is diagnosed as diabetes.[17]

These symptoms include:

- increased hunger,
- unexplained weight loss,
- increased thirst,
- fatigue,
- blurry vision,
- and sores that do not heal.

While the official criteria require that symptoms appear along with a high random blood sugar level in order for a diagnosis to be made, remember that symptoms aren't always an adequate guide. If you have a random blood glucose test of 200 or higher at any time, even without symptoms, it strongly suggests that you have blood sugar problems and should be evaluated further.

HEMOGLOBIN A1C TEST

Regularly monitoring your blood sugar level at home will reveal what it is at specific points in time. However, if you want to know how you're doing overall, the Hemoglobin A1c (HA1c) test measures your average blood sugar control for the past two to four months.[18]

Hemoglobin is a protein in red blood cells that carries oxygen throughout the body. When blood sugar levels are high, the sugar sticks to these hemoglobin proteins. The higher the blood sugars, the worse this problem becomes. Because red blood cells have a lifespan of about 120 days, by measuring the amount of sugar stuck to the hemoglobin on these cells, the HA1c test reveals the overall trend of blood sugars for the past two to four months. The HA1c test can also indicate the extent of tissue damage caused by high blood sugars and the risk for diabetes related complications.[19]

HEMOGLOBIN A1C CRITERIA[20]

Optimal = Under 5 percent
Normal = 4.5-5.6 percent
Prediabetes/at risk = 5.7-6.4 percent
Diabetes = 6.5 percent or higher

HA1c%	Blood Glucose Average
12	298
11	269
10	240
9	212
8	183
7	154
6	126
5	97

Typically, a person with optimal blood sugars will have a HA1c under 5 percent. Once it goes above 5, there is a gradual increase in risk. By the time the level hits 5.7 percent, there is definite prediabetes. When testing my patients, I caution anyone who has a HA1c over 5 percent to begin addressing the problem. If patients reach a level of 5.7 percent or higher, this is a red flag that they are already at a significantly increased risk.

In order to better understand what the HA1c levels mean, let's take a look at what the levels tell us about blood sugar. The chart above shows the correlation between HA1c levels and average blood sugar levels.[21] For example, if your HA1c level is 9 percent, your average blood sugar level for the past several months has been 212.

Lowering your HA1c level will greatly reduce your risk for diabetes related complications.[22]

Complications	Reduced risk for every 1 percentage point reduction in HA1c
Nerve Damage	37%
Vision Loss	37%
Kidney Disease	37%
Amputation or Death from Peripheral Vascular Disease	43%
Heart Attack	14%
Diabetes-related death	21%

Because the HA1c test provides such valuable information about your blood sugar control and your risk for disease and complications, it is important to have your Hemoglobin A1c checked regularly. If you are prediabetic or diabetic, or if you have a history of blood sugar problems, I recommend that you have it tested every three months. If your blood sugars are well controlled (see "The Five Stages of Blood Sugar" chart in the next chapter), but you want to make sure you stay on the right track, have the test performed at least every six months.

HEMOGLOBIN A1C AND TISSUE DAMAGE

Although the Hemoglobin A1c test is primarily used to evaluate blood sugar control, it can also help to determine the extent of damage that has occurred to cells, tissues, and organ systems as a result of high blood sugar levels.

Because the HA1c test measures how much sugar is sticking to cells, a high HA1c indicates that serious glycosylation (sticky sugar build-up) is occurring throughout the body. You may recall from Chapter 3 that glycosylation causes premature aging and serious damage to tissues.[23]

LOWERING YOUR HEMOGLOBIN A1C

The good news is that you can take action to lower your HA1c level. The body continually makes new red blood cells to replace the old ones. These new cells are not glazed with sugar. If you follow the strategies outlined in this book to keep your blood sugar levels under control, you can prevent damage to these new cells and significantly lower your HA1c level and risk for disease. Major improvements can occur within a few weeks or months. Tissues that have been damaged by glycosylation often clear up and begin to function optimally again.

LOOK AT THE BIG PICTURE

In this chapter, we've looked at multiple blood sugar tests that help us determine the presence and extent of prediabetes and diabetes. It's important to note that these tests are most valuable when considered together as a whole, instead of just individually.

For example, a person may have a normal fasting blood glucose and a normal HA1c level, but be diagnosed as diabetic after a two-hour glucose tolerance test. Another person might have a normal two-hour glucose tolerance level, but a dangerously high one-hour level. Because different tests reveal different information about the way the body responds to sugar at different times, it is important to put all the pieces together in order to discover whether there is a problem as well as to determine how to address it.

We will continue our discussion on monitoring blood sugars in the next chapter, "The Five Stages of High Blood Sugar."

CHAPTER SUMMARY

» It is important to be screened for diabetes if you have any of the following risk factors:
  - ✓ You are 45 years or older.
  - ✓ You are overweight or obese.
  - ✓ You do not exercise regularly.
  - ✓ You have elevated blood pressure.
  - ✓ Your cholesterol and/or triglyceride blood fat levels are elevated.
  - ✓ You have a family history of diabetes.
  - ✓ You are Black, Hispanic, Native American, Asian, or Pacific Islander.
  - ✓ You have had gestational diabetes or have given birth to a baby weighing more than nine pounds.
  - ✓ You have previously-identified blood sugar problems.
  - ✓ You've had a history of heart disease.
  - ✓ You've had polycystic ovary disease.

- Don't wait until you experience symptoms to be tested. Many people with prediabetes and diabetes are unaware of their condition.
- When it comes to testing, it's better to be safe than sorry!
- The fasting blood glucose test is a common test used to diagnose prediabetes.
- If your fasting blood sugar level is between 100 and 125, you have prediabetes. If your fasting blood sugar is 126 or higher, you have diabetes.
- In addition to being clinically evaluated, it is important to regularly check your blood sugar at home.
- The glucose tolerance test is also used to diagnose diabetes and often detects problems that the fasting glucose test does not.
- A blood sugar of 200 or higher two hours after drinking a glucola drink is a definitive diagnosis of diabetes. A blood sugar of 140 to 199 two hours after drinking a glucola drink indicates prediabetes.
- The one-hour glucose tolerance test is the most sensitive test for identifying early tendencies towards diabetes.
- A blood sugar of 155 or higher one hour after drinking a glucola drink is an independent risk factor for cardiovascular disease.
- The Pepsi-Jelly Bean Challenge is a modified glucose tolerance test that you can perform at home.
- A random blood sugar of 200 or higher, accompanied by symptoms, is a definitive diagnosis of diabetes.
- The Hemoglobin A1c test measures your blood sugar control for the past two to four months.

—EIGHT—

The Five Stages of High Blood Sugar

FOR MY CHRISTMAS VACATION IN 1986, I CARPOOLED from Loma Linda, California to Denver, Colorado, with my friend, Brent, and his girlfriend, Stephanie. We went to visit my brother John. After enjoying the holidays, we packed up and started back for Loma Linda. We left at about 10 p.m. on a Saturday night, planning to drive straight through the night and arrive in Loma Linda before noon the next day. (Note: I do not recommend this type of travel to my patients, as you will see in Chapter 17, "Get Sound Sleep.")

We took turns driving and sleeping as we wound through the snowy Colorado mountains into Utah. Around midnight, it was Stephanie's turn to drive. Before Brent and I went to sleep, Brent reminded Stephanie to not let the gas gauge go below a quarter of a tank. We were in a desolate area where there were sometimes more than a hundred miles between gas stations. Stephanie agreed, and Brent and I fell asleep.

We woke up to the sound of the engine losing power. Stephanie barely managed to pull off to the side of the road as the car sputtered to a stop and ran out of gas. Stephanie had forgotten to pay attention to the gas gauge.

It was 1:30 in the morning. We were in a desolate mountain pass in the freezing cold January weather. Since I was the "third wheel," so to speak,

Brent and Stephanie decided that I should be the one to go get gas. Thankfully, within 15 minutes I was able to wave down a trucker who agreed to drop me off at the nearest gas station, which was 45 minutes away. I bought a five gallon can of gas, and the gas station attendant was kind enough to radio a nearby trucker headed back the other direction. The trucker agreed to take me back to our car, and soon I was on my way.

By the time I reached the car, it had been about two hours since we'd stopped. There was already a quarter-inch of ice on the inside of the windshield. Needless to say, Brent and Stephanie were very cold. Thankfully, we soon started out again, and the rest of our trip was uneventful.

Why did we run out of gas? Was it because gas was unavailable? No. Stephanie had passed several stations while Brent and I were asleep. Was it because the gas gauge didn't work? No. The gas gauge was working fine, but it was steadily going down, down, down, until it hit empty. The gas didn't decrease all at once; it happened gradually. The problem was that Stephanie wasn't paying attention to the gas gauge (and Brent and I were asleep).

It stands to reason that, in order to prevent running out of gas, it is important to pay attention to the gas gauge *before* it hits empty.

THE BLOOD SUGAR GAUGE

It's important to pay attention to the gas guage in your car, and it is equally important to pay attention to your blood sugar levels. Although running out of gas may seem like a sudden event, it actually takes quite a while. The gas level steadily decreases until it finally runs out. Similarly, although a diagnosis of prediabetes or diabetes may seem like a sudden event, the process actually is gradual. Blood sugars have steadily been increasing for years, and possibly even decades, before they are identified and finally diagnosed.

Part of this problem is that there are no official criteria in place to define blood sugar problems before they escalate to prediabetic levels. People who do not meet the criteria for prediabetes often assume they are okay, even though they are already developing blood sugar problems that will eventually lead to prediabetes and diabetes.

A gas gauge lets you know your fuel level at every stage of the way. But the official diagnostic criteria for prediabetes and diabetes (described in the previous chapter) only identify blood sugar problems that have already reached levels of significantly increased risk. One of my goals as a clinician who treats people with blood sugar problems is to help them to identify their risk as early as possible.

In 1996, the governor of Guam established a task force to address healthcare problems on the island. One of his main goals was to prevent the development of diabetes. This was a challenging goal because diabetes is prevalent on Guam. At that time, Guam's rate of diabetes-related deaths was nearly five times higher than it was on the United States mainland.[1] Diabetes was creating a staggering health and economic burden on the island. The governor wanted to do something about it.

I was asked to co-chair the governor's diabetes prevention task force. As I thought about the enormity of the task, I asked myself, "How can we prevent a condition that is not even diagnosed until there are already complications?"

It was clear to me that the screening guidelines used to diagnose diabetes were not adequate to prevent the disease. (In fact, at that time prediabetes was not even a diagnosis. It wasn't until the following year that prediabetes was recognized as a medical diagnosis.[2]) I decided to develop a comprehensive screening system that would help healthcare professionals and clinicians on Guam detect their patients' blood sugar problems as early as possible. I called these new screening guidelines "The Five Stages of High Blood Sugar."

THE FIVE STAGES OF HIGH BLOOD SUGAR

		Stage 1	Stage 2	Stage 3	Stage 4	Stage 5
Time From Food Intake	Optimal Blood Sugar	High Blood Sugar	High Blood Sugar	Prediabetes	Advanced Prediabetes	Diabetes
Fasting	70-84	85-94	95-99	100-109	110-125	126+
1 hour	80-119	120-139	140-159	160-199	200+	
2 hours	80-99	100-119	120-139	140-159	160-199	200+

This chart outlines the five stages of high blood sugar and compares them to what optimal blood sugar levels should be. Instead of just looking at the diagnostic criteria (i.e., a fasting glucose of 126 or higher is diabetes and a fasting glucose of 100-125 is prediabetes), these guidelines help identify blood sugar problems in the earliest stages of development. This makes it possible to address these problems head-on and halt progression toward diabetes. Let's look at what the different stages mean.

OPTIMAL BLOOD SUGAR

These levels show us what ideal blood sugars should be. If your blood sugars are at optimal levels without medication, your body is sensitive to insulin and is metabolizing glucose properly. If your blood sugars remain at the optimal level, they will not increase your risk for cardiovascular disease or other prediabetic and diabetic complications.

Optimal blood sugar levels are what we should compare each of the stages of high blood sugar to. The key to understanding what each stage means is to compare it to what is truly optimal.

STAGE 1-HIGH BLOOD SUGAR

Blood sugars in stage 1 represent the beginning of risk. Most likely a person with stage 1 high blood sugars is already in a state of mild insulin resistance. If your fasting blood sugar is consistently in stage 1, it would be wise to undergo a glucose tolerance test, which will give you a better understanding of your overall blood sugar control. Because high blood sugars and insulin resistance increase the risk for cardiovascular disease, you should aggressively address these conditions and any other heart disease risk factors you may have. This stage is the easiest to reverse. The earlier you take action, the better chance you have of being successful.

STAGE 2-HIGH BLOOD SUGAR

Blood sugars in stage 2 now represent a more heightened level of risk. Frequently, people with fasting blood sugars in stage 2 who undergo a two-hour glucose tolerance test will actually be diagnosed with prediabetes or diabetes.

If your fasting blood sugars are at stage 2, it's very important to undergo additional testing and to aggressively address the underlying causes of your insulin resistance by following the comprehensive lifestyle strategies in this book. As in stage 1, it's also very important to address all of your risk factors for heart disease.

STAGE 3-HIGH BLOOD SUGAR (PREDIABETES)

A fasting glucose of 100 or higher or a two-hour blood sugar of 140 or higher fits the criteria for prediabetes. This is stage 3 of high blood sugar. If you have prediabetes, not only are you at high risk for developing diabetes in the future, but you are already at a much greater risk for developing heart disease.[3] If you have prediabetes, it is crucial that you immediately take aggressive action to undergo additional testing and to address your blood sugars, insulin resistance, and heart disease risk factors.

STAGE 4-HIGH BLOOD SUGAR (ADVANCED PREDIABETES)

If your blood sugars are at stage 4, you are just a few points away from a diagnosis of full-blown diabetes (according to the fasting blood glucose criteria). You are already at a dramatically increased risk for heart disease. At this stage, it's extremely important—actually urgent—to do everything in your power to reverse your condition before it turns into full-blown diabetes or a cardiovascular event. Be sure to undergo a glucose tolerance test, evaluate and address your other risk factors for heart disease, and diligently follow the lifestyle medicine strategies in this book.

STAGE 5-HIGH BLOOD SUGAR (DIABETES)

Once your fasting blood sugars hit 126 or higher or your two-hour blood sugar is 200 or higher, you meet the diagnostic criteria for diabetes. At this point, not only are you at an extremely increased risk for cardiovascular disease, but you are now also at risk for complications such as kidney failure, vision impairment or blindness, nerve damage, poor wound healing, amputations, and many other potential health problems.

But don't despair! Hope is available at every stage of high blood sugar. Although blood sugar problems ideally should be identified and diagnosed as early as possible, even people who already have diabetes can take aggressive action to greatly improve, and possibly even reverse, the condition.

A diagnosis of diabetes can be extremely valuable if it motivates you to take action. I frequently tell my patients that one of the best ways to improve health is to get diagnosed with a chronic condition and then do everything possible to reverse it. The sooner you start down the path toward reversal, the more likely you'll be to accomplish that goal.

A RIPPLE EFFECT

I'm thankful that the diabetes task force I was involved in proved to be beneficial to the people of Guam. I collaborated with Dr. Charles Brinegar (former director of the Diabetes Treatment Center at Loma Linda University) and several other colleagues to write *Diabetes Care on Guam: Guidelines for Prevention, Early Detection, and Treatment.*[4] These new guidelines included "The Five Stages of High Blood Sugar" and other practical information to help healthcare providers on Guam to effectively identify and address blood sugar problems in their patients. These new guidelines were published by the Guam Department of Public Health through funding from the Centers for Disease Control and Prevention. Every healthcare professional on Guam was provided with a copy of these new guidelines.

Shortly after our new guidelines were published, I had the opportunity to speak at an international conference for the prevention of diabetes throughout the lifespan. I was asked to represent the Pacific Island region and to lecture on the work that our task force had done on Guam and the new guidelines we had developed.

One of the other speakers was the chief of endocrinology for Kaiser Permanente in Southern California. After listening to my lecture, he recognized the value of having these comprehensive screening guidelines in place. A year later, our paths crossed again at another medical conference. He told me that he had introduced the new guidelines to all of the Kaiser facilities in his Southern California region. He wanted to help them better serve their patients in preventing, screening, and treating blood sugar problems.

My hope is that more health professionals and patients will become aware of the necessity of early and aggressive screening and treatment. I encourage you to use "The Five Stages of Blood Sugar" to identify and address your blood sugar problems. I also hope that you will share this information with your doctor and your loved ones.

CHAPTER SUMMARY

- The development of prediabetes and diabetes is a gradual process.
- The sooner you identify and address blood sugar problems, the better your chance for reversing them.
- By the time your blood sugars meet the official criteria for prediabetes or diabetes, you are already at a significantly increased risk for heart disease and other complications.
- It's possible to identify and address blood sugar problems early.
- "The Five Stages of High Blood Sugar" identify and explain blood sugar problems at every progressive level.
- The goal should be to gradually bring blood sugars into the optimal range.

—NINE—

How's Your Pancreas?

THE LAST TWO CHAPTERS HAVE FOCUSED ON EVALUATING and managing your blood sugars. Blood sugars are important, but they are only one piece of the puzzle. It is also important to test and pay attention to other factors, including the condition of your pancreas. In this chapter, we will look specifically at tests that evaluate pancreatic function.

LITTLE ORGAN, BIG JOB

The pancreas is a six-inch-long gland that lies slightly behind the stomach, level with the small intestine. It is shaped like a tall, thin pear, lying on its side. The pancreas gland has multiple functions. It secretes digestive enzymes into the small intestine to help break down food. It is also responsible for the secretion of several different hormones, including insulin. Insulin is produced inside of the beta cells in the pancreas.

People with type 1 diabetes have sustained damage to the beta cells of the pancreas and are no longer able to produce a significant amount of insulin. People with type 2 diabetes still have a functional pancreas, but their muscles and tissues have become resistant to the insulin their pancreas produces.

One way to measure pancreatic function is to have your insulin levels tested.

TESTING INSULIN

You already know it's important to test the amount of *sugar* in your blood, but it can also be important to test the amount of *insulin* in your blood.[1] If you are not taking insulin injections, your natural insulin level can reveal how hard your pancreas is working to stabilize your blood sugars.

If insulin levels are extremely low, especially after a meal, this indicates the presence of type 1 diabetes. The pancreas has been damaged. If insulin levels are high, this indicates that the pancreas is producing plenty of insulin, but that the body is resistant to that insulin. Often, people with type 2 diabetes have hyperinsulinemia,[2] which means that the pancreas is working extra hard to produce more insulin than is usually required, in an attempt to force glucose into cells. Eventually, the pancreas will become fatigued. When blood sugars are running high, even a normal insulin level may suggest that the pancreas is losing its ability to produce insulin. High insulin levels increase the risk of multiple diseases.

HIGH INSULIN LEVELS INCREASE THE RISK FOR MANY DISEASES, INCLUDING

- Hypertension[3]
- Heart Disease[4]
- Obesity[5]
- Prostate Cancer[6]
- Colon Cancer[7]
- Breast Cancer[8]
- Infertility[9]
- Alzheimer's Disease[10]

Because all of these conditions can be associated with high insulin levels, having your insulin tested not only provides information about your pancreatic function and your diabetes, but may also help you determine your risk for these other diseases.

THE FASTING INSULIN TEST

The fasting insulin test can be taken at the same time as the fasting blood glucose test. It measures the amount of insulin in the blood after not eating since the night before. This test is not performed for people who are taking insulin injections because the injected insulin would combine with the insulin the body produces naturally, which would skew the results.

FASTING INSULIN CRITERIA

Excellent = Below 5 (many young athletes fit in this category)
Healthy Target Range = Below 7
Increased Risk = 10 or higher
Note: measurements are in μIU/mL.

I was first introduced to the importance of insulin testing more than 20 years ago when I listened to a lecture by Nancy Bohannon, MD. Dr. Bohannon directs the Cardiovascular Risk Reduction Program at St. Luke's Hospital in San Francisco. In this lecture, she shared the importance of testing insulin levels to determine risk for heart disease. She suggested that insulin levels should be under 10 μIU/mL.[11]

Dr. Bohannon's lecture motivated me to begin testing insulin levels in my patients. If a patient's fasting insulin level was above 10 I determined that it indicated increased risk. If the level was below 10, I assumed that no risk was present. However, after carefully observing my patients and reviewing the research on this topic, I concluded that any level above seven suggested increased risk. Some functional medicine experts are even suggesting that levels should be under 5 μIU/mL. [12]

If your fasting insulin level is high, you can take action to address your insulin resistance and reduce your risk for disease. The lifestyle strategies in this book are designed to increase your body's sensitivity to insulin and to stabilize both insulin levels and blood sugar levels.

TWO-HOUR INSULIN LEVEL

Whenever I order a glucose tolerance test, I recommend a two-hour insulin level test at the same time as the two-hour blood sugar level. Sometimes people who are fasting show healthy insulin levels, but when sugar is in the system those levels rise dramatically.

An insulin level tested two hours after drinking a glucola drink should be less than 25, although less than 10 is optimal. A level over 25 indicates that the body has become resistant to the normal activity of insulin. Dr. Mark Hyman suggests aiming for a two-hour insulin level under 30.[13]

MEASURING DAMAGE TO THE PANCREAS: THE C-PEPTIDE TEST

When a person develops diabetes, it is important to determine whether they have type 1 or type 2. As we've just discovered, one way to test this is by evaluating insulin levels. Pancreatic function can also be determined by the C-peptide test.[14]

People with diabetes sometimes do not know whether they have type 1 or type 2. Patients may be prescribed insulin without knowing whether they are naturally producing any insulin or not. But once they are taking insulin injections, an insulin test won't reliably determine whether or not their pancreas is producing insulin. The test cannot tell the difference between insulin that's being produced by the pancreas and insulin that's being injected.

The C-peptide test solves this problem by evaluating natural insulin production another way. C-peptide is a protein produced by the pancreas. The pancreas releases this protein at the same time it releases insulin. For every molecule of insulin released, a molecule of C-peptide is also released. Because the level of C-peptide corresponds with the level of insulin, this test can be used to evaluate how much insulin the pancreas is producing.

NORMAL USE OF THE C-PEPTIDE TEST

The C-peptide test is normally used to help determine whether patients who are taking insulin injections have type 1 or type 2 diabetes.[15, 16] If the C-peptide level is normal or high, this means that the pancreas is producing a normal or high amount of insulin, indicating that type 2 diabetes is present, which is most frequently characterized by insulin resistance.

If the C-peptide test is very low, this means that the pancreas is producing very little—if any—insulin. This indicates type 1 diabetes, which is caused by inadequate insulin production.

EXPERIMENTAL/INNOVATIVE USE OF THE C-PEPTIDE TEST

The C-peptide test can reveal more information than just which type of diabetes is present. Because this test measures how well the pancreas is producing insulin, it actually tells how much damage has occurred to the pancreatic tissue and what the long-term chances are that a person will be able to fully control their blood sugars without the use of insulin or other medications.

Recently, a group of lifestyle medicine physicians developed a new, experimental test to evaluate the probability that diabetic patients taking multiple medications would eventually be able to control their blood sugars without medications after several months of intensive lifestyle therapy.[17] This test is an adaptation of the stimulated C-peptide test.

To perform the test, patients were given a sugary drink or carbohydrate-rich meal (similar to a glucose tolerance test). Approximately an hour later, after blood sugars had increased from the meal and the pancreas was the most likely to be producing insulin and C-peptide, the C-peptide level was measured. The amount of C-peptide in the blood revealed how effective the pancreas was at secreting insulin and C-peptide in response to rising blood sugars.

The team of physicians developed criteria to explain what the stimulated C-peptide levels meant.

INTERPRETING THE STIMULATED C-PEPTIDE TEST

Stimulated C-peptide Levels	What It Means
<2 ng/mL	The pancreas is severely damaged. There is only an estimated 5 percent chance of controlling blood sugars through lifestyle interventions alone.
2-4 ng/mL	The pancreas has undergone some damage but is still functioning. There is still a 50/50 chance of controlling blood sugars without insulin or other medication.
4+ ng/mL	The pancreas is functioning well. There is an estimated 95 percent chance that blood sugars can eventually be controlled by lifestyle interventions alone, without insulin or other medication.

It's important to note that this was simply an experimental model, and these are not official criteria. However, I believe that this new approach is a valuable way to determine the extent of pancreatic damage and to predict whether patients will be able to control their blood sugars with lifestyle approaches alone—or whether they may need to supplement their lifestyle changes with insulin.

The lines between type 1 diabetes and type 2 diabetes are not always as clear as we once thought. Many people who initially develop type 2 diabetes sustain damage to the pancreas after years of high blood sugars and unhealthy choices. Over time, the ability of the pancreas to produce insulin becomes more and more compromised.

By using these experimental guidelines to evaluate pancreatic function, we better understand a person's long-term prognosis. This helps us develop a realistic treatment plan. Luke and Patrick—two of my former patients—illustrate the usefulness of the stimulated C-peptide test.

LUKE AND THE STIMULATED C-PEPTIDE TEST

Several years ago, Luke, a 76-year-old ex-Navy SEAL, was referred to me by his family physician. He was suffering from extremely high blood sugars and a recent history of stroke and multiple heart attacks. Luke's blood sugars were well above 400. His Hemoglobin A1c was dangerously high at 13.4 percent, even though he was taking high doses of insulin multiple times each day.

I wanted to evaluate how functional Luke's pancreas was so that I could tell him what to expect if he started following a comprehensive lifestyle program. I decided to evaluate his stimulated C-peptide level. I had him go out for breakfast and eat a carbohydrate-rich meal of pancakes and orange juice. About an hour later, he went to the lab to have his C-peptide level measured.

Luke had a stimulated C-peptide level of 5 ng/mL. This was excellent news. His pancreas was still functioning well. Knowing how hopeless Luke felt about his health condition, I was thrilled to explain to him that he had an estimated 95 percent chance of getting his blood sugars into an optimal range with little, if any, medication—if he aggressively followed a new lifestyle plan.

I still remember the surprise on Luke's face when he heard the news. "Are you kidding me?" he said. "You mean to say that, even with my horrible blood sugars and poor health, it's still actually possible to undo this thing?" I reassured Luke that I believed reversal was possible if he truly wanted it and was motivated enough to give it his best shot. Luke readily agreed to make all the changes necessary to aggressively improve his health.

He started eating an optimal diet of high-nutrient, plant-based foods. He learned how different foods affected his blood sugars and how to balance his meals appropriately. He started exercising throughout the day and especially after meals (more on after-meal exercise in Chapter 15).

Luke didn't let anything get in the way of his new goal. He had suffered multiple injuries in the Navy and had shrapnel embedded in his spine. This made it difficult to exercise. When he walked, the muscles in his back would sometimes lock up, and he wouldn't be able to move for several minutes at a time. But he didn't use this as an excuse. He would wait until he could walk again and then keep going. Luke was determined to beat his diabetes!

Luke experienced dramatic results. His blood sugars normalized, and for the first time in years he didn't have to take insulin. He felt better, had more energy, and had a completely new outlook on life. He also drastically reduced his risk of another heart attack or stroke, and avoided all other diabetes-related complications.

The stimulated C-peptide test proved to be very valuable in Luke's experience. Once he realized that his pancreas was functioning and that there was hope for reversing his diabetes, Luke did everything in his power to improve his health.

The good news is that the overwhelming majority of type 2 patients I see have stimulated C-peptide levels over 4 ng/mL. This suggests that, like Luke, they still have good pancreatic function and stand an excellent chance of completely reversing their diabetes and maintaining good health without insulin.

There is, however, a small percentage of type 2 patients who have sustained damage to their pancreatic tissue and have low C-peptide levels. Patrick is one of these patients.

PATRICK AND THE STIMULATED C-PEPTIDE TEST

Patrick came to my clinic with a diagnosis of type 2 diabetes and a history of out-of-control blood sugars. Although he was incredibly fit and active—exercising between one and two hours each day—he couldn't seem to control his blood sugars without insulin.

I wanted to see how well his pancreas was functioning, so I ordered a stimulated C-peptide test. His level was 2 ng/mL. This meant that his pancreas had sustained some serious damage and that his type 2 diabetes was actually becoming more like type 1 diabetes. As I explained the results to Patrick, I encouraged him to keep exercising consistently and to also implement some additional lifestyle strategies. This would help increase his insulin sensitivity and decrease the amount of insulin he had to inject. However, I explained to him that, because the insulin-producing cells in his pancreas were so damaged, he would probably need to continue to take insulin over time in spite of his fit and healthy lifestyle. Although the news was disappointing, it gave Patrick a better understanding of his overall prognosis and helped him set realistic goals for the future.

THE VALUE OF THE TEST

We need to remember that lifestyle medicine strategies are essential *regardless* of how well the pancreas is functioning. It's just as important for type 1 diabetics, or people with extensive pancreatic damage, to make healthy lifestyle choices as it is for people with type 2 diabetes. Type 1 diabetics who eat well, exercise regularly, and take care of their health can increase their insulin sensitivity and minimize the *amount* of insulin they need to take.

However, although all diabetics (and non-diabetics) benefit from healthy lifestyle choices, some people need to take some insulin regardless of how many healthy lifestyle choices they make. The experimental model described above can be very valuable for determining your pancreatic function, which will help you set realistic treatment goals.

CHAPTER SUMMARY

» The pancreas is a small gland located behind the stomach.

» The pancreas secretes multiple enzymes and hormones, including insulin.

» Type 1 diabetics have sustained pancreatic damage and do not produce any significant amount of insulin.

» Type 2 diabetics produce insulin, but are resistant to it.

» The fasting insulin test and the two-hour insulin test measure pancreatic function.

» High insulin levels caused by insulin resistance increase the risk for many diseases, including: heart disease, obesity, and certain forms of cancer.

» The C-peptide test can be used to measure the extent of pancreatic function and/or damage.

» The C-peptide test can indirectly measure how much insulin the pancreas is producing.

» The C-peptide test can reveal whether a person has type 1 diabetes or type 2 diabetes.

» The C-peptide test helps to predict the likelihood that a diabetic person will eventually be able to manage his or her blood sugars without the need for insulin.

—TEN—

Looking at the Big Picture

SEVERAL YEARS AGO, BARBARA BEGAN COMING TO MY clinic for help with her type 2 diabetes. Her husband, Paul, came to every appointment to offer his support. They lived in a nearby retirement community. Barbara was a gregarious, social woman who was enthusiastic about improving her health. I helped her design a comprehensive plan to address her diabetes, high cholesterol, excess weight, and high blood pressure.

Barbara would frequently express how it didn't seem fair that her husband didn't struggle with the same health problems she did: "Oh, Paul is so lucky. He doesn't have to deal with diabetes. He can eat anything he wants. I wish I could be like Paul!"

Knowing that people who appear to be in good health frequently have undetected health problems, I mentioned several times that it would be a good idea for Paul to have some testing done as well. This didn't make sense to Barbara: "Oh! *He* doesn't need any of these tests. He's so healthy. *I'm* the one with all the problems." Paul was an easy-going guy and would just smile, nod, and agree with his wife.

Two years later, Paul died of colon cancer. Barbara was shocked and devastated. Her husband, who seemed perfectly healthy, was actually the one to die prematurely, while she continued to live, maintaining an improved level of health.

Barbara and Paul's sobering story demonstrates the importance of regularly evaluating our health. Health is dynamic and comprehensive. It cannot be measured by any single factor alone.

THE BIG PICTURE

Many diabetes programs focus *only* on blood sugar management. While it's extremely important to control blood sugars, it's also vital to realize that many other areas of health also need to be addressed.

Paul wasn't diabetic and had never had to worry about his blood sugar levels. Millions of people with optimal blood sugar levels are *not* healthy. Our goal isn't just to control blood sugars. *Our goal is to be healthy!* In order to do this, we need to look at the big picture.

Whether you have optimal blood sugar control or are struggling with diabetes, this chapter provides you with valuable information on other areas of your health that may need attention and outlines more of the laboratory tests I recommend to my patients. You can find more information about each of these tests online at labtestsonline.org or MayoClinic.com. Most are recommended whether or not you have diabetes. Because of the heightened risk that accompanies prediabetes and diabetes, it is even more important for anyone with these conditions to undergo these tests.

You will notice that I list both standard recommendations and optimal levels for many of the test results. After careful research, I've found that standard recommendations don't always represent optimal health. Sometimes, standard recommendations are outdated or based on national averages instead of on ideal levels. The optimal ranges listed in these charts represent what I believe are the most current and evidence-based recommendations. Many other lifestyle medicine experts also recommend these more conservative values.

It's also important to note that the standard recommended levels can vary, depending on the lab company used or the hospital or clinic administering the tests.

Let's begin by considering how to evaluate one of the most important aspects of your health—the condition of your heart.

EVALUATING YOUR HEART HEALTH

Heart disease is the leading cause of death in the United States and worldwide.[1] Every 34 seconds, someone in the U.S. has a heart attack. Every minute, someone in the U.S. dies from a heart disease-related event.[2] It's important for everyone to pay attention to cardiovascular health.

High blood sugars dramatically increase risk for heart disease. Two out of three diabetics will die prematurely from heart disease or stroke.[3] People with prediabetes are already at a 50 percent increased risk for heart attack or stroke.[4] Because of increased risk, people with prediabetes and diabetes need to be especially vigilant about monitoring their cardiovascular health.

Let's take a look at some helpful cardiovascular lab tests. I encourage you to read this section thoroughly and to take advantage of the tests outlined here. This information could save your life.

TESTS TO EVALUATE HEART HEALTH

Test	Standard Levels	Optimal Levels
Cardiac CRP This test measures inflammation throughout your body. High inflammation significantly increases the risk of heart disease, diabetes, cancer, and other diseases. See pages 24–25.	1–3 mg/L	<1.0 mg/L
Triglycerides* Triglycerides are a type of fat in your blood. High triglycerides significantly increase the risk of heart disease. See page 65.	<150 mg/dL	<100 mg/dL
Total Cholesterol* Cholesterol is a waxy, fat-like substance that can build up in the walls of your arteries. High cholesterol significantly increases the risk of heart disease. See pages 64–65.	<200 mg/dL	<160 mg/dL

Test	Standard Levels	Optimal Levels
HDL or "Good Cholesterol"* High HDL is associated with a lower risk of heart disease. Your HDL level should always be at least half your LDL level. See pages 64–65.	>40 mg/dL (men) >50 mg/dL (women)	>60 mg/dL Also consider LDL/HDL ratio (see below.)
LDL or "Bad Cholesterol"* High levels of LDL significantly increase the risk of heart disease. See pages 64–65.	<130 mg/dL	<70 mg/dL *Also consider LDL/HDL ratio (see below)*
LDL/HDL Ratio This measures the ratio of bad cholesterol to good cholesterol. It's based on dividing the LDL by the HDL. A high ratio increases the risk for cardiovascular disease.	<2:1 ratio	Same as Standard Levels
LDL Density Pattern* LDL cholesterol can be small and dense ("Pattern B") or large and buoyant ("Pattern A"). Small, dense LDL is associated with increased risk for heart disease.	You want Pattern A.	Same as Standard Levels (Pattern A)
LDL Particle Number This test is an even more sensitive indicator of heart disease than the LDL or LDL Density Pattern. It measures the actual number of LDL particles in the blood.	Total LDL particles <1,000 nmol/L Small LDL particles <500 nmol/L	Same as Standard Levels
Lp(a) or Lipoprotein a* High levels of this LDL-like particle are associated with oxidation, inflammation, and plaque formation.	<30 mg/dL	<10 mg/dL
Iron High iron levels increase risk for heart disease and diabetes. Low levels indicate anemia and fatigue.	46–175 μg/dL (men) 30-170 μg/dL (women)	70-110 μg/dL (men/women)

Test	Standard Levels	Optimal Levels
Ferritin Ferritin is a protein used to store iron. High levels represent increased risk for heart disease, certain cancers, diabetes, and diabetes-related complications.	22–322 ng/mL (men) 10–291 μg/dL (women.)	70–110 μg/dL (men/women)
Homocysteine An elevated homocysteine level increases risk of heart disease, stroke, and peripheral artery disease.	<11.4 μmol/L	<9.0 μmol/L
Uric Acid Although typically used to diagnose gout, this test can also evaluate the tendency toward insulin resistance.	3.7–9.2 mg/dL	<6.0 mg/dL

**These tests are included in one test called the VAP Profile.*
More information about these tests is available at labtestsonline.org.

EVALUATING YOUR KIDNEY FUNCTION

Kidney disease is another devastating complication of diabetes. High blood pressure and high blood sugar levels damage the tiny filters in the kidneys and can significantly impair their ability to clean and filter blood.

Approximately 35 percent of people with type 1 diabetes and 25 percent of people with type 2 diabetes have advanced kidney disease.[5] Without proper intervention, many of them will progress to end-stage renal failure, requiring either a kidney transplant or dialysis.

The CDC National Diabetes Fact sheet reports these alarming statistics:[6]

- Diabetes is the leading cause of kidney failure in the United States, accounting for 44 percent of new cases in 2008.
- In 2008, nearly 50,000 diabetic Americans began treatment for end-stage kidney disease.
- In 2008, more than 200,000 Americans with end-stage kidney disease due to diabetes were living on chronic dialysis or with a kidney transplant.

Symptoms of kidney disease do not appear until the advanced stages. By that time, the kidneys have sustained serious damage over several years or decades. The only way to detect kidney disease in its early stages is by laboratory testing. The earlier kidney disease is detected and addressed, the better the chances are for optimizing kidney function and avoiding serious complications.

If you have prediabetes or diabetes, it's very important to evaluate your kidney function.

TESTS TO EVALUATE KIDNEY FUNCTION

Test	Standard Levels	Optimal Levels
GFR or Glomerular Filtration Rate* When kidneys are functioning optimally, their filtration rate is high. When filtration rate drops, their ability to filter toxins decreases.	>60 mL/ min.	>90 mL/ min.
BUN (Blood Urea Nitrogen)* This test measures the amount of nitrogen in your blood that comes from the waste product urea. If your kidneys are compromised and are not able to properly remove urea from the blood, your BUN level rises.	9-28 mg/ dL	9–20 mg/dL
Creatinine* This substance is generated from muscle metabolism. The kidneys should filter out most of the creatinine from your blood. An elevated creatinine level signifies impaired kidney function.	<1.5 mg/ dL	<1.2 mg/dL
Microalbumin (Spot Urine Test) This test measures the amount of the protein albumin in your urine. If your kidneys are functioning properly, this level should be very low.	<30 mg/L	<20 mg/L

**These tests are all included in the Comprehensive Metabolic Panel (CMP). More information about these tests can be found at labtestsonline.org.*

EVALUATING YOUR LIVER

People with diabetes have an increased risk for developing non-alcoholic fatty liver disease. According to the Mayo Clinic, at least half of type 2 diabetics and almost half of type 1 diabetics have fatty liver disease.[7] This condition occurs when fat accumulates in the liver tissue. It impairs the liver's ability to detoxify the blood and in some cases leads to scarring (cirrhosis) of the liver and/or liver failure.

Commonly prescribed medications can also cause liver damage. It is standard practice for physicians to put diabetics on cholesterol medication, even if they don't have high cholesterol. Multiple studies have shown that cholesterol medications and other classes of diabetes medications can potentially cause damage to the liver.[8]

For these reasons, it's important to regularly evaluate your liver function if you have prediabetes or diabetes.

TESTS TO EVALUATE LIVER FUNCTION

Test	Standard Levels	Optimal Levels
ALT (Alanine Transaminase—aka SGPT)* ALT is an enzyme found primarily in liver cells, Elevated ALT levels may indicate liver damage or disease.	10–49 U/L	<30 U/L
AST (Aspartate Transaminase—aka SGOT)* AST is an enzyme found in liver cells. An increase in AST may indicate liver damage or disease. This test can also detect damage to the heart, muscle, intestines, and kidney cells.	<40 U/L	<30 U/L
GGTP (Gamma-Glutamyl Transpeptidase) Higher than normal levels may indicate damage to the liver or gallbladder.	<45 U/L	<30 U/L

**These tests are included in the Comprehensive Metabolic Panel (CMP). More information about these tests can be found at labtestsonline.org.*

EVALUATING YOUR THYROID FUNCTION

The thyroid gland, located in the neck, secretes thyroid hormones that help to regulate metabolism and optimize circulation. An estimated 27 million Americans suffer from thyroid disease—usually hypothyroidism—which means they are not producing enough thyroid hormone.[9] People with diabetes are almost twice as likely to have a thyroid problem as people without diabetes.[10]

Optimal thyroid function is essential to good circulation, and good circulation is essential to good health. Poor thyroid function increases the risk of heart disease and all diabetes-related complications.[11] Thyroid lab results require special attention. There is much debate among those in the medical community regarding optimal ranges. Your lab results should be evaluated carefully, taking into account the signs and symptoms associated with thyroid dysfunction.

TESTS TO EVALUATE THYROID FUNCTION*

Test	Standard Levels
TSH (Thyroid Stimulating Hormone) This hormone is produced by the pituitary gland and stimulates the thyroid to produce thyroid hormone. A high TSH level indicates suboptimal thyroid function. A low TSH level indicates an overactive thyroid.	0.350–5.500 µIU/mL
Free T4 or Free Thyroxine Free T4 is a thyroid hormone that can be converted to a more active form (Free T3). This test can indicate how well the thyroid gland is producing thyroid hormone.	0.89–1.76 ng/dL
Free T3 or Free Triiodothyronine Free T3 is the most active form of thyroid hormone. Your doctor will combine the results of the TSH test with the Free T3 and Free T4 tests to get a complete picture of your thyroid function.	2.3–4.2 pg/mL

Test	Standard Levels
TPOAb (Thyroid Peroxidase Antibody) There are two common antibodies that can reveal thyroid dysfunction: thyroid peroxidase and thyroglobulin. Measuring levels of these antibodies may help diagnose the cause of thyroid problems.	<61 U/mL
TgAb (Thyroglobulin Antibody) Same as above.	<41 IU/mL
Reverse T3 When the body is under stress, instead of converting T4 into T3, it conserves energy by making what is known as Reverse T3 (an inactive form of T3). High Reverse T3 levels may indicate decreased thyroid function even when T3 and T4 levels are normal.	90–350 pg/mL

* *More information about these tests can be found at labtestsonline.org.*

EVALUATING YOUR VITAMIN D LEVEL

One of the easiest and most important strategies for improving your health is to be sure you have an optimal vitamin D level. I encourage all of my patients to have their vitamin D levels tested.

According to a study published in the *Archives of Internal Medicine,* 77 percent of American adults are vitamin D deficient.[12] This is a serious national health problem. People with diabetes are even more likely to be vitamin D deficient than people without diabetes.[13]

Vitamin D can help prevent both type 1 and type 2 diabetes.[14, 15] It can also help improve those conditions once they already exist. By optimizing vitamin D levels, people with blood sugar problems can greatly reduce their risk for diabetes-related complications.

Because I strongly believe in the benefits of vitamin D, I have included an entire section on this topic in Chapter 19.

FUNCTIONS OF VITAMIN D[16]

- Boosts immunity
- Protects against infection
- Increases insulin sensitivity
- Decreases inflammation
- Lowers the risk of heart disease
- Protects against many forms of cancer
- Decreases hypertension
- Helps prevent depression
- Lowers the risk of osteoporosis
- Prevents up to 50 percent of falls in the elderly
- Prevents 50 percent of hip fractures

COMPREHENSIVE METABOLIC PANEL

The Comprehensive Metabolic Panel (CMP) is one of the most commonly ordered lab panels. It is a collection of 14 different blood tests. You can read more about it at labtestsonline.org. The CMP is frequently ordered with an annual physical exam because it provides information on a broad range of risk indicators, including kidney and liver function, electrolytes, and fasting blood glucose. The CMP includes some of the tests that we've already discussed in this chapter. I recommend a CMP for all of my patients.

EVALUATING VITAMINS AND MINERALS

Vitamins and minerals are necessary for the completion of every bodily function. From aiding digestion to fighting toxins to helping produce red blood cells, each vitamin and mineral has an important role to play.

Although many vitamins and minerals can be found in a healthy, nutrient-dense diet, sometimes it is necessary to also use supplements. Because of our biological individuality, different people need more of certain nutrients than others. Blood tests can help to determine any nutritional deficiencies, which can then be easily addressed.

Several vitamins and minerals are especially helpful for people with prediabetes and diabetes. These will be explained in more detail in Chapter 20.

HORMONES

Like vitamins and minerals, hormones have the amazing capacity to regulate a variety of body functions. People with high blood sugar levels frequently have hormone imbalances that contribute to their risk of diabetes-related complications.

For this reason, it's important to evaluate and address hormone health.

TESTS TO EVALUATE HORMONE HEALTH*

Type of Hormone Test	Recommended For
DHEA-Sulfate	Men / Women
Estradiol	Men / Women
Progesterone	Women
Total Testosterone	Men / Women
Free Testosterone	Men / Women

**More information about these tests can be found at labtestsonline.org.*

IMPORTANT TESTS IN A NUTSHELL

In addition to the tests outlined in this chapter, other lab tests are described elsewhere in this book. To make things as clear as possible, below is a concise list of the basic lab tests I generally recommend for my patients.

RECOMMENDED TESTS

- VAP Cholesterol Panel
- LDL Particle Number
- Cardiac CRP (hs CRP)
- Comprehensive Metabolic Panel
- Iron
- Ferritin
- Homocysteine
- 25 OH Vitamin D
- DHEA-Sulfate
- Testosterone
- Estradiol
- Thyroid Panel
- Hemoglobin A1c
- Four Hour Glucose Tolerance Test* (Blood sugars taken at fasting and at every hour for 4 hours, typically not used for those already diagnosed with diabetes)
- Cortisol Levels* (Taken at fasting and at 3 and 4 hours during Glucose Tolerance Test)
- Insulin Levels* (Taken at fasting and at 2 hours during Glucose Tolerance Test, not useful if taking insulin, but can substitute C-peptide test)

**These tests also help evaluate hypoglycemia and adrenal fatigue.*

HOW TO GET TESTED

Various testing options are usually available for any given test. Shop around and check out the different options. Your doctor can order the tests. Insurance companies may only cover a portion of the cost. However, you can often receive substantial discounts by paying cash directly to a laboratory. Many clinics that specialize in lifestyle medicine offer rates even cheaper than paying cash at the lab. Online services can also be used to order these tests. Regardless of which method you choose, work closely with a qualified healthcare provider to help interpret your results.

WHY TESTING MATTERS

In my opinion, the first and most important step in improving health is to undergo comprehensive testing. By broadly evaluating multiple aspects of your health, you may detect hidden problems possibly years or even decades before you would find them otherwise. Testing allows you to address those problems head-on, before they cause serious complications. Awareness of the areas in need of improvement can help motivate you to take action.

Whether or not you have diabetes, I encourage you to seek thorough evaluation before starting a wellness program. The information obtained will give you a baseline on which to base any necessary lifestyle changes. It will also help you know how to tailor your treatment plan to meet your individual needs. Once you begin making lifestyle changes, follow-up testing will help track your progress. The amazing improvements you notice in your sense of well-being should be reflected in your lab tests. It is exciting to see the results and measure the impact of your lifestyle choices.

I encourage you to take advantage of these tests to fully understand your health condition. It would be valuable to do a thorough evaluation before moving on to the final section of this book. In that section, you will begin implementing lifestyle strategies that will dramatically improve your health. Getting tested first can help you to set goals and track your progress.

While I strongly encourage you to get tested, I understand that, because of financial limitations or other reasons, people sometimes choose not to test. If that is your circumstance, go ahead and proceed with the next section of this book. Either way, you will greatly benefit from implementing the strategies outlined in the coming chapters. Although you may not be able to measure your progress clinically, you will still be getting healthier—and that's the ultimate goal.

CHAPTER SUMMARY

- » Blood sugars are important, but there are many other aspects of health that also need to be evaluated and addressed.
- » Heart disease is the leading cause of death in the United States and worldwide.
- » Diabetes and prediabetes significantly increase the risk of heart disease.
- » Kidney disease is another devastating complication of diabetes.
- » Because symptoms of kidney disease don't occur until the advanced stages, it's important to test kidney function early on.
- » Diabetes increases the risk for fatty liver disease.
- » Many commonly prescribed medications may cause damage to the liver.
- » People who are diabetic are almost twice as likely to develop thyroid problems as people who are not diabetic.
- » Optimal thyroid levels promote good circulation and decrease the risk of all diabetes-related complications.
- » The vast majority of Americans are Vitamin D deficient.
- » Diabetics are even more likely to be Vitamin D deficient than nondiabetics.
- » Vitamin D can help to prevent or improve both type 1 and type 2 diabetes, as well as many other diseases.
- » The CMP is a collection of 14 commonly ordered blood tests.
- » Vitamins and minerals are essential for all bodily functions.
- » Hormones help to regulate many specific body functions.
- » People with diabetes often have hormonal imbalances.
- » Testing should be our first strategy to improve health.

SECTION 4

Defeating Diabetes

—ELEVEN—

Think Good Thoughts

Whether you think you can, or think you can't—you're usually right.
—Henry Ford

"I'VE GOTTA FIGURE SOMETHING OUT, DOC, BECAUSE I'm losing my mind. I can't concentrate. I'm getting upset really easily. I'm nervous and shaky. I need some medication or something."

I still remember how worried and tense David was during our first visit. It was a late Friday morning at the lifestyle clinic on Guam. David had called to schedule an appointment. Luckily for him another patient had just canceled, opening up a time slot at the last minute. David was a big guy—6 feet 5 inches, and 332 pounds. As I sat across from him and listened to his story, I began to understand why he was under so much stress.

David was the residential manager of a 1,000-room exotic resort on Guam. Located on the beautiful white beaches of Tumon Bay, this resort offered a wide selection of recreational activities—swimming, scuba diving, kayaking, and more. It also hosted a variety of dining and entertainment options.

David's job was stressful. As the residential manager, David was second-in-command. At the end of each day, the general manager would walk out of the office and say, "All right, Dave. It's all yours!" and would go home to enjoy the evening with his family. Meanwhile, David was responsible for any problems that arose during the evening and night hours. He lived onsite with his wife and five-year-old daughter. Working day and night, he never got a break.

Somehow, even though David was putting in such long hours, his boss never seemed to be satisfied. He was constantly challenging David's decisions. Years of this was taking a toll on David's physical and emotional health.

The last few months had been particularly stressful. David was anxious, irritable, and edgy. He had recently had an argument with one of his 400 employees. He admitted being so angry that he almost hit the man. David realized that he was just one emotional degree away from losing his job and never being able to work in that industry again.

However, David's real wake-up call had come the night before. He had returned home after work, sat down in his chair, held his head in his hands, and started shaking uncontrollably.

Just then, he felt the little hand of his five-year-old daughter on his shoulder. She came close, hugged him, and whispered: "Daddy, I don't want you to die."

David told me that it broke his heart to realize that his little daughter was worried she was going to lose him. "I decided right then and there that I wasn't going to wait any longer; I was going to get some help first thing in the morning. So I called your clinic and somebody had just canceled, so here I am."

Fortunately for David, that Sunday we were starting a six-month wellness program, similar to the one described in Chapter 1. I told him that I highly recommended that he join. He was enthusiastic and willing to give it his best shot. I filled out a lab slip for him, and we had the tests done immediately.

On Sunday morning, he was in my office to review his labs before our program orientation began. Here are his results:

DAVID'S TEST RESULTS

Test	Results	What It Means
Weight	332	Obesity
Blood Pressure	140/100	Hypertension
Cholesterol	246	Very High
LDL	183	High
HDL	34	Low
Triglycerides	144	Higher than ideal
Fasting Blood Glucose	122	Advanced Prediabetes
Fasting Insulin	17	Hyperinsulinemia/ Insulin Resistance
Cardiac CRP	7	Heightened level of inflammation

I explained to David what his lab results meant. He had advanced prediabetes and a high risk of heart attack or stroke. David's "metabolic mess" included obesity, hypertension, high cholesterol, high blood sugars, high insulin levels, and a heightened level of inflammation.

Additionally, I shared with David that, even though the results seemed alarming, there was hope for change. A lifestyle program would give him the tools he needed to dramatically improve his health.

It's important for patients to set their own goals and to find their own motivation for change. So I encouraged David to write down specific goals he wanted to accomplish that would help motivate him to take charge of his health. David decided on three goals and shared them with me.

DAVID'S GOALS

1. To weigh less than 200 pounds
2. To run the Honolulu marathon
3. To become the general manager at a 5-star hotel in Maui

I have to admit that when I first looked at David's goals they didn't seem very realistic, given his current condition. However, I sensed that he was determined to take charge of his health, and I encouraged him to move forward with the program and do his best to reach his goals.

THE TURNING POINT

I watched David as he began the process of transforming his health. He took notes at every meeting and immediately began implementing each new health strategy he learned. He completely altered his diet and began exercising. Within a few days, he noticed a dramatic improvement in his mood and energy level.

Just one week into the program, David stuck his head in my office. "By the way," he said, "you know how I was talking about anti-anxiety meds? Well, never-mind about that. I'm feeling great."

At the end of two weeks, David had lost 11 pounds. His blood pressure had improved so much that he was able to discontinue all his anti-hypertensive medications. His cholesterol had dropped 54 points, and his blood fats had dropped by 50 percent.

David was encouraged by these improvements, but wasn't satisfied yet. He wouldn't be satisfied until he had reached his goals. David knew that if he wanted to run a marathon, he needed to start putting some miles in. At the very beginning of the program, David decided to run for 45 minutes every morning (from his home to the clinic for our session) and then 45 minutes in the evening (from the clinic back to his house).

He was also serious about losing weight. When he ate at the buffet we provided for our patients, he would go through once, fill up his plate, and sit down to eat. He wouldn't come back for seconds or thirds like many other patients did. Even though the food was healthy, he knew that if he really wanted to lose the weight, it was important to not overeat.

The resort David worked at had five different gourmet restaurants. At any time, David could ask any of the chefs to make whatever he wanted. David had done this for years—but not anymore. He resisted the urge and stuck with his new diet throughout the entire program.

By the end of six months, David had lost 79 pounds, lowered his cholesterol even further, and was no longer prediabetic. His fasting insulin had decreased from 17 to 10, and his Cardiac CRP level had decreased by 50 percent.

I continued to see David for several months after the program ended. He continued to lose weight, improve his health, and reduce his risk factors. Eventually, his health had improved so dramatically that he felt confident continuing his new lifestyle on his own. We lost touch for several months.

One day, I was in the Guam airport after returning from a medical conference in California. As I walked down the terminal, headed for the baggage claim area, I heard someone call my name. I turned around to see David, along with his wife and little girl. It took me a few seconds to recognize him. Tall, lean, and muscular, David looked like an athlete. "David!" I said. "You look great! What's your weight at?" He grinned and said, "I broke the 200 mark about a month ago." In just a year and a half, David had lost over 130 pounds!

"By the way," he continued, "guess what I did two weekends ago! Do you remember my goals? [Immediately my mind flashed back to the three goals David had set eighteen months earlier.] I ran the Honolulu marathon, and I finished it."

I congratulated David and let him know I was proud of him. "So where are you heading now?" I asked. "We're heading to Maui," he replied. "I've been offered a job as the general manager of the top resort on the island."

WHAT WAS DAVID'S SECRET?

David's story has always stuck with me. He is an inspiring example of how people with chronic health conditions can beat the odds and completely transform their health.

What was it about David that made him so successful? Many people who want to become healthy never reach that goal. What was it that enabled David to stick with his plan and experience such powerful results?

One important lesson we can learn from David's story is the importance of *setting the right goals.*

IDENTIFY YOUR GOALS

How would your life change for the better if you didn't struggle with the same health problems you're struggling with now? Why do you want to be healthy? What are the things that you want to accomplish or experience with an improved level of health?

These are important questions to answer. While different people have different motivations, I hear the following reasons quite frequently:

- I want to live a long life.
- I want to thrive, not just survive.
- I want more energy.
- I want to be around for my family.
- I want to see my children and grandchildren grow up.
- I want to be able to accomplish more.
- I want to feel better about my weight and/or appearance.
- I want to reduce my risk for disease.
- I want to keep medical costs down.
- I want my mood to improve.

I encourage you to set aside some time to write down the reasons why you want to be healthy. Constantly remind yourself of these reasons when you are tempted to give up. You can even write them on post-it notes and place them where you will see them often.

While these kinds of goals are valuable, it's important to set more specific, defined goals like David did. Examples of these goals could include:

- I want to lose 20 pounds in the next six months.
- I want to be able to walk or run five miles.
- I want to no longer fit the criteria for prediabetes.
- I want to lower my cholesterol and triglycerides.
- I want to fit into my old clothes again.

MAKE A PLAN

Once you identify the goals you want to accomplish, formulate a plan to help you reach those goals. This can be done by setting specific, short-term, action-based goals like:

- I am going to eat 40 grams of fiber each day by increasing my intake of vegetables, fruits, legumes, and whole grains.
- I am going to exercise 15 minutes after each meal, as well as 30 minutes in the morning.
- I am going to do strength training three times per week.
- I am going to eat beans and nuts with my meals to help balance my blood sugars.

Make sure that the action goals you set are **SMART** goals.[1]

Specific
Measurable
Attainable
Realistic
Time-Bound

THINK RIGHT ABOUT YOUR GOALS

David maintained a positive attitude about his potential to succeed. He believed that, regardless of his past or current health condition, there was hope for major improvements. Because he thought *right* about his goals, he was able to make good choices to reach those goals.

One of the most important strategies for improving your health is to improve your thinking. In the Bible, Proverbs 23:7 says: "For as a man thinks in his heart, so is he." We tend to become what we think about or what we identify with.

When David learned to think like a healthy person, he became a healthy person. He rejected any negative thoughts that would sabotage his success. He chose to think hopeful, encouraging, and motivating thoughts. We can do the same thing. We can replace our negative, hopeless thoughts with thoughts that will help us succeed.

EXAMPLES OF SUCCESSFUL THINKING

» My health is important to me and to the people I care about.

» I want to be healthy because...

» Taking care of my health is an investment in my future.

» I can make simple choices to improve my health.

» It's not too late. I can start today.

» Improving my health is worth the effort.

» I can overcome my risk factors.

» Little choices add up to big improvements.

» If I mess up, I can start over.

OBEY YOUR PLAN, NOT YOUR FEELINGS

In 1994, Sprite® launched a new marketing slogan: "Obey Your Thirst."[2] Commercials featured popular hip-hop artists and professional athletes promoting the beverage, as well as music with lyrics like, "Never forget yourself, 'cause first things first, grab a cold, cold can, and obey your thirst." Apparently the slogan was successful, because eighteen years later it's still being used.

But why do you think Sprite wants you to obey your thirst? Will drinking Sprite turn you into a superstar? No. A professional athlete? No. Will drinking Sprite improve your health? No. But drinking Sprite will increase the profits of *Coca Cola*®, and therefore make the marketing campaign successful.

The "Obey Your Thirst" slogan appeals to basic human desire. It is echoed in other marketing campaigns and slogans worldwide. If you're thirsty, drink it. If it tastes good, eat it. If it feels right, do it. If you want it, get it.

The problem is, what we want often isn't what we need. This is one of the reasons why we have so many problems with our health and with other aspects of our lives—we're making decisions based on our *feelings*.

When it comes to improving your health, it's important to obey your plan instead of your feelings. David didn't always *feel* like exercising. Sometimes he *felt* like cheating on his diet plan. But he chose to follow his plan instead of his feelings.

He reminded himself that the benefits he would experience from reaching his goals would far outweigh the temporary pleasure he would experience from deviating from his plan. Then, as David continued to follow his plan, his feelings eventually started to change. He realized that he actually enjoyed exercise and healthy food. He enjoyed all of the benefits he was receiving from following his plan.

David didn't look at the minimum criteria for being on the program. Instead of asking, "What's the minimum amount of exercise I can do to be successful?" he asked, "How can I best utilize exercise to improve my health and accomplish my goals?"

Instead of asking, "What foods can I sneak into this program, or how much unhealthy food can I get away with eating?" David asked: "How can I eat in a way that will best improve my health and help me lose the weight I want to lose?"

David succeeded because, instead of attempting to satisfy the *minimum* acceptable criteria for completing the program, he determined to experience the *maximum* impact his choices could have on his health. He then invested the *maximum* amount of effort to accomplish his goals.

BUT WHAT ABOUT FEELINGS?

While it's important to follow our plan instead of our feelings, this doesn't mean that emotions don't matter. Studies show that people with diabetes are twice as likely to suffer from depression as people without diabetes.[3]

The mind and the body are intimately connected. It's important to address and optimize mental and emotional wellness, while simultaneously addressing physical health.[4]

Mental health can be greatly improved by making healthy physical choices with regard to diet, exercise, and sleep. In addition to these strategies, however, some people will benefit from extra support through counseling and/or support groups. For people who need counseling, I recommend Cognitive Behavioral Therapy (CBT), which helps empower you to take responsibility for your thinking in order to improve your mood and your health.

It is also important to find supportive family members and friends who can listen to you and encourage you in your journey toward optimal health.

CHAPTER SUMMARY

- » Identify and write down the reasons why you want to improve your health.
- » Identify and write down specific health goals you want to achieve.
- » Make a plan to help you reach those goals by setting short-term goals.
- » Goals should be SMART: Specific, Measurable, Attainable, Realistic, and Time-Bound.
- » Think right about your goals and your potential to succeed.
- » Obey your plan, not your feelings.
- » Optimize your mental and emotional health through positive lifestyle choices, as well as through counseling and/or additional support if necessary.

—TWELVE—

Eat to Live

Let your food be your medicine and your medicine be your food.
—Hippocrates

THESE WISE WORDS WERE SPOKEN MORE THAN 2,300 years ago by Hippocrates, who is considered the Father of Western Medicine. Hippocrates was ahead of his time in many ways, including in his understanding of the importance of nutrition.

Healthy food is powerful medicine. When it comes to chronic diseases like diabetes, following a prescription for a healthy diet is usually much safer—and many times more effective—than simply filling a prescription at the pharmacy.

The next few chapters focus on the importance of nutrition for diabetes reversal and optimal health. This chapter explores the nutrients your body needs. Chapter 13 addresses how to develop a healthy, tasty, and easy-to-follow food plan to obtain these nutrients. Chapter 14 contains secrets to help optimize digestion and optimally benefit from your new way of eating. Let's start by taking a look at the importance of a nutrient-dense diet.

YOU ARE WHAT YOU EAT

Your house is made out of materials like wood, brick, cement, and metal. Your car is made of materials like steel, aluminum, fiberglass, and plastic. Your body is made of materials like broccoli, kale, lentils, and blueberries—or maybe pizza, pastries, white bread, and soda. It all depends on what you eat.

The foods we eat build and fuel our bodies, quite literally making us what we are. That's why it's important to pick nutrient-rich, first-class foods. In his national best-selling book *Eat to Live,* Dr. Joel Fuhrman shares a simple formula for optimal nutrition and extraordinary health. Here's how he explains it:

> "H=N/C is a concept I call the nutrient density of your diet. Food supplies us with both nutrients and calories (energy). All calories come from only three elements: carbohydrates, fats, and proteins. Nutrients are derived from non-caloric food factors—including vitamins, minerals, fiber, and phytochemicals. These non-caloric nutrients are vitally important for health. *Your key to permanent weight loss* [and health] *is to eat predominantly those foods that have a high proportion of nutrients (non-caloric food factors) to calories (carbohydrates, fats, and proteins).* Every food can be evaluated using this formula. Once you begin to learn which foods make the grade—by having a high proportion of nutrients to calories—you are on your way to lifelong weight control and improved health."[1]

HEALTH = NUTRITION/CALORIES

Simply put, in order to optimize nutrition and health, you must eat foods that are high in the nutrients your body was designed to thrive on, and avoid empty calorie foods (foods high in calories but low in nutrients). Let's take a closer look at the nutrients our bodies thrive on.

POWERFUL NON-CALORIC NUTRIENTS

Fiber If you only remember and apply one strategy from this chapter, it should be this:

Eat 35 to 50 grams of fiber every single day.

Fiber is the indigestible roughage or bulk found in plant foods—vegetables, fruits, legumes, grains, nuts, and seeds. Just like bones give your body structure, fiber gives plants their structure. The body doesn't absorb fiber but passes it through the digestive system. However, fiber does many important things along its digestive journey.

FIBER

- Stabilizes blood sugars by slowing the absorption of sugar[2]
- Lowers cholesterol[3]
- Aids in weight loss[4]
- Helps prevent or reverse cancer,[5] heart disease,[6] diabetes,[7] and many other diseases[8]
- Prevents gastrointestinal disorders[9]
- Normalizes bowel movements and prevents constipation[10]

According to the Academy of Nutrition and Dietetics, the average American eats about 15 grams of fiber each day.[11] The foods Americans predominantly eat have very little fiber. Meat, eggs, milk, and cheese do not contain any fiber. Refined grains and other popular processed foods have *very little, if any fiber*.

Research shows that the health benefits of fiber aren't optimal until a person is consuming at least 25 grams per day.[12] One study published by the *New England Journal of Medicine* showed that diabetics who began eating 50 grams of fiber per day had better blood sugar levels and improved cholesterol levels than those who followed the American Diabetes Association diet, which contains lower fiber recommendations.[13] I encourage you to gradually build up your fiber intake until you reach 35 to 50 grams per day. One way to do this is by eating at least 10 grams of fiber at breakfast and 15 grams at lunch and supper. Here are some common fiber-rich foods:

Fiber Content in Foods

Food	Examples	Serving Size	Average Fiber Content
Beans and Lentils	Navy, pinto, black, kidney, white, great northern, lima, and soy beans; chickpeas; black-eyed peas; lentils, etc.	½ c. cooked	8 grams

Non-Starchy Vegetables	Lettuce, cucumbers, tomatoes, carrots, cabbage, celery, cauliflower, etc.	1 c. raw or ½ c. cooked or chopped	2 grams
Starchy Vegetables	Sweet potatoes, yams, baked potatoes, corn, peas, etc.	½ c. cooked or chopped	3 grams
Fruits	Fresh fruit	1 medium piece of whole fruit or ½ c. chopped	3 grams
Grains	Pasta, rice, cooked cereal, bread, etc.	½ c. cooked, hot cereal, 1 slice whole wheat bread, 1/3 c. brown rice or whole-grain pasta	3 grams

Chart adapted from U.S. Department of Agriculture and U.S. Department of Health and Human Services. Dietary Guidelines for Americans, 2010. 7th Edition, Washington, DC: U.S. Government Printing Office, December 2010.

As you can see, beans and legumes are the highest sources of fiber, each containing approximately 8 grams in a half-cup serving. Think of legumes as your secret weapon in keeping blood sugars under control.[14] All whole plant foods are a good source of fiber, including a variety of whole grains, fruits, vegetables, nuts, and seeds. You may notice that there aren't any animal products on this list. That's because fiber is found only in plant foods.

VITAMINS AND MINERALS

Vitamins and minerals are vital to life and are necessary for the completion of every function in the body. From aiding in digestion, to fighting toxins, to helping to produce red blood cells—each vitamin and mineral has important roles to play. Here is information about some of these nutrients and their functions:

Vitamins and Minerals*		
Vitamin/Mineral	**Plant Sources**	**Functions**
Vitamin A (fat-soluble)	Orange/yellow fruits and vegetables (carrots, pumpkins, yams, cantaloupes, mangoes) beet greens, spinach	Vision, skin health, reproductive health, immunity, cancer prevention, antioxidant
Vitamin D (fat-soluble)	Sun exposure/fortified non-dairy milks and cereals/some mushrooms	Bone and dental health; immunity; potential role in prevention of cancer, heart disease, diabetes, and multiple sclerosis
Vitamin E (fat-soluble)	Wheat germ, green leafy vegetables, whole grains, nuts, sunflower seeds	Immunity, antioxidant, heart disease and cancer prevention, lung health
Vitamin K (fat-soluble)	Green leafy vegetables, spinach, kale, cabbage, cauliflower, broccoli	Blood coagulation
Vitamin C (water-soluble)	Oranges, lemons, grapefruits, cantaloupes, kiwis, pineapples, strawberries, broccoli, peppers	Immunity, antioxidant, circulation, skin health, collagen formation
B vitamins (water-soluble): thiamine (B1), riboflavin (B2), niacin (B3), biotin, pantothenic acid, pyridoxine (B6)	Whole grains, beans/legumes, greens, nuts, seeds	Energy metabolism, enzyme activity, skin health, nerve function, immunity
Folate (folic acid)	Green leafy vegetables, beans/legumes, broccoli, Brussels sprouts, oranges, whole grains	DNA and red blood cell synthesis, prevents heart disease and neural tube defects
Vitamin B12 (needs folate to work properly)	Fortified non-dairy milks, fortified nutritional yeast (B12 is made by bacteria and is not naturally found in plant foods*)	Nerve function, energy metabolism, enzyme activity, red blood cell synthesis
Calcium	Green leafy vegetables (kale, collard greens, mustard greens, broccoli), sesame seeds, tofu, fortified non-dairy milks	Bone and dental health, nerve transmission, muscle contraction, blood coagulation, blood pressure control
Phosphorus	Beans/legumes, whole grains, nuts, seeds	Bone and dental health, collagen formation, energy production

Potassium (sodium, chlorine, and potassium are electrolytes)	Many fruits and vegetables, beans/legumes, green leafy vegetables, potatoes, bananas, avocados, cantaloupes, melons	Fluid balance, muscle and nerve function, blood pressure control, heart function
Magnesium	Brown rice, spinach, beans/legumes, green leafy vegetables, nuts, potatoes, sunflower seeds	Enzyme activity, nerve and muscle function, heart health
Iron	Beans/legumes, dark green vegetables, spinach, beets, prunes, raisins	Hemoglobin and myoglobin synthesis, helps carry oxygen in blood, prevents anemia
Zinc	Beans/legumes, nuts, seeds, whole grains	Cell growth, immunity, wound healing, taste
Selenium	Brazil nuts, sunflower seeds, whole grains, brown rice, mushrooms	Antioxidant, immunity, potential role in heart disease and cancer prevention

* *If you intend to eat a totally plant-based diet, void of any animal products, you should include a reliable source of vitamin B12 (through vitamin supplements or fortified foods).*

The best way to benefit from these powerful nutrients is to eat a diet largely consisting of whole, plant-based foods.

PHYTOCHEMICALS

For decades, nutritionists have promoted the consumption of fruits and vegetables primarily for their vitamin, mineral, and fiber content. In more recent years, researchers have discovered that, in addition to these nutrients, plants also contain thousands of powerful micronutrients called phytochemicals—essentially "phyto" (meaning "plant") chemicals. These disease-fighting compounds have many powerful functions.

PHYTOCHEMICALS PROTECT AGAINST

- Cancer[15]
- Heart disease[16]
- Diabetes[17]
- Infection[18]

Like the name suggests, phytochemicals are only found in plant foods. They provide color, flavor, and odor to plants and serve as part of their defense system against pests and the elements. When ingested, phytochemicals can have powerful effects on our defense systems as well.

Phytochemicals		
Name	**Plant Sources**	**Potential Benefits**
Lycopene	Tomatoes, strawberries, red fruits and berries	Antioxidant, inhibits cancer cell growth, reduces risk of prostate cancer, enhances cardiovascular health, decreases blood pressure
Lignans	Flax seed and sesame seeds	Reduces risk of heart disease by decreasing oxidative stress and inflammation, improves blood pressure and lipid levels, decreases cholesterol, reduces cancer cell growth and metastasis
Resveratrol	Red grape skins, red fruits and vegetables	Antioxidant, anti-inflammatory, anti-atherogenic, reduces heart disease risk, cancer protection, decreased oxidative stress, potential protection against complications of diabetes
Quercetin	Citrus fruits, green leafy vegetables	Antioxidant, anti-inflammatory effects, reduces oxidative stress
Anthocyanins	Blueberries, many red, purple, or blue fruits	Antioxidant, anti-inflammatory, cancer protection, heart disease protection, brain health, improves memory, improves insulin sensitivity
Curcumin	Turmeric, mustard	Antioxidant, anti-inflammatory, antibacterial, antiviral, antifungal, cancer protection
Cinnamaldehyde and hydroxychalcone (insulin mimetic)	Cinnamon	Antioxidant, antimicrobial properties, blood glucose lowering effects

These are just a few of thousands of different phytochemicals being studied for their health benefits. New discoveries are made each day. The secret to getting enough of these powerful nutrients is to eat a wide variety of colorful, plant-based foods.

POWERFUL CALORIC NUTRIENTS

Carbohydrates, proteins, and fats are the three macronutrients that supply the body with energy in the form of calories. These three nutrients can be found in all different types of foods. Because they come in both healthy and unhealthy forms, it's very important for diabetics (and everyone else!) to choose *healthy* carbs, proteins, and fats.

CARBOHYDRATES

Carbohydrates provide the most abundant and readily available source of energy. Every cell in the human body needs the glucose (sugar) that comes from carbohydrates. Most adults need about 130 grams of carbohydrate per day. Unfortunately, most American adults eat twice the amount of carbs they need. Carbohydrates aren't "bad," but they do need to be managed carefully. This is especially true for people who struggle with high blood sugars, excess weight, and high triglycerides.

Not all carbs are created equal. Many whole, plant-based foods are high in carbohydrates as well as in nutrients. When used in moderation and balanced with healthy proteins and fats, these high-carb foods are much better for diabetics to consume than low-carb, fatty animal products and processed foods.

HEALTHY CARBOHYDRATES

Carbohydrates are made up of sugars, starches, and fiber. Grains, vegetables, fruit, and milk (including starchy foods such as rice, potatoes, bread, pasta, and corn) all contain carbs. Whole, plant-based foods are the best sources of healthy carbohydrates because they retain more nutrients (vitamins, minerals, phytochemicals, and fiber). The larger starch molecules found in plant-based foods take longer to digest and the fiber helps to slow sugar absorption and stabilize blood sugars. It is best to eat carbs in their original, whole-plant form, such as fresh fruits and vegetables, legumes, barley, quinoa, oatmeal, and brown rice.

ARE CARBS FATTENING?

Many people avoid even healthy carbs, believing that they will cause weight gain. Although carbs should be managed carefully, they should not be avoided altogether. Fat is the most fattening type of food. One gram of fat contains 9 calories, while one gram of carbohydrate has only 4. This makes it easier to gain weight from fat than from carbs. Unrefined, plant-based carbs are filling and nutritious. Usually, the reason people gain weight is because they consume too many refined, concentrated carbs, often accompanied by grease and fat.

UNHEALTHY CARBOHYDRATES

The majority of carbohydrates most Americans eat today are refined grains (white bread, white pasta, and white rice) and foods high in refined sugar (sweetened beverages, snacks, and desserts). These refined carbohydrates have lost their fiber and most of their nutrients. They wreak havoc on blood sugars, cause inflammation, and rob the body of important nutrients it needs. Most refined carbs are not filling but leave you wanting more, making it very easy to overeat these foods. In the next chapter, we'll take a closer look at which carbs should be eaten and which should be avoided.

PROTEINS

Protein is necessary for growth and repair of cells and tissues, as well as for many other important functions. However, the average American consumes almost 100 grams of protein each day.[19] This is at least *twice* the amount needed.[20] Excess protein causes an increased burden on the liver and kidneys, potentially leading to disease.

Most of the protein people consume comes from animal sources. A common misconception is that it's necessary to consume animal products to get adequate protein. Research shows, however, that the best kind of protein is actually found in plants.[21] Plants provide not only adequate amounts of protein, but also are the safest sources of protein.

Animal protein is linked to higher rates of diabetes, heart and kidney disease, and many forms of cancer.[22] Animal foods contain higher proportions of protein, making it easier to consume excessive amounts of protein.

THE BARLEY MEN

In 2002, archaeologists uncovered a mass cemetery in Western Turkey that contained the remains of 68 gladiators.[23] In analyzing the chemical contents of the bones, forensic anthropologists discovered that these strong, fierce gladiators had all been vegan.[24]

This explains why historically, the gladiators were called *hordearii*, which is literally translated "Barley Men." These athletes knew that, in order to survive their gruesome competitions, they needed the best optimal fuel to make them strong. Not beef—but barley.[25] Modern research supports the fact that plants contain all the protein the gladiators needed, and all the protein that you need too.

Plant sources of protein include beans/legumes, tofu, nuts, seeds, and even whole grains and vegetables. Plant proteins are far superior to animal proteins. Here are some reasons why:

Animal Protein	Plant Protein
Concentrated, no fiber; danger of eating too much	Combined with carbohydrate and fiber—more filling, less danger of overconsumption
Contains cholesterol and saturated fat	No cholesterol, mainly unsaturated fats
Requires more vitamins and minerals to metabolize	Contains the vitamins and minerals needed to metabolize
Slower digestion, higher acid requirement	Easier digestion, lower acid requirement
No phytochemicals	Rich in phytochemicals
Associated with degenerative and animal-borne diseases	Associated with good health

Source: Mitchell, Clemency, Understanding Nutrition. (Lincolnshire, UK: Stanborough Press Limited, 2011), 30.

FATS

Healthy fats give flavor to food and help provide a feeling of fullness. Fats slow down the digestion of a meal, which helps stabilize blood sugar levels.[26] Fats also aid in the absorption of certain vitamins and minerals and supply essential fatty acids.

Fats are more calorically dense than carbs and protein. As stated earlier, a gram of fat contains 9 calories, compared to a gram of carbohydrate or protein, which contains 4. It's important to have enough—but not too much— healthy fat in your diet.

HEALTHY FATS

The healthiest fats are those found in whole, plant-based foods such as avocados, olives, nuts, seeds, and coconut. Avocados, olives, and many nuts are high in monounsaturated fat, which helps decrease your LDL (bad) cholesterol. It can even help increase your HDL (good) cholesterol, especially when taking the place of saturated fats from meat and dairy products.[27]

Healthy fats like omega-3 fats have also been praised for their cardiovascular benefits. Although omega-3's are found most abundantly in fish, plant sources include flax seeds, chia seeds, hemp seeds, and walnuts.

Coconut has received bad press due to its saturated fat content. However, it's actually a very healthy fat source. Not all saturated fats are created equal. The medium-chain saturated fatty acids found in coconut function very differently than the plaque-forming saturated fat found in animal products.

The best option for healthy fat intake is to eat various plants in their natural forms, as they still contain fiber and other valuable nutrients. If you choose to use oils, use them sparingly. Refined oils are high in calories and fat, but low in nutrients.

Make sure that you are also careful about the types of oils you use. For cooking or baking, extra virgin olive, coconut, flax seed, or hemp seed oils are some of the more stable choices. Be sure to purchase the first-pressed, extra virgin forms, as they are minimally processed and closer to the form found in the original plant.

For salad dressing, you can purchase an essential fatty acid (EFA) oil blend such as Vega's Antioxidant Omega Oil Blend from your local health food store. These dressings are good sources of essential omega-3 and omega-6 fatty acids. Always keep in mind that it's best to get your fats from whole plant foods rather than oils.

LOW FAT DIETS

While some lifestyle proponents promote extremely low fat diets with 10 percent or fewer calories from fat, in my experience that isn't necessarily optimal. Such diets may not be as effective for blood sugar control as diets that allow more moderate levels of healthy fats. In addition, some people find very low fat diets to be unpalatable and difficult to maintain. Historically, people in every culture have enjoyed the flavor-enhancing benefits of fat.

I encourage my patients to aim for a healthy fat intake of 15 to 25 percent of total calories. For a person eating a 1500 calorie diet, this would be approximately 8 to 14 grams of fat per meal. Ideally, this fat would come from whole, plant-food sources.

UNHEALTHY FATS

While healthy fats can be used judiciously, some fats should be completely avoided. These include:

Animal Fats

Saturated fats found in animal products such as meat, poultry, and dairy products stimulate the production of cholesterol[28] and triglycerides,[29] promote inflammation,[30] and significantly increase the risk of heart disease,[31] cancer,[32] and diabetes.[33] There is no need to include animal fats in the diet. In fact, they should be avoided as much as possible. Even meats like chicken and turkey that are considered to be "lean meats" are high in unhealthy fats.

Trans Fats and Hydrogenated Fats

Trans fats are not typically found in natural foods (trace amounts are found in meat and dairy products). They are formed when vegetable oils are chemically modified. Trans fats were first developed to replace foods high in unhealthy saturated fats (such as butter) with chemically altered vegetable fats (such as margarine). By adding hydrogen to unsaturated vegetable oils, companies were able to produce artificial, unsaturated versions of foods formerly found only in saturated forms. These trans fats also served as preservatives to increase the shelf life of food.

We now know that these artificial trans fats are every bit as unhealthy—and probably more unhealthy—than the saturated fats they were designed to replace.[34] Trans fats increase the risk of heart disease, diabetes, and cancer even more than do saturated fats.[35] Because of the extremely harmful effects of trans fats, California, New York City, Boston, and Baltimore have all banned their use in restaurants.[36]

Trans fats are also found in all kinds of processed foods, including baking mixes, frozen entrées and waffles, fast food, canned soup, cookies, chips, crackers, and many other common snack foods. Manufacturers are only required to report trans fats if their products contain more than 0.5 grams per serving.[37] This means that some foods that are labeled "trans fat free" actually aren't. That's why you need to read the ingredients. If you see hydrogenated or partially-hydrogenated vegetable oil listed on a product's ingredients, it contains trans fats. It should be completely avoided.

PUTTING IT ALL TOGETHER

In this chapter, we've learned about the powerful nutrients designed to give us optimal health. We've also examined the harmful foods that cause disease. I like to think of nutrition as a symphony. If you are conducting an orchestra, you want the best possible musicians and instruments. There's no room for off-key notes, broken strings, or anything else that jeopardizes the quality of the music. To create a musical masterpiece, you want only the best.

The same is true with nutrition. If you want to experience optimal health, you need the best possible nutrients. By eliminating unhealthy foods from your diet and replacing them with a wide assortment of delicious, health-promoting foods, you can create a nutritional masterpiece. In the next chapter, we'll look at practical ways to make this happen.

CHAPTER SUMMARY

- » Healthy food is powerful medicine.
- » A healthy diet is high in nutrients and low in empty calories.
- » Fiber, phytochemicals, vitamins, and minerals are powerful non-caloric nutrients.
- » Fiber is a powerful tool for weight loss and disease prevention.
- » Aim for 35 to 50 grams of fiber every day.
- » Fiber is only found in plant-based foods.
- » Vitamins and minerals are essential for all body functions.
- » Phytochemicals are powerful disease-fighting compounds found in plants.
- » Whole, plant-based foods are the best sources for all of these nutrients.
- » Carbohydrates, proteins, and fats provide calories or energy.
- » Healthy carbs include whole grains, legumes, fruits, and vegetables.
- » Unhealthy carbs include refined grains (white bread, pasta, rice, etc.) and refined sugar.
- » Adequate healthy protein is abundant in plant-based foods such as beans/legumes, tofu, quinoa, nuts, seeds, whole grains, and vegetables.
- » Animal protein increases risk for many diseases, including heart and kidney disease.
- » Plant-based foods such as olives, avocados, nuts, and seeds contain a variety of healthy fats.
- » Animal fats and trans/hydrogenated fats should be completely avoided.
- » Combining a variety of healthy foods creates a nutritional masterpiece.

—THIRTEEN—

Be a First-Class Foodie

Knowledge without action is futile.
—Abu Bakr

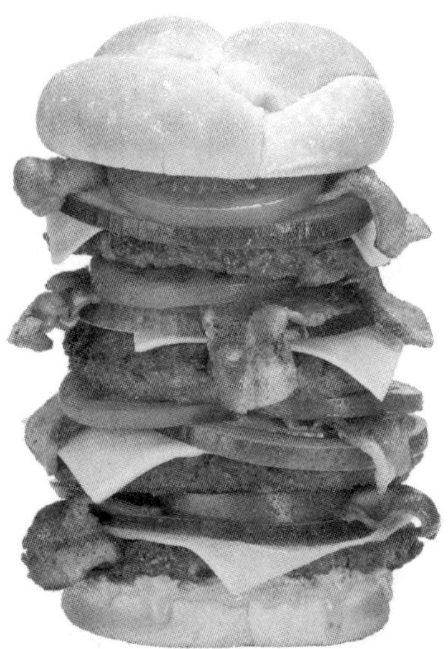

THE 9,982-CALORIE QUADRUPLE-BYPASS BURGER® contains 2 pounds of beef, 20 slices of bacon, 4 slices of cheese, and a pasty, lard-coated bun. It's often served with an unlimited side of Flatliner Fries® (deep fried in pure lard), and a Butterfat Shake® (2,000 calories).[1] These are just a few items on the menu at the Las Vegas-based Heart Attack Grill®—America's most controversial restaurant. The grill is famous for its artery-clogging, disease-promoting junk food.[2]

The grill's interior design replicates a hospital. The owner, Jon Basson, wears a lab coat and stethoscope. Claiming to be a "burgerologist," he is referred to as "Dr. Jon." The cooks dress as surgeons. The waitresses serve up fatty meals dressed as nurses. Customers (called "patients") are required to wear hospital gowns. Anyone who weighs over 350 pounds eats for free. The restaurant's motto? Taste Worth Dying For.®

The grill received considerable media attention after a male customer suffered a heart attack while eating a Triple-Bypass Burger.® Two months later a woman collapsed—unconscious after a Double-Bypass Burger® and margarita.[3]

When asked whether he feels any remorse for serving such an unhealthy menu, Jon Basson replied, "I run perhaps the only honest restaurant in America. We have been honest about exactly what we serve. 'Hey, this is bad for you, and it's gonna kill you.'"[4]

It's true that the Heart Attack Grill has put some effort into warning it's customers. There are signs on the doors that read: "Caution! This establishment is bad for your health," and "Cash only, because you might die before the check clears."[5]

Even though the Heart Attack Grill openly claims to serve unhealthy food, people continue to devour it. Customers are warned that the food causes disease, but are not motivated to avoid it. As a well-known quote says, "Knowledge without action is futile."

In the last chapter, we learned important information (knowledge) about nutrients our bodies need. This knowledge is valuable. However, it only becomes beneficial when put into practice. Unlike the patrons at the Heart Attack Grill, we want to use our knowledge to make informed, healthy choices. This chapter will help you establish an action plan to put your nutrition knowledge to work.

Eating a healthy, nutrient-dense diet is actually pretty simple. Foods can be split into three categories: first-class, second-class, and third-class. Your health is largely determined by which class of foods you primarily eat. The first step in the nutrition action plan is to start eating more first-class foods.

FIRST-CLASS FOODS

If you want first-class health, you need to eat first-class foods. First-class foods include vegetables, beans/legumes, fruits, unrefined whole grains, nuts and seeds. These plant-based foods are packed with powerful nutrients: fiber, antioxidants, phytochemicals, vitamins, and minerals. They also contain healthy carbohydrates, healthy proteins, and healthy fats.

Not only do first-class foods provide you with optimal energy and help you feel your best, but they also protect you against diabetes, heart disease, cancer, and a host of other diseases.[6, 7, 8, 9] I recommend that you eat at least 80 to 90 percent of your calories from first-class foods. Let's take a closer look at what these foods are, starting with those most dense in nutrients—green leafy vegetables.

FIRST-CLASS FOODS[10]		
Food	**Examples**	**Benefits**
Green Leafy Vegetables[11, 12]	Romaine lettuce, spinach, broccoli, kale, collards, turnip greens, mustard greens, cabbage, arugula, Swiss chard, bok choy	The most nutrient-dense of all plant foods, green leafy veggies are rich in dietary fiber, calcium, magnesium, minerals, vitamins, and other phytonutrients.
Green Vegetables	Green beans, asparagus, cucumbers, zucchini, green bell peppers, Brussels sprouts, artichokes, celery, sprouts	Green vegetables provide an abundant amount of phytonutrients for optimal health.
Colorful Vegetables	Carrots, tomatoes, purple cabbage, bell peppers, eggplant, squash, beets, cauliflower, onions, turnips, garlic, leeks	The colorful pigments of these vegetables are rich in special forms of flavonoids and antioxidants.
Beans/Legumes	Pinto beans, black beans, kidney beans, lentils, garbanzos/chick peas, lima beans, white beans, black-eyed peas, soybeans, fava beans, mung beans	Beans are rich in fiber, protein, carbohydrate, and other nutrients. Beans help control and stabilize blood sugars.
Starchy Vegetables	Sweet potatoes, yams, baked potatoes, corn, peas	Rich sources of carbohydrate, fiber, and other nutrients, these starchy vegetables need to be balanced with healthy proteins and fats.

FIRST-CLASS FOODS[10]		
Food	**Examples**	**Benefits**
Fresh Fruits	Apples, oranges, tangerines, grapefruits, pears, grapes, berries, bananas, melons, apricots, cherries, coconut, kiwis, lemons, limes, nectarines, peaches, plums, strawberries	Good sources of energy with fiber, natural antioxidants, and vitamins, these fruits need to be balanced with healthy proteins and fats.
Whole, Unrefined Grains	Barley, oatmeal, oat groats, quinoa, brown rice, wild rice, Kamut®, bulgur (cracked wheat), buckwheat, millet, amaranth, spelt	Whole grains provide fiber and other nutrients missing in refined carbohydrates. These starches need to be balanced with healthy proteins and fats.
Raw Nuts and Seeds	Walnuts, almonds, pecans, cashews, hazelnuts, macadamia nuts, pistachios, pine nuts, pumpkin seeds, sesame seeds, flax seeds, chia seeds, poppy seeds, sesame seeds, sunflower seeds, old-fashioned peanut butter, almond butter, sunflower butter	Nuts and seeds are good sources of heart-healthy fats, protein, and other nutrients. Because of their high fat content, they should be used moderately.
Whole-Food Fats	Whole olives, whole avocadoes, whole coconuts, nuts, seeds	Good sources of healthy fat and other nutrients, but high in calories. Should be used moderately.
First-Class Beverages: Water, Fresh Pressed Vegetable Juices	A wide variety of vegetables can be included in these juices. Minimal fruit can be added to enhance flavor without spiking blood sugars.	Water is your beverage of choice. Be sure to stay well-hydrated by drinking plenty of water throughout the day. Fresh pressed vegetable juices are high in nutrients and phytochemicals.

SECOND-CLASS FOODS

Second-class foods are not nearly as nutrient-rich as first-class foods. That's why I recommend that only a small percentage of calories come from these foods. Not all second-class foods are created equal. I have attempted to list them in order of decreasing nutritional value. Depending on your current health status and dietary preferences, you may want to avoid some second-class foods altogether.

SECOND-CLASS FOODS		
Food	**Example**	**Benefits/Dangers**
Processed Whole Grains	Whole wheat or whole grain bread or pasta (or other whole wheat flour products), whole grain cereal, couscous	These refined whole grain foods are healthier than foods made with white flour. However, they are still processed foods and generally spike blood sugars more than unrefined whole grains.
Processed Fruits or Vegetables (with added sugar, salt, or fat)	Applesauce, canned fruits with added sugar, dried fruits with added sugar, canned and salted vegetables	Processed fruits are not as healthy as fresh fruits and can raise blood sugars more dramatically. Processed vegetables lose many of their nutrients and can be high in sodium and fat.
Milk Alternatives	Soy milk, almond and other nut milks	These milk-replacement products are healthier alternatives to real milk. They can be used in cereal, smoothies, etc. Be sure to choose unsweetened varieties.
Meat Substitutes	Soy burgers, veggie burgers, soy hot dogs, textured vegetable protein	Imitation meats are lower in saturated fat and cholesterol than real meats. However, it's important to be selective and read the labels! These are processed foods and should be used moderately.
Organic, Fat-free Dairy and Free-range Eggs	Organic, fat-free milk, yogurt, and cottage cheese	These foods are lower in saturated fat and cholesterol than regular dairy products. Organic forms are safer to eat. However, dairy is not an optimal food for humans. If it's consumed, it should be on a limited basis. Free-range eggs are high in saturated fat and cholesterol, but are safer to eat than regular eggs. Using only egg whites removes the fat and cholesterol.
Cold-water Fish	Mackerel, trout, herring, water-packed tuna, and salmon	These fish are high in omega-3 fatty acids. However, many fish contain mercury and other dangerous toxins.[13] A better option is to take a DHA/EPA- rich, microalgae supplement or an omega-rich purified fish oil. Flax seeds and walnuts also contain some omega-3 fatty acids. Pregnant and lactating women are especially encouraged to limit fish intake.

SECOND-CLASS FOODS		
Food	**Example**	**Benefits/Dangers**
White Meat	Chicken and turkey	White meat contains less saturated fat than red meat, but it contains the same amount of cholesterol. If you choose to eat these meats, it's best to use organic products to avoid contamination associated with hormones, antibiotics, etc. [14]
Virgin Oils (use sparingly)	Extra virgin, cold-pressed olive oil, coconut oil, flax seed oil, hemp seed oil, EFA oil blends	It's best to get fats from whole plant sources such as olives, avocadoes, coconuts, nuts, and seeds. However, if you choose to use oil, use extra virgin, cold-pressed forms for baking, and try an essential oil blend for salad dressings.
Second-class Beverages: Fruit Juices	100% fruit juice	Fruit juice contains vitamins and minerals. However, even 100%, all-natural juice can spike blood sugars and contribute to weight gain. It's better to eat whole fruit than to drink fruit juice. Use juices sparingly and only on special occasions.

My personal goal is to primarily eat a balanced variety of first-class foods. I also incorporate into my diet some second-class foods, such as whole wheat bread and pasta, small amounts of virgin oils, non-dairy milks, meat substitutes, and egg whites. I avoid dairy as much as possible. I do not eat fish or meat. My diet isn't perfect, but I strive to make healthy choices. However, I recognize that different people have different dietary habits. My goal is not to make you eat exactly like I do, but to encourage you to move toward optimal health.

If you are regularly eating third-class foods, such as processed or red meats, it would be a step in the right direction to switch to second-class organic chicken and only have it a few times a week, combined with first-class foods. While I personally believe that moving toward a whole-food, total vegetarian diet is the best option for preventing and reversing disease, I understand that not everyone will choose to completely avoid meat and animal products. If you fall into this category, I want to give you healthier options that work for you.

If you're a vegetarian (you don't eat meat, fish, or poultry) or vegan (you don't eat meat, fish, poultry, dairy, or eggs), then the animal products listed in second-class foods obviously aren't the best choices for you. You will benefit greatly from focusing primarily on first-class foods, eating vegetarian second-class foods sparingly, and avoiding vegetarian third-class foods such as refined grains and sweets. Remember, while a vegetarian diet can be extremely healthy and beneficial, there are many unhealthy foods (and unhealthy people) that are vegetarian. Dr. Joel Fuhrman encourages his patients to be "nutritarians" by eating a nutrient-rich diet.[15] If you're a vegetarian, make sure you're a nutritarian too!

THIRD-CLASS FOODS

There's no getting around it—third-class foods are simply bad for your health. These foods have been shown to promote inflammation, raise triglycerides and cholesterol, increase insulin resistance, and significantly raise your risk for disease. Ideally, these foods should be completely avoided, but if included in your diet, it should be on a *very* limited basis.

THIRD-CLASS/NUTRIENT-BARREN FOODS		
Food	**Example**	**Dangers**
Refined Grains	White breads (or any bread that doesn't say "100% whole grain"), white flour, white rice, white pasta, etc.	Refined grains promote inflammation,[16] raise triglycerides, and spike blood sugars.[17] They are also low in nutrients.
Refined Sweets	Cakes, pies, pastries, cookies, candy, sodas, artificially-sweetened candy and desserts	Refined sweets have an even worse impact on inflammation, triglycerides, and blood sugars than refined grains alone. Most artificially sweetened foods contain damaging, disease-promoting chemicals.
Cheese/Dairy	Cheese, yogurt, cottage cheese, sour cream	These foods are full of saturated fat and cholesterol.
Regular Oils	Non-virgin vegetable oils, shortening, lard	Major sources of empty calories. Lard and shortening contain high amounts of either saturated or hydrogenated fat.

THIRD-CLASS/NUTRIENT-BARREN FOODS		
Food	**Example**	**Dangers**
Processed, Packaged Foods	Margarines, baking mixes, frozen entrees and waffles, fast food, canned soup, potato chips, cookies, microwave popcorn, and many other snack foods.	Besides the high sodium, fat, and sugar often found in these products, they can also be a source of trans fat. These harmful fats increase the risk of heart disease, diabetes, and cancer even more than saturated fats. Read the ingredients and avoid products that contain hydrogenated or partially hydrogenated oils.
Deep-fried Foods, Fast Food, and Restaurant Fried Foods	French fries, onion rings, chicken nuggets, fried chicken, fried fish, egg rolls, samosas	These foods are notorious for their high fat, sugar, and sodium content. Deep-fried animal products are also laden with saturated fat and cholesterol.
Red Meat	Beef, lamb, pork, veal	Very high in saturated fat and cholesterol. Known to significantly increase risk of diabetes, heart disease, cancer, and other diseases.[18, 19]
Processed Meats	Hot dogs, hamburgers, salami, sausage, SPAM®, jerky, ground beef	Processed meats are even worse than red meats. They dramatically increase risk of many diseases, including diabetes, cancer, and heart disease.[20]
Third-class Beverages: Sodas, Natural and Artificially Sweetened Beverages, and Caffeinated Beverages	Sodas, fruit drinks, sports drinks, energy drinks, coffee, caffeinated tea, artificially sweetened beverages	These beverages are loaded with sugar and calories, but depleted in nutrients. Avoid these over-stimulating beverages. Low- or zero-calorie, artificially-sweetened beverages contain unhealthy chemicals and should be completely avoided.

QUALITY AND QUANTITY

You now have a basic understanding of what an optimal diet consists of. You know what nutrients your body needs and what foods contain those nutrients. You also know which harmful foods should be avoided. In essence, you have learned about the *quality* of foods. First-class foods are the best, and third-class foods are the worst. Choosing high-quality first-class foods will start you on your path to better health. In addition to choosing the best *quality* of food, however, you also need to eat the right *quantity* of food. This is where meal balancing comes in.

MEAL BALANCING

I used to believe that, as long as a diabetic ate first-class foods, his or her blood sugar levels would remain stable. In the early years of my wellness classes, I encouraged patients to eat a wide variety of first-class foods of any type—assuring them that their sugars would be okay. It didn't take long to figure out that just wasn't true. Unless first-class foods are properly balanced in the right proportions, blood sugar levels will remain high.

In all aspects of health, but especially when it comes to blood sugar management, it's crucial to pay attention to the amounts of different foods eaten and to the way that those foods are combined.

Imagine that you are trying to make a loaf of bread for dinner guests. The recipe calls for the following ingredients:

3 cups whole wheat flour

1 cup water

2 tablespoons olive oil

1 teaspoon salt

2 tablespoons active dry yeast

You collect your ingredients and you realize you only have one cup of flour. You're in a hurry, so you decide to add two extra cups of salt to substitute for the missing flour. How will your bread turn out? Will you want to serve it to your guests?

The obvious answer is no. The bread would taste terrible and wouldn't be fit to eat. Why? Because you didn't have the right ingredients? No, you had all the ingredients on the list. But you didn't have the right amount of each of those ingredients. To successfully follow a recipe, you need to have both the *right ingredients* and the *right amounts*.

It's the same when it comes to health. A recipe for optimal health requires that you eat both the right quality of foods and the right quantity of those foods. This is what meal balancing is all about. To balance your meals, you need to consume the right amounts of healthy proteins, healthy carbohydrates, and healthy fats that come from first-class foods. The key here is that all three nutrients should be present at each meal.

THREE MEALS A DAY

I encourage my patients to eat three meals a day, including a light supper early in the evening. I find this especially helpful for people who are trying to lose weight or improve sleep. I also advise patients to avoid snacking and to follow a consistent mealtime schedule. These suggestions are discussed further in Chapter 14.

BALANCING HEALTHY PROTEINS

Every meal should include a source of healthy protein. When healthy proteins are added to carbohydrate-rich foods, they help slow sugar absorption and balance blood sugar levels. First-class, protein-rich foods such as beans, lentils, nuts and seeds should be added to meals containing carbohydrates. Second-class protein foods, such as meat substitutes, eggs, dairy, and white meats do not control blood sugars nearly as well as first-class protein foods, even though they have similar amounts of protein. Many of my patients have found that eating beans or lentils with a meal helps to control blood sugars—not just for that meal but for up to the next three meals. Aim for two servings of healthy protein per meal, or a total of six servings per day (more about serving sizes later).

BALANCING HEALTHY CARBOHYDRATES

Every meal should include healthy carbs. Carbohydrate-rich foods like whole grains, starchy vegetables, and fruits contain a variety of powerful nutrients. However, carbohydrates are made up of glucose (sugar) molecules that can very easily affect blood sugars. Not all carbs are created equal. First-class carbs are better for blood sugars than second-class carbs, which are better than third-class carbs. Because there are so many types of carb foods, it is often a challenge for people to control carb portions, and, in turn, to control blood sugars. Carbohydrate foods include:

- Grains (rice, bread, pasta, noodles, cereal, etc.)
- Starchy vegetables (potatoes, sweet potatoes, corn, etc.)

- Fruit
- Sugars (white sugar, cakes, cookies, candy, sodas, etc.)
- Non-starchy vegetables (these are in a special category, which we'll discuss later)
- Legumes (beans, peas, and lentils)

Several methods are available to help you keep track of your carbohydrate intake. One of the most common methods is carb counting. This involves counting the number of carbohydrate servings consumed in each meal and limiting them to healthy amounts that will help you control your weight and blood sugar levels.

CARB COUNTING

Because not all carbs are created equal, they aren't all counted the same. Some foods that contain carbohydrates should be counted, while other don't need to be. I recommend keeping track of:

1. Your starchy carbohydrate intake
2. Your fruit intake

COUNTING STARCHY CARBS

Depending on your current health status, I recommend eating one to three servings of starchy carbohydrates per meal. These foods include grains and starchy vegetables.

One serving of carbohydrate = 15 grams of carbohydrate

This equates to 15 to 45 grams (or 1 to 3 servings) of starchy carbohydrates per meal.

Here are examples of one serving of starchy carbohydrates:

- 1 slice whole wheat bread
- 1/2 cup oatmeal
- 1/3 cup rice or pasta
- 1 six-inch tortilla
- 1/4 baked potato (3 ounces)
- 1/2 cup corn, sweet potatoes, winter squash, or mashed or boiled potatoes

If you are diabetic or prediabetic, overweight, or struggling with high triglycerides, the lower end of this 1 to 3 serving range is ideal for you. Cutting out excess starchy carbs will help you lose weight and lower your blood sugars and triglycerides. Be sure to check your blood sugar levels frequently to monitor how carbohydrates affect you. If your after-meal sugar levels are spiking after eating 3 servings per meal, you need to cut back. The amount of carbs you can handle may increase somewhat once your health has stabilized.

Remember that the whole, unrefined grains mentioned in the first-class foods section (oatmeal, barley, quinoa, wild rice, etc.) are better for blood sugar control than second-class processed whole grains (processed brown rice, whole grain bread or pasta, and other whole wheat flour products). Third-class refined grains (white rice, white bread, white pasta, etc.) and refined sweets (cookies, pastries, etc.) are the worst for blood sugar control. These carbs should be greatly minimized or avoided completely.

COUNTING FRUIT

In addition to starchy carbs, you also need to count your fruit intake. I recommend eating 3 to 5 servings of fruit per day (roughly 1 to 2 servings per meal).

Examples of single servings of fruit (15 grams of carbs per serving):

1 small fresh fruit (4 ounces)
½ cup canned fruit (in its own juice)
¼ cup dried fruit (2 tablespoons)
17 small grapes (3 ounces)
1 cup melon or berries

If you eat half a cup of oatmeal with apple slices for breakfast, this would equate to one serving of starchy carb and one serving of fruit. For another starchy carb serving, you could add a slice of whole wheat toast. To add healthy protein to your meal, you could spread peanut butter on your toast.

Remember, there are many carbohydrate foods. Servings add up quickly. Anytime you eat starches, grain products, fruits, sweetened beverages, sweets, or desserts, they all need to be counted towards your carbohydrate limits. Individual needs vary, depending on caloric needs and blood sugar control. Some people may need to stay in the lower end of these ranges, while others may stay closer to the higher end. Those who are more metabolically active may be able to exceed these recommended limits. It's crucial to monitor your blood sugars to determine how different amounts of various carbs affect you.

CARBS THAT DON'T COUNT (THE SAME WAY)

Beans and legumes are high in carbohydrates. However, they also are high in fiber and protein, and have a remarkable ability to help stabilize blood sugars. For this reason, their carbohydrate content doesn't have to be included in the usual carbohydrate count. Beans and legumes only need to be counted as protein servings. Beans and legumes that contain added sugar (such as baked beans) are an exception to this rule.

Non-starchy vegetables are high in fiber and low in carbohydrates. These veggies don't need to be counted, but can be eaten liberally. Try to eat at least six servings of non-starchy veggies a day. If you're still hungry at the end of your meal, you can reach for more veggies—like kale, broccoli, greens, cabbage, cauliflower, cucumbers, or tomatoes. The list goes on and on! I encourage you to maximize your non-starchy vegetable intake as much as possible.

BALANCING HEALTHY FATS

Healthy fats slow digestion, which slows the release of sugar into the bloodstream. The healthy fats contained in olives, avocados, nuts, and seeds should be combined with healthy carbohydrates and proteins for optimal blood sugar control. Aim for 15 to 25 percent of your total calories from fat. This amount varies by individual, but a person on a 1,500-calorie diet would consume approximately 25 to 42 grams of fat per day, or 8 to 14 grams of fat per meal. In the breakfast example above, you might add almonds or ground flax seed to your oatmeal.

FIBER—THE SECRET WEAPON

Fiber is key to blood sugar control. As we learned in the last chapter, the fiber contained in plant foods helps naturally slow the absorption of sugar into the bloodstream. Your goal should be to eat at least 35 to 50 grams of fiber every day. Healthy proteins like beans and legumes, healthy carbs like whole grains and fruit, and healthy fats like nuts and seeds all contain this secret weapon. That's why choosing first-class foods is an important strategy for blood sugar control.

The table below gives you a basic idea of how to balance your meals. You can also learn more by reviewing the "Food Lists" appendix at the back of the book.

A DAY IN THE LIFE OF A FIRST-CLASS FOODIE

Food	Servings Per Day/Meal	Serving Size
Non-Starchy Vegetables (including green leafy and colored non-starchy vegetables)	6 or more servings (usually split between lunch and dinner)	1 cup raw or 1/2 cup cooked or chopped
Healthy Carbohydrates (whole-grain starches, starchy vegetables, fruits)	1–3 servings per meal (15–45 grams of carbohydrate). Carbohydrate needs can vary and may be increased for people who are more metabolically active.	1 serving = 15 grams of carbohydrate 1 slice whole-grain bread 1/2 cup cooked whole-grain cereal 1/2 cup corn, squash, or potato 1/3 cup brown rice
Healthy Carbohydrates (fruit)	1–2 servings per meal (3–5 servings per day.)	1 piece small fruit (apple, orange, pear, etc.), 1/2 banana, or 1/2 cup chopped fruit
Healthy Proteins	2 servings per meal (6 servings per day)	1 serving = 7 grams protein 1/2 cup beans or lentils 1 ounce nuts or 2 tablespoons nut butter 1/2 cup (4 ounces) tofu
Healthy Fats	No more than 15–25% of your total calories should come from fat. 2–3 servings per meal (25–42 grams per day on 1,500 calories) 3–4 servings per meal (33–55 grams per day on 2,000 calories)	1 serving = 5 grams fat 1/8 large avocado, 1 teaspoon oil, 7 large olives, 1/4 ounce nuts, 2 teaspoons old-fashioned peanut or almond butter, 1 teaspoon extra virgin oil.

THE PLATE METHOD

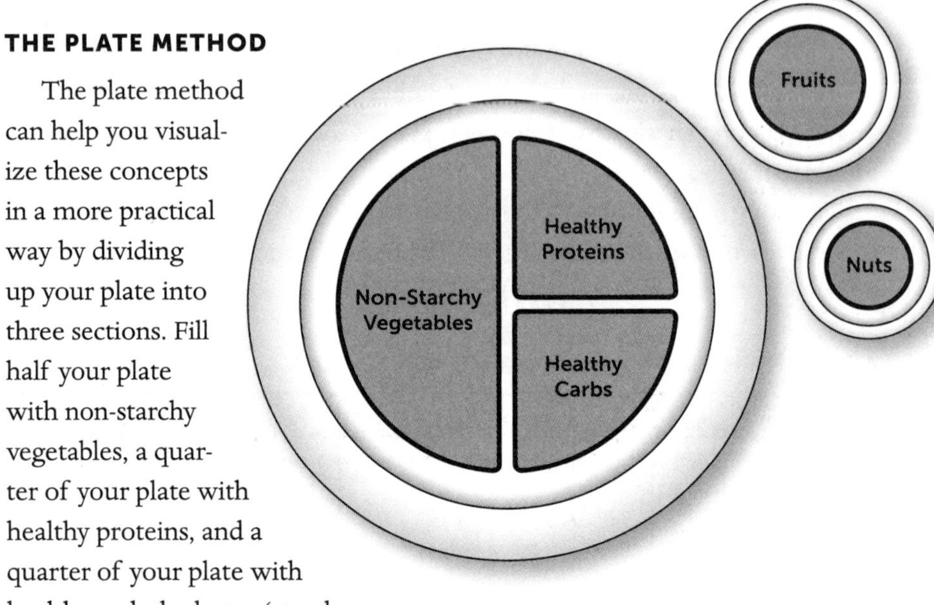

The plate method can help you visualize these concepts in a more practical way by dividing up your plate into three sections. Fill half your plate with non-starchy vegetables, a quarter of your plate with healthy proteins, and a quarter of your plate with healthy carbohydrates (starches and/or whole grain carbohydrates). Fruit, also a carbohydrate, can be reserved as a healthy dessert option. Healthy fats and nuts can be incorporated to any part of your plate as appropriate. The illustration above shows the plate method in practice.

GLYCEMIC INDEX AND GLYCEMIC LOAD

If you're choosing first-class foods and controlling portion sizes, but still struggling with high blood sugar levels, there are other tools available to help. You will benefit from using the glycemic index and glycemic load for further fine-tuning.

Glycemic Index

The glycemic index (GI) is a tool designed to measure how quickly your blood sugar will rise after eating a particular type of food. Foods are classified on a scale from 0 to 100.

The GI of each food is measured by feeding a human subject 50 grams of carbohydrate from a particular food. For example, 50 grams of the carbohydrate glucose has a GI of 100—the highest level. The GI of black beans (which is 30) is measured by feeding someone enough beans to equal 50 grams of carbohydrate (almost a cup-and-a-half of beans). Their blood sugar is then monitored for two hours after the meal.

Every food is numbered based on how it compares to pure glucose, which raises blood sugars the most rapidly of any food (to a GI of 100.) The higher the GI value, the more rapidly a particular type of food raises blood sugar levels.

A GI of 70 or more is considered high, a GI of 56 to 69 is medium, and a GI of 55 or less is considered low. Foods with high GI values typically cause quick rises in blood sugar, which lead to poor blood sugar control. Foods with low GI values typically release sugar into the blood slowly, which helps with blood sugar control. Fruit, pasta, breads, breakfast cereals, and snack products have both high and low GI foods. Not surprisingly, beans and legumes have a low GI.

The GI system isn't foolproof. Some high-fat dessert items (like chocolate cake) have a low GI, but that doesn't mean that they are healthy. The high fat content in these foods delays blood sugar absorption. However, these foods still drive the metabolic mess that causes diabetes. The GI table should always be used in conjunction with the first-class food table.

Glycemic Load

Another limitation of the Glycemic Index is that it doesn't take into account actual serving sizes typically consumed. The system assumes that a person will eat 50 grams of carbohydrate from any given food. In reality, consumption varies considerably.

For example, watermelon has a high GI of 72. This would indicate that watermelon is bad for blood sugars. However, how much watermelon would a person have to eat to consume 50 grams of carbohydrate? Approximately half a watermelon! That is unlikely to happen. The GI system fails to account for the amounts of food people actually eat.

For this reason, a new classification system called the Glycemic Load has been developed. The Glycemic Load (GL) takes serving sizes into account to give a more complete picture of how various foods affect blood sugars. The GL is calculated by multiplying the Glycemic Index by the number of carbohydrate grams in the actual serving, then dividing this number by 100. For one serving of food, a GL of 20 or higher is considered high, a GL of 11 to 19 is considered medium, and a GL of 10 or less is considered low.

Now back to our watermelon example. Watermelon has a high GI of 72 but a low GL of 4. In this case the GL is a more accurate predictor than the GI. However, the GI can still be a useful tool for comparing different foods, as well as for calculating the GL.

Numerous charts are available online that contain the Glycemic Index and Glycemic Load values for various types of foods. You can easily find this information by doing a Google search. I encourage you to pay attention to these values and to replace high GL foods with first-class foods that have low GL values. Keep in mind that these values use averages tested on other people and may vary somewhat among individuals.

Check your blood sugar levels regularly to see how various foods affect you personally. Use a table like the sample below to track your blood sugar levels before and after you eat. Evaluate your results by comparing your blood sugars to the guidelines outlined in Chapter 8.

Blood Sugar Levels			
	Breakfast	Lunch	Supper
Pre-meal			
One Hour After			
Two Hours After			

PUTTING IT ALL TOGETHER

You now have several tools available to help you achieve optimal nutrition. First, choose first-class, nutrient-dense foods. Second, balance healthy carbs, proteins, and fats in appropriate portions and serving sizes. Third, use the plate method to fill your plate. And finally, use the Glycemic Index and Glycemic Load systems to fine-tune your choices for optimal blood sugar control.

ADDITIONAL RESOURCES

Becoming a first-class foodie may seem overwhelming at first, but there are many excellent resources available. Here are just a few:

I highly recommend *Defeating Diabetes*, an excellent book by registered dietitian Brenda Davis.[21] This book contains a wealth of nutritional information for diabetics, as well as a collection of first-class recipes.

Another great resource is *Eat to Live*, by Joel Fuhrman, MD.[22] This *New York Times* bestseller explains the importance of quality nutrition for disease reversal.

I enjoy co-hosting the *Naturally Gourmet* television cooking show series with Karen Houghton, RN, author of the *Naturally Gourmet* cookbook.[23] Although not specifically designed for diabetics, Karen's cookbook contains a variety of delicious plant-based recipes. My wife, Betsy, enjoys using this cookbook for holidays and special events.

Regardless of what nutritional resources you use, you can apply the principles outlined in this chapter to control your blood sugar levels and optimize your health.

CHAPTER SUMMARY

- Nutrition information is only valuable when put into practice.
- If you want first-class health, you need to eat first-class foods.
- First-class foods include vegetables, legumes, fruits, unrefined whole grains, nuts, and seeds.
- Second-class foods are not nearly as nutritious as first-class foods and should be limited.
- Third-class foods promote disease and should be limited or eliminated as much as possible.
- You can become a first-class foodie!
- It's important to balance healthy carbohydrates, healthy proteins, and healthy fats.
- Carb counting, the plate method, Glycemic Index, and Glycemic Load systems can all be used to help you monitor your carbohydrate intake.
- Remember to monitor your blood sugar levels frequently.

—FOURTEEN—

Optimize Digestion

When I prayed for success, I forgot to ask for sound sleep and good digestion.
—Mason Cooley

I WAS REQUIRED TO READ *THE GLASS MENAGERIE*[1] FOR a literature class my freshman year of college. This classic play tells the story of a low income family in Saint Louis—struggling to survive the Great Depression.

Tom, the main character, works at a shoe factory to support his mother and disabled sister. Tom's father abandoned the family years before. Life is challenging, and Tom has to put up with Amanda, his overbearing and controlling mother. In one scene, Tom arrives home after a long day of work, and the family sits down at the table for dinner. Tom is very hungry and quickly begins devouring his food—using his hand to push the food onto his fork. His mother is horrified by his behavior and attempts to intervene:

> **AMANDA:** Honey, don't push with your fingers. If you have to push with something, the thing to push with is a crust of bread. And chew! Chew! Animals have sections in their stomachs which enable them to digest food without mastication, [chewing] but human beings are supposed to chew their food before they swallow it down. Eat food

leisurely, son, and really enjoy it. A well-cooked meal has lots of delicate flavours that have to be held in the mouth for appreciation. So chew your food and give your salivary glands a chance to function!

[Tom deliberately lays his imaginary fork down and pushes his chair back from the table.]

TOM: I haven't enjoyed one bite of this dinner because of your constant directions on how to eat it. It's you that makes me rush through meals with your hawk-like attention to every bite I take. Sickening—spoils my appetite—all this discussion of—animals—secretion—salivary glands—mastication!

It's been over 30 years since my freshman literature class, but I still remember my first impression of that particular scene of the play. Because I was already interested in health and digestion, I knew that Tom's mother was actually giving him good advice. However, I felt sorry for Tom. He was so frustrated with his mom's constant nagging that he didn't want to listen to anything she said!

In this chapter, we will look at some simple, yet powerful strategies for optimizing digestive health. One of those strategies is exactly what Tom's mother shared—the importance of chewing thoroughly. But there are also many simple things you can do to improve your digestion.

DOES IT REALLY MATTER?

Why is digestion important? If you're like most people (including Tom), you probably haven't given it a second thought. As long as you're eating nutritious food, your body can worry about what to do with it, right?

You may be surprised to discover that it's actually critically important for you to pay attention to your digestion. When it comes to optimizing health and preventing disease, digestion is arguably one of the most overlooked and underemphasized topics.

Diabetes. Cancer. Heart Disease. Arthritis. Fibromyalgia. These diseases and many others are often exacerbated, or even caused, by digestive problems.

I see patients with a wide variety of health conditions and concerns. Regardless of the diagnosis, I always make sure to address each patient's digestive health early on in the treatment plan. Digestion impacts every aspect of health. In my experience, the majority of people experiencing health problems can greatly benefit from making simple changes to improve digestion.

In the past few chapters, we've talked about the importance of choosing nutrient-dense, first-class foods. In addition to eating adequate nutrients, we need to make sure that our bodies are optimally absorbing these nutrients. Proper digestion is a fundamental part of the body's ability to heal from any condition, including diabetes.

Here's one example: magnesium is an important mineral found in plant-based foods. This nutrient plays many critical roles. One function is to reduce cholesterol and plaque build-up in the arteries. Multiple studies have shown that people who have low magnesium levels are much more likely to develop arterial plaque.[2] Having adequate amounts of magnesium in the blood helps to prevent high blood pressure,[3] heart disease,[4] and all diabetes-related complications.[5] (You'll learn more about magnesium in Chapter 20.)

However, just because you eat magnesium-rich foods doesn't mean you are necessarily absorbing *all* of the magnesium. If you have digestive problems, your ability to effectively use magnesium—and many other important nutrients—may be impaired.

The good news is that there are easy strategies you can implement to improve and optimize your digestive health. These strategies apply to everyone. Whether you have a known digestion problem, or whether you've never given digestion a second thought, you can greatly benefit from putting these into practice.

Let's begin by taking an imaginary tour through the digestive journey. We'll start where it all begins—the mouth.

DIGESTION STRATEGY #1: CHEW YOUR FOOD.

The table is set. Dinner is served. You've filled your plate with first-class foods. You sink your fork into your non-starchy vegetables and place them in your mouth. Now it's time to chew. If you're in a hurry, you may be tempted to wolf down your food. However, it's very important that you take the time to chew your food properly. This is the first phase of digestion.

Your saliva contains the digestive enzyme called "amylase." Amylase breaks down carbohydrates and starches into a digestible form. This enzyme is first produced in the mouth. As you chew your food thoroughly, your mouth continues to release salivary amylase. This enzyme mixes well with the carbohydrates that you eat. It makes it easier for the stomach to further process the food before sending it to the small intestine.

If you've ever made a loaf of bread by hand, you know the importance of kneading. Unless bread is properly and patiently kneaded and the yeast is given time to leaven (raise) the bread, the bread won't turn out the way it should. If you go through the above steps but rush them, it won't work very well. The yeast takes time to activate. In the same way, the enzymes in your saliva need enough time to thoroughly mix with your food to optimize digestion.

When you take a bite of food, make sure you chew it thoroughly and let it remain in your mouth long enough to mix with your saliva. Not only does this aid digestion, but it also helps you enjoy your food more and feel satisfied sooner. (Just ask Tom's mother!)

Foods containing protein and fat also need to be thoroughly chewed. Pepsin is a digestive enzyme released by the stomach to break down protein. Lipase is the primary enzyme that breaks down fat. The more thoroughly you chew, the easier it is for these enzymes to accomplish their task.

One of the many benefits of eating plant-based, first-class foods is that they naturally require more chewing than processed foods. This explains why many of my patients experience dramatic improvements in their digestion just by eating more vegetables and other plant foods.

What is the best way to start chewing thoroughly? While some guidelines recommend that each bite be chewed a certain number of times, I don't give a specific number to my patients. Counting bites can be tedious. The best way to chew properly is to set aside enough time for a meal and to slowly and mindfully chew, taste, savor, and enjoy your food. Try to get the most taste and enjoyment you can out of every single bite!

DIGESTION STRATEGY #2: UNDERSTAND YOUR ACID.

It is important to have a proper understanding of your stomach acid and how it works. If you are part of the 25 to 35 percent of Americans who suffer from heartburn or acid reflux,[6] this information can be especially helpful. Even if you aren't suffering with these problems, learning about the acidity of the stomach will help other digestive strategies make more sense.

You've probably seen TV commercials for antacids like Tums® and Rolaids®, as well as acid blockers such as Nexium® and Prevacid®. These drugs minimize discomfort associated with heartburn and acid reflux by decreasing acidity in the stomach.

Heartburn and acid reflux occur when the acidic stomach contents splash up or reflux into the esophagus, causing a sharp, burning sensation. Over time, the acid can erode and damage the esophageal lining, causing severe pain and ulcers, and increasing the risk of esophageal cancer. This explains why medications that reduce stomach acidity are so popular.

The idea that stomach acid is a bad thing is not supported by science, however. It's actually just a popular myth. The stomach is designed to be extremely acidic. The hydrochloric acid that the stomach produces has many important functions.[7] It activates pepsin, which is the enzyme necessary for protein digestion. It aids in the absorption of vitamins and minerals. Hydrochloric acid also serves as a protective barrier, killing harmful bacteria and microorganisms found in food.

While many believe that heartburn and acid reflux are caused by too much hydrochloric acid in the stomach, most people with these conditions actually don't have *enough* hydrochloric acid.[8] This may seem illogical, but allow me to explain.

Consider a person with *hypochlorhydria* (low hydrochloric acid in the stomach) who has just eaten a meal. The food is now in the stomach. Normally, hydrochloric acid would help break the food into smaller pieces, and would also activate pepsin to begin digesting the protein. This would help the meal digest properly and pass from the stomach into the small intestine.

However, because not enough stomach acid is present, this process is impaired and slowed. The food remains in the stomach where the carbohydrates ferment and the proteins putrefy (rot) producing gassy acids. Unlike hydrochloric acid, gassy acids are not good for you. Often the pressure, bloating, and pain associated with acid reflux actually are caused by the buildup of fermented foods and gassy acids. Most of the time, adequate levels of hydrochloric acid prevent these problems from occurring.[9]

Medications that lower the acidity of the stomach may provide temporary pain relief, but they have drawbacks. Not only do they fail to address the underlying cause of the problem, but they also come with dangerous side effects. Because low acid levels cause malabsorption of nutrients and decreased immune protection, they are associated with a significant increase in fractures, osteoporosis, Alzheimer's, bacterial and fungal infections, chronic diarrhea, and other digestive issues.[10] Because malabsorption of nutrients contributes to many diseases, I believe further studies will show that these drugs have even more adverse effects than we now realize.

Because of the adverse effects of these drugs, the instructions for proton-pump inhibitors (acid blockers) clearly state that they should only be used for two weeks at a time and no more than three times per year.[11] These instructions are often ignored by both patients and physicians, however. Many people take proton pump inhibitors habitually. Because these drugs don't address the underlying cause of the problem, symptoms reappear as soon as the drugs are discontinued, and patients turn to the drug again for temporary relief. (If you are taking acid blockers but would like to get off of these drugs, the guidelines at the end of this chapter can help.)

If it's not a good idea to take these drugs, how can heartburn and acid reflux be resolved? The good news is that the simple digestive strategies discussed in this chapter will not only help improve digestion in general, but they also will help people with heartburn and acid reflux to naturally recover from these conditions.

DIGESTION STRATEGY #3: KEEP HYDRATED, BUT DON'T DROWN YOUR MEALS!

You may be used to washing down your meals with water, juice, and other beverages. While it is important to stay well hydrated, it is my personal belief that drinking a large amount of fluid with your meals can impair digestion.[12] I have experienced this first hand, and have observed it among my patients.

This should make sense when you understand the importance of stomach acid and digestive enzymes. If you drink a lot of fluid with your meals, it dilutes the acid and enzymes needed for digestion. Your stomach has to work longer and harder to do its job.[13]

While the stomach does need some fluid in the mix, it can actually extract this fluid from the blood plasma. If you stay well hydrated in between your meals, your stomach can "decide" how much fluid it needs, and you won't need to drink with your meals.

However, if you come to a meal already thirsty and dehydrated, it's better to drink with the meal and avoid further dehydration than not to drink with that meal for digestive reasons. The key is to plan ahead and stay well hydrated throughout the day.

STAYING HYDRATED

- Drink 1-2 cups of warm water when you first wake up. (This will help to wake up your body and cleanse your digestive tract.)
- Hydrate between meals. Drink 2 cups of water midmorning and midafternoon.
- Drink water between dinner and bedtime, but not enough to keep you up all night!
- Stop drinking water 20-30 minutes before your meal.
- Wait 90 minutes after your meal to drink again.

You may not need to completely give up drinking fluids with your meal. Drinking a small amount of fluid with a meal will not have nearly as negative an impact as drinking several cups.

Temperature is also an important consideration.[14] If you choose to take liquids with your meals, a small amount of warm tea, water, or broth actually helps to stimulate digestion. Because the inside of your stomach is warm, when you drink ice water or cold beverages, your stomach has to work extra hard to warm it up and absorb it before continuing the digestive process.

DIGESTION STRATEGY #4: GO FOR A WALK.

After you consume a good, healthy-sized meal, your stomach goes to work to churn, mix, and break down the foods you've eaten. Your circulatory system sends extra blood to your digestive organs to enhance the process.

Because blood is congregating in your digestive organs, less blood is flowing to your brain and muscles. This can leave you feeling sluggish and tired after a meal, or not able to concentrate as well as you would like.

Some people respond by taking a nap. However, this slows digestion and allows blood sugars to spike. The best thing to do after a meal is to take a walk.

If you engage in light to moderate exercise right after eating, blood is drawn back out of your digestive organs to circulate more fully to your muscles and brain. It carries with it those nutrients that have already been absorbed into your bloodstream. This improves digestion, minimizes bloating and gassiness, boosts your energy, and helps you to think more clearly. It also helps prevent your blood sugars from spiking. We'll talk more about after-meal exercise in the next chapter.

DIGESTION STRATEGY #5: DON'T EAT BETWEEN MEALS.

Imagine that you're doing a load of laundry. After sorting your colors and emptying pockets, you fill the washing machine, add soap, and start the 40-minute cycle. Thirty minutes later, you realize that you forgot to put in a muddy pair of jeans. You think to yourself, *Oh well, the cycle isn't over!* So you open the washer, throw in the jeans, and expect to find a clean load of laundry in 10 minutes. Obviously this doesn't work. The mud on your jeans mixes in with the clean clothes, and the entire load needs to be washed again.

Think of your stomach as a washing machine. You fill your stomach with food. Just as soap mixes with clothes, the acids and digestive enzymes mix with your food and the stomach spins and churns it around and around. Just as throwing in a pair of jeans at the end of the cycle messes up the entire wash, eating extra food between meals messes up digestion.

When you eat a snack, the contents in your stomach—already carefully churned and broken down—combine with new food that still needs to be digested. This delays stomach emptying and slows digestion.[15, 16]

It takes the stomach about four or five hours to digest a meal and produce enough hydrochloric acid and digestive enzymes in time for the next meal. People with bloating, gas, discomfort, and other digestive problems may need six or even seven hours to fully empty the stomach.[17] If you eat a snack two hours after a meal, your stomach isn't ready to digest new food. Neither the snack, nor the next meal, will be digested as well as if they were eaten together at the appropriate time. Because snacking minimizes the effect of hydrochloric acid, it impairs the absorption of nutrients.

Because diabetics often suffer from low blood sugar levels, (as well as high blood sugar spikes), many health professionals encourage them to eat small, frequent meals and to snack anytime their blood sugars run low. While this can provide a quick fix to a specific blood sugar reading, it doesn't address the actual cause of the hypoglycemia, and it further impairs digestion.

The reason blood sugars drop so low between meals is generally because they spike earlier, after meals. Along with the after-meal sugar spike comes an insulin spike that drives the blood sugar too low. Yes, eating a snack raises the blood sugar— but it is only a temporary fix.

Hypoglycemia can also occur from taking too much insulin and other diabetic medications. Regardless of the cause of hypoglycemia, if your blood sugar drops dangerously low and you're having trouble functioning, you obviously need to eat a healthy snack to avoid a hypoglycemic crisis. If you must snack, try to incorporate the meal balancing strategies discussed previously. For example, eat half an apple or half a banana with some peanut butter or nuts. This type of balanced snack helps to prevent your blood sugars from spiking.

Many of my patients who follow the strategies in this book to decrease insulin resistance and stabilize blood sugars naturally soon find that they do not need or want to snack anymore. This helps improve their digestion. Proper meal balancing and after-meal exercise are especially useful for keeping blood sugars stable—preventing both hyperglycemia and hypoglycemia. If you take advantage of these strategies, with time you should be able to wait at least four or five hours between each meal.

DIGESTION STRATEGY #6: EAT A BIG BREAKFAST, A MEDIUM LUNCH, AND A SMALL DINNER.

If you aren't already a breakfast eater, it's time to become one. Eating a good-sized breakfast is one of the most important strategies for optimizing digestion. Breakfast literally means "breaking the fast." If you eat dinner at 6 p.m. and then eat breakfast at 7 a.m. the next morning, you've gone 13 hours without food. Your body needs adequate nutrients and energy to begin the new day.

Eating a good breakfast jump-starts your metabolism and helps you to burn more calories all day long. It also helps to stabilize your blood sugars throughout the rest of the day. Breakfast eaters have increased mental ability[18*] and are less likely to overeat at lunch and dinner. Make sure you eat a healthy, balanced, first-class breakfast every day.

Four to five hours after breakfast, you should be ready for lunch, which should be a good-sized, balanced meal full of first-class foods. Be sure to include lots of non-starchy vegetables and some legumes or nuts to help balance your blood sugars. After breakfast, the majority of your calories for the rest of the day should come from lunch. Because breakfast and lunch generally are eaten when the body is most active, they should be larger than the supper meal.

One of the biggest mistakes people make when it comes to weight loss, digestion, and overall health is to eat a large supper too late in the day. At the end of the day, the body's work is nearly complete. There is no need to consume a large amount of food. When you lie down to sleep, your stomach and digestive organs also need to rest. A large evening meal interferes with sleep, and is much more likely to be stored as fat than food eaten earlier in the day.

Supper should be the smallest meal of the day. Many of my patients find that skipping supper altogether is extremely effective for weight loss. If you do eat supper, you should allow at least three, but preferably four or five hours in between supper time and the time you go to sleep. This gives your digestive organs time to rest, and you will be more likely to get a good, sound sleep.

Many people who have a difficult time eating breakfast find that by eating a lighter supper, or by skipping it all together, they are hungry for breakfast the next morning. When it comes to meal spacing and size, remember, "Eat like a king for breakfast, a prince for lunch, and a poor pauper for supper."

DIGESTION STRATEGY #7: LIMIT THE VARIETY OF FOODS PER MEAL.

Have you ever eaten at a potluck or all-you-can-eat buffet and sampled just about every dish in sight? Even if the foods were healthy, you may have felt lousy later on. While it's important to eat a wide variety of first-class foods, it's best to limit any given meal to just a few choices.

The more types of foods that you put into your stomach at once, the more challenging it is for your body to break down and assimilate the nutrients.

While it's important to incorporate the meal-balancing strategies found in the previous chapter—healthy carbohydrates, healthy proteins, and healthy fats with each meal—it isn't necessary to eat an excessive variety of foods to accomplish this.

In my clinical experience, my patients benefit from selecting no more than 3 to 5 different types of foods per meal (fewer for supper), and then eating reasonable amounts of those foods.

DIGESTION STRATEGY #8: AVOID IRRITATING FOODS.

One day at the clinic on Guam, Tasi—a tall, beautiful woman in her early 30s—came in for a consultation. She was seen by my colleague, Dr. Horinouchi.

Ten days later, Tasi returned to the clinic for a follow-up visit. Dr. Horinouchi was away, so she visited with me instead. She described to me the health problems she had been experiencing and the treatment that Dr. Horinouchi had suggested.

When she was 15 years old, Tasi had started having deep pelvic pain. Her parents and doctor were very concerned. After being referred to a gynecologist, she underwent multiple expensive tests to determine a diagnosis, but nothing could be detected. "There's nothing wrong with you," the doctors told Tasi. But still the pain remained.

For 15 years she had suffered with this pain almost daily. Additional tests provided no further information. Tasi lived in constant fear that she had some rare, deadly disease.

Tasi's gynecologist had finally suggested that she give our lifestyle clinic a try: "There's nothing else I can do for you, Tasi. I don't know if they can help you or not, but I'm out of ideas." After years of wasted medical visits, tests, and bills, Tasi didn't have much hope that we would be able to help her. But she made an appointment anyway.

Tasi told me that she had been surprised by Dr. Horinouchi's response to her story. "I think I know exactly what the problem is," he had told her after just a ten-minute visit. After 13 years of doctor's visits, she was naturally skeptical. *How could he know what's wrong?* she thought. *He hasn't even run any tests. If the other doctors couldn't find anything, how would he be able to know just from talking to me?*

The reason Dr. Horinouchi thought he knew what was wrong was because he had asked Tasi a question he often asked his patients: "What's your favorite food?" Tasi explained that, when she got sick, she had started going to her high school library to learn as much about health as she could. After reading about the benefits of a vegetarian diet, she decided to give up meat. Her parents were worried that she wouldn't be getting enough protein. So she began increasing her consumption of dairy products—especially cheese. "My very favorite food," she responded, "is deep-dish, extra-cheese spinach pizza. I love that!"

"Tasi," Dr. Horinouchi responded, "if you thought there were any chance that you could get rid of your pain, would you be willing to give up cheese?"

This caught her off guard. "Are you serious?" she responded. "I've already given up meat, and now you're telling me I can never eat cheese again?"

"No, I'm not saying you have to do anything forever," he said. "Let's just do an experiment. Will you avoid cheese and dairy products for three weeks to see if it helps you feel better?"

Tasi negotiated with him, and they agreed on two weeks instead of three. At the end of the two weeks, Tasi would do a challenge test, which means that she would eat a large amount of cheese again to see what effect it had on her body.

"So what happened?" I asked Tasi. "It hasn't even been two weeks since your visit."

"Well, I went home determined to follow Dr. Horinouchi's advice" she said. "I stopped eating all dairy. I was surprised that, by the next evening, I wasn't noticing any pain. At first I thought it was just a coincidence, but sure enough, as long as I avoided dairy, the pain didn't come back. After a week of no pain, I decided to go ahead and do the challenge test early. I heated up my favorite extra-cheese, deep-dish spinach pizza and ate several slices. About 20 minutes later, the pain came back, very severely. I can't believe it! For 15 years I've been battling this mysterious problem, when all along it's been something so simple."

Tasi had finally learned that her pain wasn't caused by a strange disease; it was caused by eating cheese.

Throughout my practice, I've noticed that dairy is often particularly offensive to people's digestion. Dairy acts like an antacid—decreasing the acidity of the stomach.[19] This can impair the body's ability to digest and absorb nutrients. Many of my patients with autoimmune diseases and other health problems have greatly benefited by eliminating dairy from their diets.

Other patients have sensitivities to other types of foods. In general, first-class foods tend to be much less irritating to the body than second- and third-class foods. It's important to avoid foods that you know are unhealthy, and to then pay attention to how healthy foods make you feel. Reason from cause to effect and eliminate foods to which you are particularly sensitive.

DIGESTION STRATEGY #9: CONSIDER SUPPLEMENTS.

We've already discussed the danger of antacids and acid blockers—the drugs most commonly used to treat indigestion. There are, however, several valuable supplements that can safely and effectively help to heal digestive problems. I will describe them here. I will also provide instructions for people who are currently taking acid blockers but want to eliminate them safely.

DIGESTIVE ENZYMES

The body produces several different enzymes that help break down nutrients and optimize absorption. Elderly people and people with digestive problems often do not produce as many digestive enzymes as they need.[20]

If you experience gas, bloating, or pressure after your meals, you may benefit from taking digestive enzymes. These are available in both non-vegetarian and vegetarian forms.

PROBIOTICS

Probiotics are tiny organisms such as healthy bacteria that are similar to the bacteria found in a healthy gut. Probiotics can help enhance digestion and immunity by colonizing the gut with these healthy bacteria.[21]

BETAINE HCL

Betaine HCL is a natural supplement that helps to increase stomach acidity and promote digestion.

More than half of American adults over age 60 have inadequate stomach acid production.[22] Burping, belching, or bloating after a meal (especially within

45 minutes after eating), are strong indicators of inadequate acid production. Many people with low acid do not experience symptoms, however.

While all of the strategies outlined in this chapter can help to restore the natural acidic balance of the stomach, betaine HCL can help to jump-start this process. This supplement is also available in both non-vegetarian and vegetarian forms.

HEALING THE STOMACH AND THE ESOPHAGUS

If you have suffered damage to the mucosal lining of your esophagus and/or stomach, you may benefit from products like Gastrozyme™ (from Biotics Research) and/or Gastro Care™ (produced by Karuna Health). These products contain multiple nutrients and herbs shown to be beneficial for healing and soothing the lining of the esophagus and stomach.

If you have an ulcer or any inflammation in the stomach or esophagus, it's very important to let your gastrointestinal (GI) lining heal before starting betaine HCL. Adding acid to an ulcer can be very painful. I recommend taking Gastrozyme or Gastro Care for a week or two before starting betaine HCL supplement. Even if you don't have an ulcer or inflammation, these supplements can still be beneficial. I recommend that any patient who begins taking betaine HCL also take Gastrozyme and Gastro Care for at least two weeks. (If you don't have a stomach ulcer, gastritis, or esophagitis, you can begin taking betaine HCL at the same time that you begin these products.)

Gastrozyme and Gastro Care are chewable tablets and should be taken on an empty stomach at least 30 minutes before a meal.

GALLBLADDER SUPPORT

Most people who have their gallbladders removed are told that this organ is unnecessary and that there's no need to be concerned about living without it. The truth is that the gallbladder actually has a very important function for healthy digestion. It releases bile that aids in the digestion of fats and helps the body absorb many fat-soluble nutrients.

If you've had your gallbladder removed or have a sluggish gallbladder, addressing this problem should be one of your main digestive concerns. I highly recommend taking products that provide the same benefit the gallbladder was designed to provide. For patients who do not require only vegetarian supplements, I recommend Ortho Digestzyme™ (by Ortho Molecular Products). Vegetarian options are also available.

ACTIVATED CHARCOAL

I wish I could write an entire book on the many different health benefits of activated charcoal, but for the sake of this chapter I will briefly mention some of its digestive benefits.

Activated charcoal absorbs toxins. When taken orally, it can help with digestive problems such as bloating, gas, diarrhea, and stomach flu. It can also be taken a few times a week just to help cleanse out the GI system. Activated charcoal comes in powder form and is much more potent than charcoal tablets.

You can take advantage of activated charcoal by mixing a teaspoon of the powder with a glass of cold water—making what my family calls a "black shake." Make sure you take charcoal at least 2 to 3 hours after taking medication, or it may interfere with the medication's absorption. If you're interested in learning more about the many benefits of charcoal, I recommend the book *Rx: Charcoal,* by Agatha Thrash, MD.[23]

ELIMINATING ACID BLOCKERS

We've already discussed the multiple risks associated with acid blocking medications. If you take these medications, this section is for you. If not, you may wish to skip to the end of the chapter.

Many people who become aware of the dangers of acid blockers (and the inability of these medications to address the underlying causes of digestive problems) want to stop taking them. It's important to do this safely and effectively. You don't want to quit cold turkey.

After even just a few weeks of taking an acid blocker, your stomach lining realizes that you have too little acid, and it begins releasing gastrin, a hormone that signals your stomach to produce more acid. As long as you are on an acid blocker, your stomach will ignore this signal. If you stop the acid blocker, however, your stomach will soon start producing high levels of acid—higher than the body needs. This can cause severe burning and pain in the stomach, which explains why so many people become dependent on these drugs.

There is, however, a way to break the cycle that doesn't damage you or burn your stomach. This can be accomplished in three phases. Please note that weaning from the acid blocker does not occur until stage four.

PHASE 1: HEAL THE STOMACH NATURALLY.

The first step to eliminating acid blockers is to help the stomach heal naturally. This can be done by following all of the digestive strategies we've discussed in this chapter, and also by using Gastrozyme™ and Gastro Care™ supplements. Begin by taking these supplements for two weeks to help heal damage to the lining of the esophagus and stomach. Chew one to two tablets of each of these products at least 30 minutes before each meal and also at bedtime. Continue to take these products as you move through the additional phases.

PHASE 2: ADD DIGESTIVE ENZYMES AND PROBIOTICS.

Now that your stomach has begun to heal, it's time to add digestive enzymes and probiotics to your routine. We've already discussed the benefits of these supplements earlier in this chapter.

PHASE 3: GRADUALLY BEGIN TAKING BETAINE HCL.

The third phase in this process is to slowly begin taking betaine HCL with your meals. This gradually will reintroduce acid into your stomach. As you begin this step, it's important to work with a qualified health professional who is knowledgeable about nutritional therapies.

While it may seem illogical to take betaine HCL while taking an acid blocker, it actually makes sense. If the acid blocker were discontinued immediately, your stomach would quickly begin producing too much acid. (Remember, your stomach has sensed low acid, so it wants to make extra.) By starting betaine HCL while you're still taking the acid blocker, your stomach begins to sense that there is enough acid. This will decrease the amount of gastrin produced, and you will eventually be able to start gradually weaning off of the acid blocker—without your body overreacting and producing too much acid.

Begin by taking one betaine HCL tablet with each meal. Every few days, add one additional tablet at every meal. Continue to increase the dose until you reach 7 tablets per meal, or until you feel a warm sensation in your stomach, (whichever comes first). This warm sensation means that you have taken too many tablets for that size of a meal. At the next meal, take one less. After you have determined the largest dose that you can take at your large meals without feeling any warmth, maintain that dose at all meals of similar size. You may find that you need to take fewer tablets with smaller meals. Most patients end up taking 2 to 4 tablets with normal-sized meals, but everyone needs to establish their own optimal dose.

Be sure to take the tablets during your meal—not before or after. When taking several tablets per meal, it's best to spread them throughout the course of the meal, rather than take them all at once.

If taking betaine HCL results in stomach pain or burning, this suggests that you have an ulcer or gastritis. In this case, discontinue the betaine HCL and focus only on phase 1—stomach healing (Gastrozyme and Gastro Care). When you begin taking the betaine HCL again, do it gradually, like before.

PHASE 4: BEGIN WEANING OFF OF THE ACID BLOCKER.

Once your stomach has had time to heal and you've been taking betaine HCL with no burning feeling for at least a week, you can consider slowly weaning off of your acid blocker.

Discontinuing any medicine can be a complex process. As in phase 3, it's important to work with a healthcare professional who is knowledgeable about the digestive process and who knows how to use natural strategies to promote digestive healing.

A general strategy that has worked for many of my patients is to begin by skipping your acid-blocker dose every fourth day. (Take it for three days, and skip the fourth.) Once you've done that for approximately 10 to 12 days, you can try skipping every third day if you aren't experiencing any pain or burning. (Take it for two days, and skip the third.) Once you've been comfortable with this for at least seven to ten days, try skipping every other day.

If at any time you experience pain and burning, you have the option to slow the process by taking your acid blocker. There are natural things you can do to minimize the pain, however, such as chewing extra tablets of Gastro Care (one to two). Of course, all of the strategies outlined in this chapter should help to optimize digestion and to promote healing in the stomach.

PUTTING IT ALL TOGETHER

In this chapter, we've looked at multiple strategies for optimizing your digestion and health. This information may be new to you, and may seem overwhelming at first. I hope you don't feel like Tom felt after his mother's nagging advice: "I haven't enjoyed one bite of this dinner because of your constant directions on how to eat it."

My goal in sharing this information hasn't been to nag you or to present you with a list of rules you must follow. Instead, it has been to provide you with practical opportunities to improve your health. I encourage you to maintain a positive frame of mind while putting these strategies into practice. Don't regard them as a tedious list of do's and don'ts, but as an exciting way to help your body function optimally.

When it comes to digestion and many other aspects of health, maintaining a positive attitude is one of the most healing things you can do. In fact, depression, anxiety, and anger may harm digestion more than anything else. We can learn an important digestive lesson from the early Christians. The New Testament says they "ate their food with gladness and sincerity of heart."[24]

CHAPTER SUMMARY

» It's important to optimize your digestive health.

» Many diseases are caused or worsened by digestive problems.

» Employ the following simple strategies to improve your digestion and optimize your absorption of nutrients:

1. Chew your food well.
2. Understand the importance of stomach acid.
3. Keep hydrated, but don't drown your meals.
4. Go for a walk after you eat.
5. As far as possible, avoid eating between meals.
6. Eat a big breakfast, a medium lunch, and a small supper.
7. Limit the different types of foods per meal.
8. Avoid irritating foods.
9. Consider supplements.
10. Eat your food with gladness and sincerity of heart.

—FIFTEEN—

Get a Move-On

A man's health can be judged by
which he takes two at a time—pills or stairs.
—Joan Welsh

I STILL REMEMBER THE DAY MICHAEL FIRST LIMPED INTO my class. I was in the middle of a lecture, discussing the importance of exercise for blood sugar management. Michael showed up late and began the challenging process of getting to a seat. He slowly crept across the room with his walker—moving in front of the rest of the audience to get to the nearest seat. It took several minutes before he finally sat down.

I continued my lecture, discussing the importance of after-meal exercise to prevent blood sugar spikes. As I shared the information, I thought to myself: *If anyone has an excuse not to exercise, it's this guy. He can barely make it across the room.*

Michael had been referred to my class by his primary care physician. He set up an appointment to meet with me one-on-one. I ordered some lab tests for him and we went over them together:

MICHAEL'S BASELINE LABS

- Fasting Blood Glucose: 278
- Hemoglobin A1c: 10.8%
- Cholesterol: 230
- Triglycerides: 166
- Blood Pressure: 150/100 (with medication)
- Weight: 230 pounds

The wellness program continued, and Michael kept coming, each time limping across the room to find his seat. Just three-and-a-half weeks later, I again met with Michael to review his new lab tests and to compare them with his baseline tests. I was completely surprised by the results.

THREE-AND-A-HALF WEEKS LATER

- Fasting Blood Glucose: 90
- Hemoglobin A1c: 8.2%
- Cholesterol: 157 (no medication)
- Triglycerides: 102
- Blood Pressure: 120/90 (with medication)
- Weight: 221 pounds

I was shocked that Michael had made such remarkable progress in so little time. "Michael," I said, "These are tremendous results. Whatever you're doing is working. What *are* you doing?"

"What do you mean?" he said. "I'm just doing what you told me to do. The first thing I heard you talking about when I started coming to your class was how important it is to exercise after meals. My diabetes was out of control. My doctor had made it clear to me that, unless something drastic changed, diabetes would shorten my life and destroy my kidneys. When I heard you talk about walking after meals, I knew that's what I needed to do."

"How long after each meal do you walk?" I asked.

"Half an hour after every meal," Michael replied.

Michael explained to me that ever since he had been in a car accident, he had experienced pain while walking. "I go for a few minutes with my walker.

Then if my leg or hip gets sore, I just stop and exercise my arms by making big circles like this [he showed me]. Then I walk some more."

I was impressed and challenged by Michael's attitude. He sincerely wanted to improve his health. Instead of making excuses as to why he couldn't exercise, he let nothing get in the way of his goal.

Over the next several months, Michael continued to improve dramatically. Within months after his initial visit, Michael no longer fit the diagnosable criteria for diabetes. His Hemoglobin A1c had dropped to a much healthier 5.7 percent, which dramatically reduced his risk for heart disease and stroke and eliminated his risk for diabetes-related complications.

While Michael made multiple lifestyle changes to accomplish his goal, exercise was one of his most effective strategies. Exercise has a powerful influence on blood sugars, diabetes reversal, and health.

Studies from Harvard University have shown that regular exercise could prevent 30 to 50 percent of all new cases of diabetes.[1] Exercise can also powerfully help to reverse or improve diabetes once it's already present. In this chapter, I will explain the importance of exercise and help you to set up an exercise plan that works for you.

EXERCISE AND INSULIN

You will recall from previous chapters that insulin resistance is the main driver of diabetes and prediabetes. This simply means that the cells (especially the muscle and liver cells) don't want to allow insulin to unlock them for sugar storage. The cells have become "fat and sassy." These muscles are full of energy but they have no expectation of using that energy anytime soon. They generally have not been involved in adequate physical activity. The muscles essentially say, "We already have all the sugar we need, why would we want to store more?"

When this occurs, glucose continues to build up in your bloodstream and damage your body. Medications attempt to force sugar into your cells, but they usually don't address the actual cause of insulin resistance.

But how can you address the cause? How can you deal with your "fat and sassy" cells? One of the most powerful ways to do this is by exercising.[2,3] When you exercise, your muscle cells naturally require more glucose for energy. Realizing this need, these cells become much more sensitive to insulin, allowing it to unlock them for sugar storage. This dramatically helps to lower and control blood sugars. Let's examine the most effective forms of exercise and how they help in blood sugar management.

AFTER-MEAL EXERCISE

One of the most powerful things you can do to lower and manage your blood sugars is to exercise immediately after meals.[4] After-meal exercise is a little-known secret in the diabetes world, but people (like Michael) who take advantage of this strategy find that it can work wonders.

After testing patients for over twenty years, I've found that most people's blood sugars are typically the highest 45 minutes to 1 hour after the beginning of a meal.[5] These blood sugar spikes are what cause damage to tissue by glycosylation.[6] They also trigger an excessive spike in insulin, which raises blood pressure, promotes fat (as well as sugar) storage, and increases the risk of many diseases. These sugar and insulin spikes also make it much more likely that hypoglycemia will occur within the next few hours, creating an unhealthy roller-coaster ride of blood sugar levels. It's important to minimize these after-meal spikes as much as possible.

After-meal exercise can greatly minimize these sugar spikes.[7] I have found that my patients with blood sugar problems can reduce their blood sugar spikes by 1 to 3 points for every minute of light to moderate exercise that they engage in immediately following a meal.

For example, if your after-meal blood sugar typically spikes to 200, you could potentially prevent that spike and lower it to somewhere between 140 to 180 by taking a 20-minute walk after eating. By lowering this spike, you will minimize blood sugar damage, which will be reflected on your next Hemoglobin A1c test. You also reduce the amount of insulin your body needs to secrete—which may lower your risk for obesity, heart disease, cancer, and other diseases.

AFTER-MEAL EXERCISE AND REDUCED DISEASE RISK

Bill scheduled an appointment at my clinic—not because he had noticed any health problems, but because he had just retired and wanted to use some free time to make sure he was properly addressing his health. Bill was fit and lean. He exercised regularly. He also tried to eat a healthy diet. Bill didn't appear to be at risk for diabetes.

But, as I evaluated Bill's records from previous lab tests, I noticed that his fasting blood sugars were a little high. They were in the low 90s—not yet in the prediabetic range, but still not optimal. I wanted to further evaluate Bill's blood sugars, so I ordered a two-hour glucose tolerance test.

Bill's two-hour blood sugar reading was 162, indicating advanced prediabetes. His corresponding insulin levels were also high. Shocked to discover that he was at risk, Bill determined to make any necessary changes to turn his health around.

Bill was already exercising regularly, but I shared with him the value of after-meal exercise to lower blood sugar and insulin spikes. Bill put this new knowledge to work, and soon found that it had been the missing piece in his fitness routine. After a few months, Bill's blood sugar management had improved dramatically and his insulin levels had normalized. By taking advantage of the simple strategy of after-meal exercise, Bill had reversed his prediabetes and dramatically lowered his risk of heart disease, cancer, and other diseases.

WHY TIMING MATTERS

Do you really have to exercise right after your meal to get this benefit? Actually, yes. If you wait an hour after a meal to go for a walk, your blood sugar and insulin have already spiked. The exercise may help lower your blood sugar then, but the sugar spike has already caused damage to your tissues, and the excess insulin has already been released. Exercising right after a meal allows your body to stop these spikes in their tracks.

When done consistently, after-meal exercise can have a profound impact on blood sugar management, weight loss, and disease prevention. To get the maximum benefit, aim to exercise after as many meals as possible. I usually tell my patients to aim for at least 10-15 minutes after every meal. However, patients like Michael prove that 30 minutes can be even more effective. On the other hand, five minutes is better than zero minutes. The principle is to set aside as much time as you can.

This exercise should not be as intense as regular aerobic exercise. The goal is just to get moving. Walking is an ideal after-meal exercise, but other forms of light exercise can work as well. You should be able to do this in your regular clothes, without getting sweaty or needing to shower or change afterwards. If it's raining outside or too hot or cold, you can even walk indoors.

I encourage you to take advantage of this powerful strategy and to exercise after as many meals as you can.

AEROBIC EXERCISE

In addition to after-meal exercise, it's important to incorporate aerobic or cardio exercise into your plan. Aerobic exercise involves continuous, rhythmic movements of your large muscle groups. It elevates your heart rate and increases your need for oxygen. Aerobic exercise makes the heart stronger and enhances cardiorespiratory fitness. It helps to improve blood sugars, burn fat, and lower triglycerides.

Examples of aerobic exercise include:

- Brisk walking
- Hiking
- Jogging
- Biking
- Swimming
- Cycling
- Aerobic workout videos

A good goal is to build up to 45 minutes of aerobic exercise, at least 5 times per week.[8] Find an activity that you enjoy (or at least can tolerate). It may be helpful to have an exercise buddy, to join a gym or health club, or to let other people know about your exercise goals.

Depending on your fitness level, it may take you a few weeks or months to build up to 45 minutes of aerobic exercise. If you find that you are huffing and puffing when doing your light, after-meal exercise, be sure to build up your aerobic exercise slowly. You might even start with just 5 or 10 minutes a day and then gradually build up.

Aerobic exercise should be either before breakfast or at least several hours after any given meal. This exercise should get you huffing, puffing, and sweating—but at a healthy level. You should not be in pain or to the point of collapse.

Some people like to use heart rate monitors to carefully track their level of exertion. While this can be valuable, I find that most people don't have time for it. As long as you are exerting yourself and getting your heart rate up, you will get the benefits of aerobic exercise.

An easy way to monitor the intensity of your workout is to pay attention to your voice. You should be able to talk or hold a conversation while exercising (it's okay if you're slightly winded), but you shouldn't be able to whistle or sing.

Aerobic exercise strengthens the heart and reduces the risk for cardiovascular disease.[9] Because heart disease is one of the most common—and the most deadly—complications associated with diabetes, it's very important to protect the heart through every possible strategy. Ralph Paffenbarger, MD, was the lead investigator of the Harvard Alumni Heath Study,[10] which examined the effect of aerobic exercise on cardiovascular health. This study followed over 12,000 middle-aged participants for 16 years. Those who regularly engaged in vigorous aerobic activity were between 25 percent and 33 percent less likely to die of heart disease.

The study also analyzed the longevity benefits of exercise. Dr. Paffenbarger summarized his findings with the following formula: For every hour that you exercise, you can add two to three hours to your lifespan.[11] (For reasonable amounts of exercise, of course.) I encourage you to incorporate aerobic exercise into your routine. You can begin experiencing the benefits today.

BENEFITS OF AEROBIC EXERCISE

- Lowers blood sugars
- Lowers blood pressure
- Helps control weight
- Increases stamina

(continued)

- Reduces the risk of many diseases, including:
  - Heart Disease
  - Stroke
  - Diabetes
  - Obesity
  - Hypertension
  - Osteoporosis
  - Alzheimer's
  - Some forms of cancer
- Improves mood and mental functioning
- Increases longevity

STRENGTH TRAINING

Once you are consistently benefiting from after-meal and aerobic exercise, it's time to begin strength (resistance) training. This type of exercise strengthens all the major muscle groups in the body. Studies show that people who combine both aerobic exercise and strength training have better blood sugar control and Hemoglobin A1c improvement than those who only participate in one or the other.[12]

Muscle is much more metabolically active than fat. When muscles are strengthened, they burn up glycogen stores (glucose stored in the muscle). The muscles are then more willing to accept more glucose from the bloodstream. Strength training can powerfully reduce insulin resistance and help balance blood sugars.[13] The stronger a muscle is, the better capacity it has to hold sugar. As you increase your lean muscle mass, you naturally decrease insulin resistance.

BENEFITS OF STRENGTH TRAINING

- Improves insulin sensitivity
- Helps lower blood sugars
- Increases metabolism

- Strengthens bones
- Strengthens muscles for everyday use
- Improves posture and balance
- Prevents age-related mobility problems

I recommend getting 20 minutes of strength training exercise two to three times per week.[14] As with aerobic exercise, start out slowly and build up gradually. Depending on your fitness level, you may need to start with just 5 to 10 minutes, a couple of times a week. Because your muscles need time to rest and recover between workouts, it's not necessary (or healthy) to do strength training more frequently than every other day.

There are several strength training activities to choose from. You can buy dumbbells or other free weights to lift at home. You can join a gym and use their weights and strength training machines. It may be valuable for you to work with a personal trainer or physical therapist who can help teach you safe and effective strength training exercises. In addition to regular gyms, many physical therapy centers have gyms that are open to the public. There are also a variety of strength training exercise videos available that you can do in the comfort of your own home. Strength training doesn't have to include weights. Some exercises use bands. Other exercises don't require any equipment at all but utilize the resistance or weight of your own body.

I encourage you to enjoy the benefits of strength training as you make it a part of your weekly routine.

INTERMITTENT TRAINING (IT)

Once you have become consistently comfortable with after-meal, aerobic, and strength training exercise for at least a month or two, you may want to consider intermittent training, or IT. IT exercise involves alternating short bursts of intense physical activity with intervals of lighter activity. For example, it could include running or jogging for 30 seconds, then walking slower for 90 seconds, then repeating this cycle multiple times.

IT boosts the metabolism and helps the body to burn more fat.[15] It increases the secretion of the human growth hormone, the fitness hormone for adults.[16] Growth hormone helps make the body more toned and lean. It can dramatically improve strength, endurance, and overall fitness. IT also improves thyroid function and can help to lower triglycerides.[17, 18]

It's important to start IT gradually. It can be done at the same time as your usual aerobic exercise. Pick an aerobic activity that you enjoy, and that can be done at both a low and high intensity. Do the activity at a relatively slow, relaxed pace for 90 seconds, then at an intense pace for 30 seconds. The intense bursts should raise your heart rate and leave you out of breath. Follow this with another 90 seconds of low-intensity exercise.

Be sure to ease into IT, gradually building up the intensity and the number of repetitions over time to avoid injury or illness. Overexercising can make you susceptible to a cold or flu. Start by incorporating just one or two sets of IT, no more than one or two times per week, as part of your normal aerobic workout. You can gradually increase your repetitions to up to eight sets (low intensity and high intensity), two to three times per week. However, you may prefer fewer sets, which is okay.

EXERCISE AND WEIGHT

Weight loss is one of the most popular benefits of exercise. Exercise burns calories and helps increase metabolism. It also helps balance and optimize several of the key hormones that regulate weight loss.[19,20] These hormones include insulin, cortisol, growth hormone, and thyroid hormone.

Many people have over-simplified views of weight loss, believing that weight is only determined by the amount of calories consumed and the amount of calories burned. While calories certainly are important, body weight and body fat are affected by multiple factors, such as meal timing (as discussed in the previous chapter) and hormonal balance. Regular exercise can help decrease hormones that promote weight gain and increase hormones that promote weight loss.

Of course, exercise must be coupled with a healthy diet for optimal weight-loss results. By combining the nutrition and exercise strategies you've learned, you should have the tools you need to gradually achieve, and then maintain, your ideal weight. A healthy weight is a byproduct of a healthy lifestyle.

THE IMPORTANCE OF CONSISTENCY

When I ask my patients if they are on an exercise program, they frequently reply, "Oh, yes. I exercise. I'm on a walking program." I ask a few more questions, only to discover that their "walking program" consists of just a leisurely stroll once or twice per week. While any exercise is better than no exercise, exercising only a few times a week simply does not provide significant health improvements. To be effective, exercise needs to be consistent.

If you want to see a dramatic improvement in your health, you need to make a dramatic effort to make that happen. In order to encourage my patients to exercise consistently, I often tell them an embarrassing story about myself.

DR. YOUNGBERG AND THE PEANUT BUSTER PARFAIT™

It had been a busy week. Struggling to balance multiple work and family responsibilities, I had not prioritized my health. At the end of the week, I realized I hadn't exercised at all. *At least I'm scheduled to play basketball on Sunday,* I thought. *That will be a great workout.*

Sunday came, and I played a very aggressive, fun, high-intensity game of basketball. Then another game. Then another. This continued for two and a half hours. *Well, I definitely got my exercise in today!* I thought. *In fact, I pretty much made up for not exercising all last week.*

But my body didn't seem to agree. For the next few days, I could tell something was wrong. Not only was I stiff and sore, but I also felt like eating everything in sight. I wasn't satisfied with my usual types or amounts of food.

That Tuesday night, I was driving home after giving a nutrition wellness seminar. I was in the fast lane, looking forward to seeing my wife and kids after a long day at work. And that's when I saw it. There, in all its splendor, was a billboard displaying milkshakes, chocolate-dipped ice cream cones, banana splits, sundaes, and my long-forgotten favorite childhood dessert—the Peanut Buster Parfait. "Dairy Queen®—Exit Ahead," the billboard commanded. I decided to obey.

With no time to think, I quickly crossed six lanes of traffic, racing to get to the exit in time. I parked at Dairy Queen, went inside, and unabashedly ordered a Peanut Buster Parfait. I quickly devoured the gooey, chocolaty, peanuty ice cream—and the 730 calories, 31 grams of fat, and 85 grams of sugar that went along with it. As I threw my trash away and headed to the parking lot, I started to think about what had just happened. *Why did I DO that?* I thought to myself. *I just gave a lecture on the importance of eating first-class foods. I've driven past this Dairy Queen almost every day for the past eight years, and I've never even thought about stopping. I haven't had a Peanut Buster Parfait for at least 20 years. Why did I think I needed one now?*

Looking back, I realize that my dessert fiasco on Tuesday actually started a lot earlier. By failing to exercise the week before, then trying to make up for it by over-exercising on Sunday, I set myself up for unhealthy cravings and Peanut Buster problems.

I share this story with you for two reasons. One is so that you will realize that, as a lifestyle educator, I am still human and, like you, sometimes struggle to make healthy choices.

The second reason I share this story is to encourage you to stay away from the "weekend warrior" mentality—exercising only when it's convenient, or overdoing exercise to make up for lost time. This mentality can totally sabotage your goals. Your body was designed to benefit from *daily* exercise, not weekly or bi-weekly. In order to truly experience the benefits of healthy habits like exercise and proper nutrition, it's important to be consistent.

IT'S NOT TOO LATE

Regardless of your age or current activity level, it's not too late to start exercising! The story of Hulda Crooks powerfully illustrates this lesson.[21, 22, 23]

Hulda was born in 1896 in Saskatchewan, Canada. She was one of 18 children. Raised on a farm, Hulda feasted on the typical farm menu—meat, eggs, potatoes, milk, butter, biscuits, and pie. By age 16, the food was already showing on Hulda's waistline, and her brothers teased her that, by the time she turned 20, she would be wider than she was tall. As you can imagine, this was very embarrassing.

Once in college, Hulda became more concerned about her health. She decided to give up meat and become a vegetarian. However, despite her improved diet and resulting weight loss, Hulda began struggling with multiple health problems.

After her first year in college, Hulda developed pneumonia. She had to take a year off of school to recover, but later reported that it had taken her more than 20 years to fully regain her strength after her bout with the illness.

Hulda married Dr. Samuel Crooks, an anatomy professor at Loma Linda University. She also worked for the university, first as a dean and then in research. Hulda's husband had a congenital heart defect, and Hulda was devastated when he died while she was still in her early 50s.

To help recover from her grief, Hulda turned to hiking outdoors. Hulda noticed that this exercise significantly improved her mood. She enjoyed it so much that she began to climb mountains. She climbed every major peak in California. At age 66, she climbed Mount Whitney for the first time. She enjoyed the hike so much that she repeated it almost every year. By the time she was 91, Hulda Crooks had summited Mount Whitney 23 times. She also hiked the John Muir Trail, climbed Mt. Fuji in Japan at age 91, and beat 8 world records for women over age 80 in marathon and road races.

Hulda Crooks was affectionately dubbed "Grandma Whitney," and in 1990 Congress voted to rename one of the peaks closest to Mount Whitney "Crooks Peak" in her honor.[24]

Hulda's inspiring story teaches us that you're never too old to exercise. She lived to be 101, inspiring senior citizens and young people alike to experience the benefits of exercise. I had the privilege of hearing Mrs. Crooks speak when I was in high school, and also was able to meet her personally. Her story inspired me to be consistent with exercise and to help encourage others to do the same—regardless of age.

THE IMPORTANCE OF SYNERGY

For my twenty-first birthday, my dad gave me a copy of Jim Fixx's new book, *The Complete Book of Running.*[25] Jim Fixx was a famous runner who helped to promote America's 1980s fitness revolution. The book sold over a million copies and remained the number one national best seller for 11 weeks.

Jim Fixx's story is inspiring. He had transformed from a 240-pound, two-pack a day smoker to an extremely fit athlete—simply by running. Fixx avidly promoted the health and longevity benefits of running, and inspired thousands of people to take up the sport.

I enjoyed the book very much. It included Fixx's story, motivational quotes, running instructions, and an exercise journal. The cover featured a picture of Fixx's muscular running legs.

The next summer (1982), I was listening to Chicago WBBM Newsradio as I painted a hallway at my parents' house. Radio hosts Bob and Betty Sanders were interviewing Jim Fixx, who was promoting an upcoming race in Chicago. Betty Sanders began the discussion by asking Jim a question.

"Jim, we understand you run 10 miles every day. What kind of *craziness* is that?"

Without missing a beat, Jim Fixx replied: "Well you know, Bob and Betty, when I run 10 miles every day, *I can eat anything I want!*"

While I considered myself to be a fan of Jim Fixx, his response troubled me. *Jim's sure going to have some health problems down the road if he's got that philosophy,* I thought.

Just two years later, I was in my first year of professional training at Loma Linda University. Driving home after class, I turned the radio on to hear the news. I was stunned by the announcer's report: "Jim Fixx, avid marathoner and best-selling author of numerous running books, was found dead this morning on the path of his morning run."

Jim Fixx had died of a massive heart attack. His autopsy showed three blocked coronary arteries. This totally shocked and rocked the foundation of the running movement. At that time, little was known about the connection between diet and heart disease. Many people assumed that runners and other athletes were immune to such problems.

Throughout the 1970s and 1980s, the popular opinion was that, as long as you exercised every day, there was no need to worry about what types of food you were eating. You were going to burn it all off anyway. As long as you exercised enough, *you could eat anything you wanted.* But Jim Fixx's tragic death didn't seem to support this philosophy. Within a few short years, the medical world began to understand why.

Jim Fixx's story is a sobering reminder of the importance of combining *multiple* strategies to improve health and prevent disease. Yes, exercise is important—critically important. But exercise alone is not enough. It must be combined with a healthy diet, adequate rest, and all of the other principles discussed in this book.

The word synergy is defined as: "The interaction or cooperation of two or more agents to produce a combined effect greater than the sum of their separate effects."[26] For example, one strong workhorse can pull an estimated 4,000 pounds. But two workhorses together can pull 12,000 pounds. Instead of merely doubling their impact, the horses triple their impact by working together. 1+1=3. The same is true when it comes to health. The more health strategies you incorporate into your wellness plan, the more powerful the results will be.

CHAPTER SUMMARY

- Exercise greatly improves health and blood sugar management.
- Exercise increases insulin sensitivity, which naturally lowers blood sugars.
- After-meal exercise helps prevent damaging blood sugar and insulin spikes.
- You can lower your after-meal sugar spike by 1 to 3 points for every minute you engage in light exercise after a meal.
- Consistent, after-meal exercise lowers HA1c levels and promotes weight loss.
- Aim to exercise at least 10 to 15 minutes after each meal.
- Aerobic exercise improves cardiovascular health, lowers blood sugars and triglycerides, and burns fat.
- People who get regular, vigorous aerobic exercise are much less likely to have a heart attack or stroke.
- Try to build up to 45 minutes of aerobic exercise at least 5 times per week.
- Strength training increases lean muscle mass and can dramatically lower blood sugars.
- Aim for 20 minutes of strength training 2 to 3 times per week.
- Intermittent Training improves thyroid function, builds endurance, and helps to strengthen and tone the body.

- Exercise helps in weight management both by increasing the metabolism and by balancing hormones related to weight.
- It's important to be regular and consistent with your exercise program.
- Your body was designed to benefit from exercise every day.
- You're never too old to become active.
- Exercise is most effective when combined with other healthy habits, including good nutrition, regular sleep, and adequate hydration.

—SIXTEEN—

What About Weight?

The journey of a thousand miles begins with a single step.
—Lao-tzu (ancient Chinese philosopher)

I STILL REMEMBER THE DAY WHEN JASON'S PANTS FELL off. It was one of the most embarrassing, yet also one of the most encouraging, moments of his life. Jason came to our group wellness session that night, eager to share the good news. In the middle of a crowded public gym, Jason's pants had fallen to his ankles, reassuring him that he was becoming lean again.

About a month earlier, Jason had been referred to me by his diabetologist. He had multiple serious health problems. He was diabetic. He was a heavy smoker. His cholesterol, triglycerides, and blood pressure were out of control. At 6 feet 4 inches tall, Jason weighed almost 300 pounds. He also struggled with depression and anxiety.

Jason had been an athlete in college. He wondered how he had allowed his health to fall apart over the past 20 years. His diagnosis of diabetes was a wake-up call. He was also alarmed to discover that he already had chronic kidney disease and was at risk for kidney failure. Knowing that, unless something drastically changed, his condition would only get worse, Jason was determined to take control of his health. He made the decision to join our three-month diabetes reversal program.

Jason was highly motivated to change his lifestyle. He started balancing his meals and eating first-class foods. He started exercising consistently—using after-meal, aerobic, and strength training exercises to improve his insulin sensitivity and his overall health.

Two weeks into the program, Jason noticed tremendous results. Before starting, Jason had been taking 140 units of insulin each day. Just two weeks later, he was completely off his insulin. Jason's triglycerides had dropped from 320 to 115. His cholesterol and blood pressure had also normalized. His kidney function had improved. Jason also noticed an increased level of energy.

Three weeks into the program, Jason's lab results looked even better. He reported that his chronic headaches were gone. He had quit smoking. His sleep had dramatically improved. Jason was excited to see what would happen next.

Four weeks after the program started, I was surprised when Jason came to my office looking discouraged and defeated. "I don't think this is working for me, Dr. Youngberg," he said. "It's already been a month, and I'm not really getting better." In my estimation, Jason's health was improving dramatically, so I was surprised at his discouragement.

"What do you mean you're not getting better?" I asked. "We've been seeing so many improvements."

Jason sighed and looked down at his shoes. "I haven't lost any weight at all," he said. "I've been doing all these things for an entire month, and I haven't lost a single pound. When I was diagnosed with diabetes, they told me that if I just lost 30-40 pounds it would dramatically improve my health, but I haven't lost any weight at all!" Depressed by his situation, Jason was almost ready to quit the program altogether.

"Jason," I said. "Remember all the problems you were experiencing a month ago? Out-of-control diabetes, high triglycerides, high cholesterol, insomnia, headaches, smoking, and chronic kidney disease? For the past several weeks, all of those conditions have improved dramatically. You've shared your excitement about your increased level of energy and the improvements in your lab results. And now you want to quit the program because you haven't lost weight? Do you really think that makes sense?"

"Well...no, I guess it doesn't," Jason admitted. "But I just don't understand. If I'm getting healthy, how come I'm not losing weight?"

"Jason, the weight will come off," I said. "Weight loss is an important goal. But as long as you keep making healthy choices, you don't need to stress about it. The important thing is to keep improving your health by doing what you're doing. I know you've been exercising consistently. It's possible that you've lost quite a bit of fat weight and gained muscle weight instead. Muscle is more dense than fat. A pound of muscle is only half as big as a pound of fat. The fact that you haven't lost weight doesn't mean you aren't getting smaller—or more importantly, more lean and fit."

Jason left my office that morning feeling somewhat better, but still disappointed that he hadn't lost weight. That afternoon, he went to the gym for his strength training workout. In college, Jason had been able to bench-press over 300 pounds. Now he was slowly building back up. He went to the weight rack and picked up a 45-pound barbell, then turned to slide it onto the bench press bar—and that's when it happened.

Jason felt his gym pants slide off his hips, all the way down to his ankles. He was standing in the middle of the gym, with people working out all around him. Although he wanted to immediately pull his pants back up, he was still holding the 45-pound weight. He had to set it back on the rack before he could free his hands.

Thankfully, Jason had a good sense of humor and chuckled along with his audience. Jason had never been so happy to be embarrassed. He realized that, even though his scale didn't show the results, his body was becoming leaner. The program really was working! Jason came to our group session that night in much better spirits, eager to brag about how his pants had fallen off. In the coming weeks and months, Jason did lose a significant amount of weight and continued to become more lean and fit. Jason's story illustrates several important lessons for anyone struggling with weight.

IT'S ABOUT HEALTH

Like most people, Jason had some misconceptions about weight loss. He believed that his health couldn't improve until he lost a specific amount of weight.

Jason was obese and certainly did need to lose weight. However, many aspects of his health improved quickly and dramatically before the scale ever started to show results. His blood sugars improved. His kidney function improved. His risk for cardiovascular disease was dramatically reduced. Jason's story is not unusual. Many of my patients experience dramatic changes in their health before losing any significant amount of weight. Why is this?

While it's true that people who are overweight are at a higher risk for developing diabetes and other degenerative diseases than people who maintain a healthy weight, it's important to understand why. These diseases are not caused as much by the excess weight itself as by the underlying "metabolic mess" that accompanies an unhealthy lifestyle. For example, while obesity contributes to atherosclerosis, it isn't the primary cause of the condition. Obesity and atherosclerosis are both symptoms of an unhealthy lifestyle—namely, an unhealthy diet. That's why it's important to address the underlying cause of disease instead of just targeting symptoms. By addressing the cause, multiple symptoms will improve.

This is good news. People who are overweight, even obese, can begin to experience dramatic health improvements within weeks of beginning a healthy lifestyle program. As they continue to make healthy choices, the weight will naturally and steadily come off.

Weight is an important aspect of health, but it's not synonymous with health. There are many people who are thin but unhealthy. That's why I encourage my patients to focus on improving their health rather than just on "getting thin." Thankfully, the same healthy choices that promote overall wellness also promote a healthy weight.

It's important to be patient with your weight loss. While cholesterol, triglycerides, blood sugars, and other lab values can improve within just days or weeks, losing a large amount of weight takes some patience and perseverance.

REMEMBER DAVID?

Remember the story of David from Chapter 11? David was highly motivated to accomplish his three goals:

1. To weigh less than 200 pounds
2. To run the Honolulu marathon
3. To become the general manager of a 5-star hotel in Maui

These goals didn't happen overnight, but David did notice immediate improvements. Within just one week, his energy had increased and his mood had improved dramatically.

Within two weeks, his blood pressure, blood sugars, cholesterol, and triglycerides had dropped significantly. He had lost 11 of the 130 pounds he wanted to lose. David realized that he was heading in the right direction, and he didn't allow his goal to overwhelm him. He continued to make healthy choices. He gave his body the time it needed to get rid of all the excess weight. Within a year and a half, David had reached his goal.

If weight loss is one of your goals too, there's hope for you. In this chapter, I'll show you how to optimize the lifestyle strategies you've learned to reach and maintain your ideal weight. But let's start by looking at some common methods used to understand weight and fat.

WEIGHING IN

Without question, there's a connection between diabetes and weight. As mentioned in Chapter 6, being obese or overweight is one of the most significant risk factors for developing type 2 diabetes. Excess fat increases insulin resistance. Harvard studies suggest that 50 to 70 percent of all new cases of diabetes could be prevented by maintaining a normal weight or by losing weight if necessary.[1]

The National Diabetes Education Program has created a chart to help people to determine whether or not their weight puts them at risk for diabetes.[2]

AT-RISK WEIGHT CHART FOR DIABETES

Not Asian or a Pacific Islander: AT RISK=BMI > 25		Asian: AT RISK=BMI > 23		Pacific Islander: AT RISK=BMI > 26	
Height	Weight	Height	Weight	Height	Weight
4'10"	119	4'10"	110	4'10"	124
4'11"	124	4'11"	114	4'11"	128
5'0"	128	5'0"	118	5'0"	133
5'1"	132	5'1"	122	5'1"	137
5'2"	136	5'2"	126	5'2"	142
5'3"	141	5'3"	130	5'3"	146
5'4'	145	5'4'	134	5'4'	151
5'5"	150	5'5"	138	5'5"	156
5'6"	155	5'6"	142	5'6"	161
5'7"	159	5'7"	146	5'7"	166
5'8"	164	5'8"	151	5'8"	171
5'9'	169	5'9'	155	5'9'	176
5'10"	174	5'10"	160	5'10"	181
5'11"	179	5'11"	165	5'11"	186
6'0"	184	6'0"	169	6'0"	191
6'1"	189	6'1"	174	6'1"	197
6'2"	194	6'2"	179	6'2"	202
6'3'	200	6'3'	184	6'3'	208
6'4"	205	6'4"	189	6'4"	213

This chart can be valuable for helping people identify their risk. However, it allows some who are at risk to fall through the cracks, undetected. It's important to remember that weight is only *one of many* risk factors for diabetes.

This chart is based on Body Mass Index calculations. The Body Mass Index, or BMI, is calculated from a person's weight and height. Many doctors use the Body Mass Index and other weight charts to monitor their patient's weight.

While this method has a purpose, it is incomplete. For one thing, it is not gender specific. Typically, males carry more weight than females of the same height, but BMI standards do not take this into account.

There's another potential problem with the BMI. While it focuses on how much a person weighs, it doesn't take into account how much of that weight is lean muscle mass versus how much is fat. Because excess *fat*, not muscle, is what increases risk for disease, a more accurate method for assessing weight and health is to measure body composition.[3]

BODY COMPOSITION

When Jason's pants fell down at the gym, he learned the importance of body composition. The scale can tell you the number of total pounds you weigh, but it can't tell you what those pounds are made of. Jason was depressed because he hadn't lost weight, but once his pants fell off he realized he had lost fat and gained muscle. His body composition had changed dramatically.

The lean muscle tissue that Jason built helped him to lower and control his blood sugar. By losing fat (particularly the abdominal fat that used to hold his pants up), Jason lost several inches and lowered his risk for disease. Jason was still overweight, but he was less "overfat" than before. It's possible for people who are at a normal, "healthy" weight to be overfat (i.e. have a higher percentage of body fat than is healthy). It's also possible to be overweight but not overfat.

For example, imagine a small-framed, 5 foot 5 inch, Asian woman who weighs 120 pounds. Her BMI is within the healthy range. According to the "At Risk Weight Chart," her weight does not place her at risk for developing diabetes; but even though she appears to be healthy, this woman has a high percentage of body fat. She is carrying a few pounds of dangerous visceral fat in her abdomen. This significantly increases her risk of developing metabolic problems—including diabetes. This woman is not overweight, but she is overfat. Her case is not unusual. Many people who are thin in appearance actually have a high percentage of body fat.

On the other hand, a fit and lean athlete might be "overweight" according to Body Mass Index calculations and weight charts. However, he might have a very low body fat percentage. People who weigh more than average, but are lean and carry a lot of muscle weight, are much less likely to develop diabetes than those who are thin but have a high body fat percentage.[4] That's why it's important to measure your body fat percentage.

Numerous military personnel have come to the clinics where I've worked, frustrated after failing their annual physical exam because their weight was too high. These men are lean and fit. They weigh more than average because of increased muscle mass. In order to prove that they are healthy, these men come in for an exam so they can take a letter back to their supervisors, explaining that their weight will not interfere with their performance. My colleagues and I test their body composition. Even though the men are overweight or obese based on the BMI scale, their low body-fat percentages prove that they are just highly fit. This teaches us the importance of paying attention to body composition. After all, do we want our military personnel to fit into a certain weight category—or to be fit and strong?

TESTING BODY FAT PERCENTAGE

Now that you understand the importance of body composition, it's time to test your body fat percentage. This test will give you valuable information about your risk for disease and overall fitness level. Body fat percentage can be calculated several different ways, including bioelectrical impedance, skin-fold calipers, and underwater weighing. These methods vary in accuracy, convenience, and price. Talk to your doctor, physical therapist, or someone at your local gym or sports medicine clinic about the options available to you for accurate body fat percentage testing.

The World Health Organization and the National Institutes of Health have developed body fat percentage guidelines that will help you determine whether your body composition places you at risk for diabetes, heart disease, cancer, and many other diseases.

BODY FAT PERCENTAGE GUIDELINES[5]

WOMEN

Age	Underfat	Healthy	Overweight	Obese
20-40 yrs	Under 21%	21-33%	33-39%	Over 39%
41-60 yrs	Under 23%	23-35%	35-40%	Over 40%
61-79 yrs	Under 24%	24-36%	36-42%	Over 42%

MEN

Age	Underfat	Healthy	Overweight	Obese
20-40 yrs	Under 8%	8-19%	19-25%	Over 25%
41-60 yrs	Under 11%	11-22%	22-27%	Over 27%
61-79 yrs	Under 13%	13-25%	25-30%	Over 30%

Your goal—at the very minimum—should be to keep your body fat percentage within the "Healthy" range. However, because people with low (but not too low) amounts of body fat have such a reduced risk for disease, ideally you should aim for the lower end of the "Healthy" range.[6, 7] Regardless of your current body composition, there is hope for improvement. By consistently following the nutrition and exercise principles outlined in previous chapters, you are sure to see results.

WAIST CIRCUMFERENCE

In addition to knowing your body fat percentage, it's also important to know how your fat weight is distributed throughout your body.

As mentioned in Chapter 6, although any excess fat can increase diabetes risk, fat in the mid section (i.e. belly fat) is the most dangerous. People who are "pear-shaped" tend to carry more weight in the lower body, particularly in the hips and thighs. People who are "apple-shaped" carry more weight in their abdominal region. This contributes to increased visceral fat (i.e. fat surrounding the organs) and increases the risk for heart disease, diabetes, several forms of cancer, and numerous other diseases.

If you don't know your waist circumference, it's time to pull the measuring tape out. Research has shown that, for many people, waist circumference is typically a more accurate indicator of increased risk than BMI.[8]

To measure your waist circumference, use a flexible tape measure. Be sure to measure around the smallest part of your waist. This should be midway between the lowest portion of your rib cage and the top of your hipbone. Don't pull the tape measure too tight, and don't hold your breath while measuring.

Most guidelines state that men should have a waist circumference less than 40 inches, and women less than 35 inches.[9] However, recent research has shown that these guidelines are not stringent enough. Even people with smaller waist sizes can still be at risk because of excess abdominal fat. These are the results of a study that followed more than 27,000 men for 13 years:[10]

WAIST SIZE AND DIABETES RISK*

A waist size of 34-36 inches doubled diabetes risk.
A waist size of 36-38 inches tripled diabetes risk.
A waist size of 38-40 inches was associated with five times the risk.
A waist size of 40-62 inches was associated with twelve times the risk.
**Compared to men who had a waist size under 34 inches*

The American Institute for Cancer Research has suggested more conservative guidelines that recommend men keep their waist circumference under 37 inches and women under 31.5 inches in order to minimize disease risk.[11] While these guidelines are more evidence-based than the standard guidelines, it's important to remember that even a 34 to 36 inch waist size doubled the diabetes risk in men who participated in the above study.

Don't let the numbers fool you. If you have a small frame, your waist may need to be even smaller than these conservative guidelines suggest. One way to determine your optimal waist size is to consider your past. If you were a healthy weight and size in your late teens or early twenties, your ideal waist size would be the size you were then. Of course, very few people are the same size today that they were in their twenties. Don't let that discourage you. If you have excess abdominal fat, any reduction in waist size will be beneficial to your health.

WAIST TO HIP RATIO

Don't put that tape measurer away quite yet! Next, you need to compare your waist circumference to your hip circumference. This is called the waist-to-hip ratio. Because excess weight in the buttocks, hips, and thighs does not pose nearly as much risk as excess weight in the abdomen, the waist-to-hip ratio helps reveal your risk by taking into account your weight distribution.[12]

Measure your hip circumference by placing the tape measure around the widest portion of your hips (without clothes on). For women, this is usually at groin level. For men, it's usually two to four inches below the navel. You can then calculate your waist-to-hip ratio:

Waist-to-Hip Ratio = Waist Circumference / Hip Circumference

For example, if your waist is 34 inches and your hips are 37 inches, your waist-to-hip ratio is 0.92 (34/37=0.92) In other words, your waist is 8 percent smaller than your hips.

If you are a female, your optimal waist-to-hip ratio is less than 0.75 (with your waist at least 25 percent smaller than your hips). If you are a male, your optimal waist-to-hip ratio is less than 0.85 (with your waist at least 15 percent smaller than your hips).[13] Keeping your waist-to-hip ratio at or near these levels will help to reduce your risk for diabetes and heart disease.[14]

There are, of course, exceptions. For instance, this test may not accurately reveal risk for people with very wide hips. Even though their waist-to-hip ratio may be low, they still may carry a large amount of excess abdominal fat. That's why it's important to also evaluate waist circumference, independent of the waist-to-hip ratio.

REACHING A HEALTHY WEIGHT AND BODY COMPOSITION

Now that you know how to assess your weight and determine your body composition, you need to know how to improve your results. We've already discussed numerous lifestyle strategies for improving blood sugar management and reducing your risk for many diseases. The good news is that these same strategies also help you achieve and maintain a healthy weight and body fat percentage.

NUTRITION

Good nutrition is your most powerful weight-loss weapon. In Chapters 12 and 13, you learned about the power of eating nutrient-dense, first-class foods. The suggestions in those chapters will help you lose weight, manage your blood sugars, and improve your overall health. Nutrient-dense, high-fiber foods will satisfy your hunger and help you to feel full longer. Well-balanced, first-class meals provide your body with the energy it needs while allowing you to shed excess fat weight. You can optimize your weight loss potential by following the nutrition strategies in those chapters.

Avoid restrictive diets that promise quick results. These weight-loss plans rarely lead to long-term success. They promote muscle loss and are not sustainable for long periods of time. Because these plans are unrealistic, it's only natural that people become frustrated and give up. Instead of trying a new diet, try a new lifestyle. The only weight management plan that works in the long run is the one you can stick with over time.

DIGESTION

The digestion principles outlined in Chapter 14 can help you to achieve a healthy weight. Taking time to chew your food thoroughly and to savor each bite helps you feel satisfied sooner and ultimately helps you to eat less.

Eating a big breakfast jump-starts your metabolism and helps you burn more calories all day long. Eating a small supper prevents you from storing excess calories as fat and enables you to get a good night's sleep—which is very important for weight loss.[15] Many of my patients have experienced dramatic weight-loss results simply by downsizing their evening meal.

EXERCISE

After-meal exercise, aerobic exercise, and strength training all powerfully influence weight and body composition. After-meal exercise lowers insulin spikes, which makes the body less likely to store fat. Aerobic exercise burns calories and increases metabolism. Strength training builds muscle mass—which significantly increases metabolism and makes the body more fit and lean. Strength training is especially important for anyone trying to lose weight, because it stimulates fat loss and helps prevent muscle loss.

A powerful benefit of exercise is the release of "feel-good" endorphins into the bloodstream. These chemicals enhance mood and diminish unhealthy cravings. They provide the body with a sense of satisfaction and pleasure. This makes it easier for you to make healthy choices, decreasing your desire to get pleasure from unhealthy or excess foods.

WATER AND WEIGHT

Are you drinking enough water to lose weight? Water can help reduce cravings and keep you satisfied between meals. People who are dehydrated often mistake their thirst for hunger, and respond by eating. When you feel the urge to eat something between your regularly scheduled meals, drink a tall glass of water instead. Wait at least five to ten minutes. If your body was asking for water instead of food, your craving will diminish. In Chapter 18, I will further discuss the importance of water for weight loss and diabetes control or reversal.

SLEEP AND WEIGHT

Allow me to introduce the "Dream Diet," a program that allows you to lose weight while you sleep. While it may sound too good to be true, sleep actually influences weight loss. Not only do people who go to bed early consume fewer calories by avoiding the late night "munchies," but they also optimize the hormones that influence weight.

Ghrelin is a hormone that stimulates the appetite by sending hunger signals to the brain. Leptin is a hormone that stimulates a sensation of fullness by telling the brain that it's time to stop eating after a meal. Sleep deprivation causes ghrelin levels to increase (which increases hunger) and leptin levels to decrease (which decreases fullness). This double whammy of hormonal chaos can cause increased calorie consumption and weight gain.

In one Stanford University study where more than 1,000 people were evaluated, researchers found that those who slept less than eight hours per night had lower levels of leptin and higher levels of ghrelin than those who slept eight or more hours.[16] They also had higher body fat percentages. People with the highest body fat percentages were those who got the least amount of sleep.

Learn more about the importance of sleep for weight loss and overall health in Chapter 17.

SUNSHINE AND WEIGHT

Adequate sun exposure can improve your mood and increase your overall sense of wellness, which can reduce unhealthy food cravings. Sunlight also influences several hormones related to weight.

Early morning sunlight is especially helpful. Early light stimulates the pineal gland to produce more melatonin at night.[17] Melatonin is the hormone that promotes a healthy sleep cycle, which rejuvenates the body and helps to optimize the metabolism. Inadequate melatonin means inadequate rest, and inadequate rest means metabolic problems and increased weight. Take advantage of the sun to improve your sleep, and then take advantage of your sleep to improve your weight! Early morning sunlight also helps to balance and optimize other hormones related to weight.[18, 19]

Intense, mid-day sunlight is also beneficial. During the late morning and early afternoon (when the sun is at least 45 degrees above the horizon), the sunlight is intense enough to stimulate vitamin D production.[20] Studies have shown that people with adequate vitamin D levels are able to lose weight more easily than people with low vitamin D levels.[21]

Vitamin D also plays other important roles in the body. It's important to have your vitamin D level tested. You can learn more information about sunlight and vitamin D in Chapter 19.

EMOTIONS AND WEIGHT

Although food was designed to satisfy physical hunger, we often turn to it to satisfy emotional hunger. It is easy to overeat (or to eat the wrong types of foods) in response to stress, anger, loneliness, and other negative emotions. This is called emotional eating. Emotional eating can provide a temporary sense of comfort and satisfaction, but the results are short-lived. Soon, guilt and remorse set in, and you feel even worse than you did before.

The good news is that you can learn to eat in response to true hunger instead of in response to emotions. In order to do this, you need to learn practical ways to address your emotional concerns without turning to food when you don't need it. This takes some prior planning. If you're stressed, take a short walk, listen to music, or call a friend. If you're lonely, find someone to spend time with, journal, or pray. If you're angry, allow yourself time to cool down without immediately turning to food.

You were designed to experience optimal health in every facet of life—body, mind, and spirit. The things that affect your physical health also affect your mental health, and vice versa. It's important to make sure you are taking the time to improve your health—physically, mentally, and spiritually. Not only will this prevent emotional eating, it will improve every aspect of your life and health.

THYROID

If you consistently follow all of the health strategies in this chapter but do not see an improvement in your weight after several weeks or months, consider having your thyroid function evaluated. Decreased thyroid function slows the metabolism and makes it very difficult to lose weight. There are multiple strategies you can follow to improve your thyroid function. For more information on evaluating your thyroid function, read Chapter 10.

CHAPTER SUMMARY

- A normal weight is one important indicator of good health. However, your health can improve dramatically before weight loss ever occurs.
- A healthy weight is a byproduct of a healthy lifestyle. Focus on your health, and your weight will also improve.
- Living an overweight or obese lifestyle significantly increases the risk of diabetes, heart disease, and cancer.
- Weight loss takes time and perseverance. It's important to be patient with the process.
- Body Mass Index is a measurement relating weight and height. While it can help some people identify their risk, it does not take body fat percentage, gender, or weight distribution into account.
- Not all weight is created equal. Weight from lean muscle mass is very different from excess fat weight. Body composition is another important factor to evaluate.
- It is important to evaluate and optimize your body fat percentage.
- People with optimal body fat percentages are at much lower risk for disease than people who carry extra fat.
- Excess abdominal weight significantly increases risk for diabetes, heart disease, and cancer.
- Identifying waist circumference helps you know whether your abdominal weight puts you at risk.

- The waist-to-hip ratio identifies risk by evaluating fat distribution.
- The same strategies that improve overall health also improve weight.
- To optimize your weight and health:
    1. Eat balanced, nutrient-dense, first-class foods.
    2. Avoid restrictive diets that promise quick results.
    3. Eat slowly, chewing your food thoroughly and savoring every bite.
    4. Eat a large breakfast to jump-start your metabolism.
    5. Eat a small supper, several hours before bedtime, or skip it altogether.
    6. Consistently take advantage of after-meal, aerobic, and strength-training exercise.
    7. Drink water to promote hydration and prevent false hunger signals.
    8. Get adequate sleep to balance weight-related hormones.
    9. Go outside in the early morning sunlight to improve sleep.
    10. Get adequate sunlight exposure to improve hormonal health.
    11. Consider evaluating your thyroid function if you aren't seeing weight loss results.

—SEVENTEEN—

Get Sound Sleep

A problem difficult at night is resolved in the morning after the committee of sleep has worked on it.
—John Steinbeck

I'VE ALWAYS FELT SORRY FOR RIP VAN WINKLE, A FICTITIOUS character from a classic short story by Washington Irving.[1] Rip was a lazy man who "would rather starve on a penny than work for a pound." Although he was friendly and helpful to his neighbors and members of the community, Rip felt no responsibility to provide for his family. This frustrated his poor wife, who constantly accused him of being idle. To escape his wife's lectures, Rip would hike into the mountains with his dog, Wolf. They spent countless hours together—hiking, fishing, and hunting for pigeons and squirrels.

During one such hike, Rip heard someone calling his name and turned to see a short, stout, elderly Dutchman carrying a heavy load. The man asked for help. Rip agreed and helped the man carry his load up the mountain. Soon they reached a small, mysterious village where Rip met a group of strangely-dressed, peculiar-looking people. Eventually, Rip grew exhausted and fell asleep on the grass.

When he woke up, Rip was surprised to discover that it was morning. Knowing that his wife would be upset at his absence, Rip began gathering his belongings. He was surprised to find that his gun was old and rusty. He assumed that the villagers had replaced his new gun with an old one. His dog, Wolf, had also disappeared. He whistled and called, but Wolf was nowhere to be found.

As he moved around, Rip realized that his joints were stiff. He didn't have his usual strength. Even more disturbing was the realization that his beard had grown a foot long. Confused and disturbed, he slowly made his way down the mountain.

When he reached his village, everything seemed different. There were people he didn't recognize, dressed in fashions he had never seen. The village was larger than before, with new houses and buildings replacing those he remembered. Upon reaching his house, Rip was horrified to discover it abandoned, with broken windows, a sunken roof, and doors off the hinges. There was no sign of his family.

Returning to the village, Rip inquired about the whereabouts of his friends and family. Many reportedly had died during a war, and others had moved away years before. Rip's wife had recently died after bursting a blood vessel in an argument with a peddler.

Rip was bewildered at the long period of time that seemed to have passed since he'd last left his village. He thought he'd been gone only one night, and wondered if he had gone crazy.

"I'm not myself. I'm somebody else...I was myself last night, but I fell asleep on the mountain, and they've changed my gun, and everything's changed, and I'm changed, and I can't tell what's my name, or who I am! Does anybody know poor Rip Van Winkle?"

An old woman hobbled forward to take a closer look, and then exclaimed: "Sure enough! It is Rip Van Winkle—it is himself! Welcome home again, old neighbor. Why, where have you been these twenty long years?"

WASTED TIME

Rip Van Winkle slept away 20 years of his existence. He missed watching his children grow up, interacting with friends, and experiencing the joys and challenges of life. Although it's a make-believe story, I feel sorry for a man who wasted his time sleeping.

But is sleep really a waste of time? As we manage busy schedules and deadlines, it's easy to skimp on sleep. We "don't have enough time to sleep." We think it will decrease our productivity. We're tempted to stay up late in order to accomplish our goals.

Unlike Rip's 20-year slumber, adequate sleep is never a waste of time. In fact, the average 60-year-old person should have already spent 20 years asleep (not all at once, of course). Sleep does not rob us of time—it improves our time. It helps us to function optimally and to enjoy our time awake.

Sleep is powerful medicine. It dramatically influences health. It also affects diabetes. In this chapter, we'll explore the significance of sleep and discuss how to fully benefit from it.

WHILE YOU ARE SLEEPING

Sleep may seem like an inactive process—a time when the body simply shuts down to rest. When you're sleeping, you are unconscious and unaware of what is happening inside your body. However, a multitude of important activities occur inside your body during sleep. Your muscles and tissues repair themselves. Your short-term memory consolidates and files as long-term memory. Your body produces a variety of different hormones that impact your mood, appetite, and overall sense of well-being the next day. Your immune system is recharged to protect your body from sickness. Your brain is rested and renewed. Sleep is like a physical and emotional makeover to help you to prepare for each new day.

SLEEP DEPRIVATION AND DISEASE

Not only does adequate sleep help you feel better on a day-to-day basis, it also lowers your risk for many diseases. Studies show that people who get an inadequate amount of sleep have increased risk for developing diabetes,[2] heart disease,[3] obesity,[4] and many other health problems.[5, 6] An article from Harvard School of Medicine explains a connection: "The thread that ties these together may be inflammation—the body's response to injury, infection, irritation, or disease. Poor sleep increases levels of C-reactive protein (CRP) and other substances that reflect active inflammation."[7]

Inadequate sleep increases the amount of calcium build-up in the arteries, promoting atherosclerosis.[8] Sleep deprivation also elevates blood pressure. One study found that missing just one hour of needed sleep each night increases the risk of high blood pressure by 37 percent.[9] Sleep deprivation also raises cortisol levels. This promotes high blood sugars, and increases insulin resistance.[10, 11]

Sleep deprivation also affects mental health. People who get adequate sleep are not as likely to suffer from mental illness, including depression or anxiety.[12] Sleep improves memory and mood, and helps promote an overall sense of mental well-being. Sleep also improves attention and mental processing.[13]

In general, good sound sleep reduces inflammation, lowers your risk of disease, boosts your immunity, and helps you to function optimally each day. Let's take a look at simple strategies you can follow to benefit from the powerful medicine of sleep.

1. SET THE RIGHT BEDTIME.

With regard to sleep, your two main goals should be *quality* and *quantity*. Not only do you need a certain amount of sleep, but you also need that sleep to be of the best possible quality. Benjamin Franklin hit the nail on the head when he wrote, "Early to bed and early to rise makes a man healthy, wealthy, and wise." Writing in the 1700s, Franklin didn't have our modern scientific evidence to support an early bedtime—he just knew from experience that it was true.

My personal bedtime is 10 p.m. I can tell a big difference in how I feel the next day, depending on whether I stick to that bedtime. Sleeping from 10 p.m. to 6 a.m. leaves me much more rested than sleeping from 11 p.m. to 7 a.m. The hours of sleep before midnight are deeper and more valuable to the body than the hours after midnight.

Sleep is a complex process that involves multiple stages and cycles. Going to bed early will increase the amount of time you spend in stage 3 and 4 sleep—the deepest and most restorative sleep.[14] During these stages tissues repair and grow and important hormones are released. Because sleep before midnight is so valuable, I recommend that my adult patients choose a bedtime somewhere between 9 p.m. and 10 p.m.

In one study, people who were accustomed to going to bed at 10 p.m. went to bed at 3 a.m. instead. The next morning, the participants' immune function was suppressed by more than 50 percent.[15] This made them much more susceptible to illness.

In addition to setting an early bedtime, it's also important to set a wake-up time. Most adults need between seven and eight hours of sleep per night. Children need roughly ten hours of sleep and teenagers need about nine.

Once you pick a bedtime and a waking time, it's important to stick to it. The body thrives on consistency and regularity. Just like the earth rotates on a 24-hour cycle, the body is also designed to follow a 24-hour pattern. This pattern is called the circadian rhythm. It's an internal body clock that helps to regulate sleep, activity, energy levels, and more. Following regularly scheduled patterns for eating, sleeping, exercising, and other activities helps you stay in sync with your circadian rhythm, optimizing your energy and effectiveness.

2. OPTIMIZE YOUR SLEEP ENVIRONMENT.

The best place to sleep is in a dark room that is slightly cool and quiet. Sleeping in the dark boosts the body's production of melatonin,[16] a hormone that enhances sleep and immunity. Melatonin must be produced each night since it is not stored.

Sleeping with a light on at night, or sleeping during the daytime instead of at night, significantly suppresses the production of melatonin.[17] This helps explain why people who work late-night shifts and sleep during the day are at a significantly higher risk for developing diabetes,[18] cancer,[19, 20] and many other diseases.[21]

Room temperature is also important. Studies have shown that 60 to 68 degrees Fahrenheit is the best temperature for sleep.[22] It helps to decrease the core temperature of the body, inducing sleepiness. When possible, it's better to breathe in cold air while using extra blankets than to sleep in a warm room.

Be sure that your sleep environment is quiet. If circumstances beyond your control cause extra noise (i.e., noisy neighbors or kids), try using "white noise" to help drown out the other noise. For example, you might turn on your ceiling fan or use a white noise machine to help you sleep.

3. WIND DOWN BEFORE BEDTIME.

One reason so many people find it difficult to sleep is that their minds are over-stimulated—still processing and thinking about the events of the day. It's important to allow both your body and your mind to relax before bedtime. Try to end your usual responsibilities at least 30 minutes to an hour before bedtime. You might take a warm bath, read a book, or dim the lights to prepare for sleep. Avoid watching TV or working on your computer or smart phone before sleep, as backlit devices stimulate the brain and decrease the amount of melatonin production.[23]

4. EXERCISE.

While many insomniacs turn to sleeping pills to induce rest, exercise offers a safer, healthier way to improve sleep. Aerobic exercise is especially beneficial. It puts a healthy strain on the heart and muscles, which helps induce tiredness when it's time to go to sleep. Exercise also helps boost melatonin production and optimize the circadian rhythm. Studies have shown that exercise helps people to fall asleep faster, stay asleep easier, and remain in stage 4 sleep—deep, restorative sleep—for longer periods of time.[24, 25]

To get these benefits, it's best to exercise in the morning or early afternoon. Exercising in the evening close to bedtime actually interferes with sleep for most people. Aim to complete any vigorous exercise at least a few hours before going to sleep. Light evening exercise such as walking will not interfere with sleep as will vigorous exercise.

5. AVOID A LATE MEAL.

In Chapter 14, I discussed the importance of eating a big breakfast, a medium lunch, and a small supper. Many people eat the majority of their calories at the evening meal, however, which is a recipe for weight gain and sleep disturbances.

At the end of the day, the body's energy requirements are low. The digestive organs, along with the other organs, need rest. A large meal late in the day impairs sleep quality and digestion, and may leave you feeling groggy the next morning. Try to make your evening meal the smallest of all your meals, and eat it no later than three to four hours before bedtime. (For those who have digestive concerns, five hours might be even better.)

6. GET BRIGHT LIGHT.

Exposure to bright, natural light, especially early in the morning, can powerfully influence the time you spend asleep, as well as the time you spend awake! Early morning bright light exposure increases alertness, energy, and mental performance. If you are not a morning person and tend to feel tired or sluggish unless you've had a cup of coffee, try going outside instead. You can energize your day naturally with early morning sunlight. The best thing to do when you wake up is to immediately go outside and get some sunshine. This sunlight sends a signal to your body's internal clock that the day has started and it's time to wake up. That same internal clock will remind you that it's bedtime about 16 hours later.[26]

Natural light in the day—especially in the morning—stimulates more melatonin production at night, causing sleep to be deep and restorative.[27]

THE CURE FOR JET LAG

As part of my professional training, I completed an internship in the small country of Singapore. Because Singapore was 15 hours ahead of the Pacific Time Zone where I was from, I knew I was headed for some serious jet lag. I flew out of Los Angeles, had a layover in Seoul, Korea, and finally made it to Singapore late at night—local time. I was exhausted and eager to go to sleep.

A doctor from the hospital picked me up at the airport and took me to where I would be staying. "Tomorrow morning we're having a 5K race to promote wellness in the community and to raise money for the hospital," he told me. "You're welcome to join us. It starts at 7 a.m.!"

On the inside, I groaned. After an exhausting trip, the thought of waking up early to go running sounded utterly miserable. However, I had come to the hospital as a lifestyle medicine intern, and I knew that not participating would make a bad first impression. "Sure, that sounds great!" I said. "I'll see you bright and early."

The next morning, I slowly rolled out of bed and headed to the race. It was one of the most miserable short runs of my life. Singapore is close to the equator, and the weather is hot and humid. The president of the hospital was there, as well as several other influential people. I didn't want to look like a wimp, so I ran hard and tried to make it look easy. But on the inside I felt like my chest was going to explode. It was a relief to cross the finish line.

Although the run was tiring, it was the best thing I could have done. It essentially eliminated my jet lag. That night I was ready to go to sleep, and the next morning I woke up refreshed and ready to start the day. My body was right on schedule. I didn't even notice the time difference.

I later learned that exercising in the bright light first thing in the morning is the best way to reset your circadian rhythm. It's a simple cure for jet lag. Even more importantly, because many people have circadian rhythm disturbances even when they aren't traveling, this strategy can help to optimize your sleep/wake cycles regardless of where you are.

7. TAKE A CAT NAP—OR NO NAP AT ALL.

If you are doing your best to optimize your sleep at night but still find that you are tired during the day, short power naps may boost your energy and improve your concentration and mood. Long naps, especially late in the afternoon, are a recipe for sleeplessness at bedtime. If you are going to nap, it's best to do it in the late morning or early afternoon, and it's important not to sleep too long. A short 20 to 30 minute nap at the right time of day can boost your energy without interfering with your night-time sleep.

8. AVOID STIMULANTS AND DEPRESSANTS.

I grew up in a health-conscious family that didn't drink caffeine. Because I was interested in wellness, this never bothered me, and I was thankful that my parents raised me that way. Once I was old enough to make my own decisions, I still chose to avoid caffeinated drinks.

My freshman year of college I took a class called "Drugs, Society, and Behavior." In that class, I learned that caffeine is actually a speed learning drug that helps its users learn a large amount of information at once. Although I found that information interesting, I still knew that caffeine wasn't healthy, so I continued to avoid it.

As my first quarter was coming to a close, however, I was troubled to realize that I had B's in all my classes. It had been an exciting transition switching from high school to college, and I hadn't put enough effort into school. Because my goal was to go on to professional training after college, I wanted to keep my GPA high, so I knew I needed to get my grades up. Final exams were coming up soon, and I knew I needed to do well to make up for being a slacker.

I remembered the information about caffeine and speed learning, and I made a hasty decision to see if it would work for me. Finals week arrived, and I was fortunate enough to have my exams spread throughout the week. I had five morning exams, one each day. The afternoon before my first exam, I went to the grocery store and bought six-packs of several varieties of soda—Mountain Dew,® Coke,® Pepsi,® etc. I sat down to study and feverishly crammed an enormous amount of information into my head while sipping on my soda. I studied until 2 a.m. After sleeping for a few short hours, I got up and went to take my test. I was relieved to know that I knew almost all of the answers from cramming the previous day.

After heading back to my room and crashing for a few hours, I started the process all over again for my second test. I repeated this cycle for the entire week—cramming with caffeine late into the night, and doing very well on all my tests. In fact, I did so well that all my grades came up to A's.

But it didn't come without a cost. As each day went by, I realized that it was getting more and more difficult to bounce back. By the end of my last test, I felt like a zombie. For more than a week after the tests were over, I was completely burned out. Normally a very structured person, I couldn't understand why I had lost my ambition and determination to be healthy and productive. All I wanted to do was to sit around, watch TV, and eat junk food. I was depressed and irritable—not enjoying life at all.

I promised myself that I would never repeat the same mistake. I knew the reason I had B's in the first place was because I hadn't put enough effort into my classes over the past several months. Although my final exams boosted my grades, it was at the expense of my health. I had borrowed energy and vitality from my future to use it up for my tests. A week later, I still felt terrible.

I also realized that I hadn't really learned anything. Even two days after the tests, I couldn't remember what I had studied. While caffeine is a speed-learning drug, the information stays only in the short-term memory. I made a decision then that I never wanted to sell my health or my education to buy a good grade. Instead, I would earn good grades consistently and healthfully.

I did my best to follow that rule from that point on, and was much happier with the results.

Nine years later, as I was finishing the last quarter of my doctoral program, I watched my friends and classmates make the same mistake I had previously made. As we prepared for final exams, many of them loaded up on caffeine to survive. Remembering my previous experience, I decided to remain caffeine free. After taking my last test, I went home and relaxed in our backyard pool. A friend came by, carrying a 32-ounce Coke and a candy bar. As I watched him enjoy his junk food, I started feeling sorry for myself. I'd been missing out. Tests were over and I'd been "good" for so long. It was time to reward all my hard work. "Just this once," I told myself.

I went to the gas station down the street and bought a 32-ounce bottle of Pepsi and a candy bar. Heading back to the pool, I relaxed in the sun—chugging down the soda and savoring every gooey, chocolaty, candy-bar bite. It went down so easy.

Within minutes, I realized I'd made a big mistake. I could tell things were about to go sour. I couldn't sleep that night. I felt anxious and antsy. The following day I felt drained. The cycle continued for the next three days. I was once again reminded of the negative effects of caffeine in robbing me of my health and vitality.

CAFFEINE AND CREDIT

"But I drink caffeine all the time," you may say. "That's never happened to me." I admit that my caffeine symptoms may have been a bit more dramatic than most people experience. However, if you consume caffeine, you too are robbing your body of health and vitality. Caffeine compromises your quality of sleep and damages your body.[28]

Drinking caffeine is like living on credit. Instead of living within your means, you are borrowing from your future. Chronic use of caffeine and other stimulants forces the adrenal glands to overwork.[29] The adrenals are the "fight-or-flight" organs. They produce hormones that provide us with energy and help us respond to stressful situations. When the adrenal glands are overworked they eventually become fatigued. And when they become fatigued, so do you.

I've seen many patients whose adrenal glands are so fatigued that they barely have the energy to make it through a normal day, much less a crisis. This decreases immunity and energy and increases the risk of infection and disease.

The regular use of caffeine and other stimulants is a slow and insidious way to compromise health. While sleep is designed to restore the body and improve immunity, caffeine is the antithesis of sleep. It may provide a short-lived pick-me-up, but it eventually leads to fatigue and premature aging.

ALCOHOL AND SLEEP

The idea that alcohol improves sleep is simply a myth. Although alcohol may induce sleep initially, it interferes with the quality of sleep and prevents deep, restorative stages of sleep from occurring.[30] It also causes people to awaken more frequently after the relaxing effect of the drug has worn off. Nighttime alcohol consumption leads to daytime fatigue. People who struggle with alcoholism are more likely to suffer from a sleep disorder than people who do not drink.[31]

Not only does alcohol interfere with sleep, but it also has other negative effects on blood sugar management and health. Drinking may lead to a severe hypoglycemic crisis for people on insulin or oral diabetes medications.[32] Excess alcohol consumption contributes to the "metabolic mess" we discussed in Chapter 3 by raising triglyceride levels and promoting abdominal obesity. [33]

But perhaps the most damaging effect of alcohol is how it impacts the mind. Alcohol lowers inhibition and causes people to make poor choices they wouldn't otherwise have made if they were sober. To be in control of your health, you need to be in control of your mind. For this reason, I encourage my patients to avoid the use of alcohol.

SMOKING/TOBACCO

Nicotine also contributes to sleep disturbance and insomnia. Smokers are four times more likely to report feeling unrested after sleep than people who don't smoke.[34] Like alcohol, smoking decreases the amount of time spent in deep, restorative sleep, causing sleep to be shallow and less beneficial.

Tobacco also wreaks havoc on the body in numerous other ways. Smokers are 50 percent more likely to develop diabetes than nonsmokers, and heavy smokers are at an even higher risk.[35] According to the CDC, more deaths are caused each year by smoking than by HIV, illegal drug use, alcohol use, car accidents, suicides, and murders—*combined*.[36] Smoking more than doubles the risk for heart disease and stroke.[37] It accounts for 80 to 90 percent of all lung cancer deaths and 90 percent of all COPD deaths.[38] Smoking is bad news for diabetes and for health in general. Interestingly, the same strategies that help with diabetes reversal also help with smoking cessation.

MANAGING STRESS

We live in a society of stress. Many of us suffer from insomnia because our lives are burdened with anxiety and pressure. Sleep and stress are closely connected. Lack of sleep can cause stress, and stress can cause a lack of sleep. It's important to learn healthy ways to cope with stress. If your worries keep you up at night, it's time to address the problem. You may need to cut back on your responsibilities, or to find a friend or counselor you can talk to. These are a few stress management strategies that have helped me personally:

- Sound sleep
- Regular exercise
- Good nutrition
- Sunlight
- Social support
- Time management
- Learning to say "no" when necessary
- Taking time to do things I enjoy
- Faith and prayer
- Regularly scheduled rest (not just sleep, but rest)

REST

Sleep and rest are not the same thing. Sleep is one form of rest, but there are other important ways to rest and relax. It's important to take time to rest even when you are awake. Rest doesn't necessarily mean that you have to be still. It simply means that you allow your brain to unplug and unwind while doing things that help restore you physically, emotionally, and spiritually. I encourage you to set aside a little time each day for a restful, relaxing activity that you enjoy. It could be reading a book, taking a bath, sitting in the sun, journaling, praying, or spending time with someone you love.

One of my favorite health strategies is to devote one day out of each week to rest. I call this my Sabbath and observe it each Saturday. On that day, I don't do any of my usual work or activities. Instead, I enjoy spending time with God, with my family, and in nature. I have found it to be a very rewarding habit that has significantly improved my health.

CHAPTER SUMMARY

- Sleep is powerful medicine. Adequate sleep is never a waste of time.
- Sleep is an active process. During sleep:
  - Muscles and tissues are repaired.
  - Memory is stored.
  - Important hormones are released.
  - The immune system is recharged.
  - The brain and other organs are rested and renewed.
- Sleep deprivation increases the risk of many diseases, including heart disease and diabetes.
- Sleep deprivation promotes insulin resistance, raises blood sugars, and causes inflammation.
- There are simple things you can do to optimize your sleep:
  - Set a regular bedtime and waking time.
  - Get to sleep early.
  - Optimize your sleeping environment.
  - Wind down and relax before bedtime.
  - Exercise early in the day.
  - Avoid eating a late meal.
  - Get bright light exposure, especially in the early morning.
  - Keep naps short and take them in the morning or early afternoon.
  - Avoid stimulants such as caffeine and energy drinks or pills.
  - Find healthy ways to manage your stress.
  - Find ways to rest—physically, emotionally, and spiritually.

—EIGHTEEN—

Stay Well Hydrated

Water is the only drink for a wise man.
—Henry David Thoreau

IT WAS A PARENT'S WORST NIGHTMARE. FIFTEEN-YEAR-old Troy Driscoll and seventeen-year-old Josh Long were lost at sea.[1,2] The best friends had set out on Sunday morning, April 24, 2005, in a small sailboat to fish for sharks off the coast of Sullivan's Island, South Carolina. They were unaware that the Coast Guard had forecasted a powerful rip tide in that very spot. Shortly after launching, they were caught in the current and carried far out into the ocean. With no food, no water, and no way to communicate for help, the boys were in serious trouble.

For the next six days, Troy and Josh survived cold weather, extreme hunger, lurking sharks, severe sunburn, and dehydration. Day after day they struggled to survive. They prayed and sang hymns. Troy ate jellyfish he caught, while Josh gargled salt water just to get some moisture in his mouth. Losing hope for a rescue, they began carving goodbye messages to family and friends into the wood of the boat.

Miraculously, on April 30—almost a week after they had set out—the boys were discovered by a fishing vessel. They were rushed to emergency medical care and treated for severe dehydration. Josh had lost over 40 pounds.

Physicians reported that the boys couldn't have survived more than a few more hours at sea.

The average person can survive approximately four to six weeks without eating, but only one week without water. Troy and Josh almost lost their lives to dehydration. Their story reminds us how very fragile life is, and how absolutely necessary it is to drink adequate amounts of water.

WATER—THE MIRACLE MOLECULE

The human body is made up of 60 percent water.[3] Every cell, tissue, and organ in your body needs water to survive. According to the Mayo Clinic, the average adult loses 10 cups of water each day through breathing, sweating, urinating, and eliminating waste.[4] This water must be continually replaced to prevent dehydration. Virtually all of the body's systems depend on water. It is the most important of all nutrients. Eighty-three percent of your blood is water, and adequate hydration is essential for proper circulation and health.[5]

ADEQUATE HYDRATION:

- Cleanses the body and removes wastes
- Optimizes circulation
- Lowers inflammation
- Carries nutrients and oxygen to cells
- Improves digestion
- Helps manage weight
- Increases alertness and memory
- Aids in immunity and prevents sickness
- Helps regulate body temperature
- Lubricates and cushions joints

THE DEHYDRATION EPIDEMIC

Many Americans suffer from symptoms of chronic, mild dehydration. It isn't because they don't have access to clean drinking water (like 20 percent of the world's population).[6] It's because they simply forget to drink it. Chronic dehydration causes a variety of physical problems, including a significantly increased risk for heart attack or stroke.

EFFECTS OF DEHYDRATION

- Increased risk for heart attack or stroke
- Fatigue or sluggishness
- Irritability
- Headaches
- Constipation
- Decreased mental performance
- Dry skin and lips
- Overeating / unhealthy cravings
- Increased build up of toxins
- Urinary tract infections
- Stress on kidneys
- Increased risk for injury
- Joint pain
- Premature aging

WATER AND YOUR HEART

People who are dehydrated are twice as likely to have a heart attack or stroke as people who are well hydrated.[7] This helps to explain why heart attacks are three times more likely to occur in the morning hours, when the body is the most dehydrated.[8]

Dehydration increases the viscosity (thickness) of the blood. Thick, sludgy blood is much more likely to form clots than well-hydrated blood. These clots can cause obstructions in the blood vessels—causing a heart attack or stroke.

Because heart disease is the number one (and most dangerous) complication associated with diabetes, it's especially important for people with diabetes or prediabetes to drink plenty of water. Adequate hydration also helps to prevent or reduce other diabetes-related complications.

WATER AND BLOOD SUGARS

People with very high blood sugars have increased risk of dehydration. When the body detects excess sugar in the blood, it dumps this sugar into the urine. The sugar takes water with it, leaving the body dehydrated. That's why diabetics have increased risk for dehydration and its complications—just one more reason why it's important to follow natural strategies to manage your blood sugars!

Not only can high blood sugars cause dehydration, but dehydration may also contribute to high blood sugars. In one French study following over 3,600 people, those who drank 34 ounces of water each day were 21 percent less likely to develop diabetes over 9 years than those who drank 16 ounces or less.[9] This may be explained in part by the hormone vasopressin. When you are dehydrated, your body releases vasopressin, an anti-diuretic hormone that causes your body to conserve water. Some studies have shown that vasopressin also increases blood sugars.[10] The connection between dehydration and high blood sugars needs to be researched further, but these findings suggest that adequate water intake will help lower your blood sugars.

WATER AND WEIGHT

In Chapter 16, I mentioned the connection between water and weight. Water helps reduce cravings and keeps you satisfied between meals. People who are dehydrated often mistake thirst for hunger and respond by eating. When you feel the urge to eat something between your regular meals, drink water instead. Chances are your cravings will soon diminish. This will also help you to manage your weight and blood sugar levels.

HOW MUCH WATER TO DRINK

Your body loses water every day as you breathe, sweat, and go to the bathroom. This water must be consistently replaced to prevent dehydration. But how much water is enough? And is it possible to drink too much water?

One day an urgent care doctor who works near my office stopped by for a casual visit between patients. He asked, "How much water do you tell your patients to drink?" I replied that it depends on the patient and how healthy their diet is, but that an optimal amount for most people is 8 to 10 cups per day.

"That's good," he replied. "I just had a patient come into urgent care who was fasting from food and only drinking water. She had drunk so much water that her blood was diluted and she had an electrolyte imbalance. After giving her electrolytes in an IV, I told her about water intoxication and advised her not to drown herself."

Water intoxication does exist, but it's very rare. Almost all water intoxication deaths are caused by people competing in water-drinking contests, or by extreme athletes who did not replace lost electrolytes during long periods of exercise, but kept hydrating. It's almost unheard of to get water intoxication by accidentally drinking too much water, especially if you're eating a healthy diet. In fact, most of us have the opposite problem. Far more deaths are caused by, or related to, dehydration than water intoxication.

Most adults need about 8 to 10 cups of water per day to function optimally. This amount can vary, however, depending on your size, activity level, and environment. If you are exercising heavily or are in a hot climate, your water need will be higher.

One rule of thumb is to drink half an ounce of water for every pound that you weigh. For example, a 150-pound person should drink 75 ounces (about 9 cups) of water each day, while a 90-pound person should drink 45 ounces (about 6 cups). Again, this amount varies somewhat for each person.

The amount of water you need also depends on your diet. A healthy diet helps you stay well hydrated. Fruits and vegetables have high water content, while junk foods tend to dehydrate the body and introduce toxins into the system. People who eat a lot of junk food need to drink even more water than those who eat healthfully.

One way to evaluate whether you're adequately hydrated is to pay attention to the color of your urine. It should be clear or slightly yellow. Dark yellow or amber urine indicates dehydration.

WHEN TO DRINK

We've discussed optimal times for eating and sleeping. There are also optimal (and not so optimal) times for drinking water. The two most important tips to remember are:

1. Drink water when you wake up.
2. Drink water between meals.

DRINK WATER WHEN YOU WAKE UP

The body is least hydrated in the morning. This is the most important time to drink water. During the night, we lose water from sweating, breathing, and urine production. Nighttime dehydration increases risk for heart attack (as well as all other potential side effects of dehydration).

The best way to combat morning dehydration is to drink water as soon as you wake up. I encourage my patients to drink 1 to 2 cups of warm water first thing in the morning. This helps optimize your circulation and cleanse your body. It also boosts your energy and alertness throughout the morning.

Another benefit of drinking water early in the morning is that it helps prevent constipation. Drinking warm water first thing in the morning often stimulates a bowel movement and helps you stay regular all day.

Several years ago, I was giving a lecture on the value of water for optimizing immune function and improving circulation. A man in the back of the room raised his hand and made an interesting comment. "My father was a railroad engineer," he said. "He had a strict schedule with brief stops at multiple train stations. He was always required to be on time and didn't have time for bathroom breaks. My father and the other people he worked with knew that if they were going to have a bowel movement that day, they needed to do it before getting on the train. Their secret was to drink a tall glass of hot water first thing in the morning."

DRINK BETWEEN MEALS

In Chapter 14, I mentioned the importance of drinking water between meals instead of with meals. Many of my patients have experienced digestive improvements by minimizing the amount of fluid they drink with meals. If you stay hydrated between meals, you won't need to drink water at mealtime.

However, if you come to a meal and know that you are dehydrated, it's better to drink with the meal and avoid further dehydration than not to drink with the meal for digestive reasons. The key is to plan ahead and stay hydrated enough throughout the day so you don't need to drink with your meals. You may not need to give up fluids with your meal completely. Drinking a small amount of fluid with a meal should not have as negative an impact as drinking several cups.

After drinking your morning water, wait at least 20 to 30 minutes before eating breakfast. Drink two to three cups of water mid-morning (at least 90 minutes after breakfast), and then mid-afternoon (at least 90 minutes after lunch). You can also drink water in the evening, but don't drink so much right before bed that it interferes with your sleep.

STAYING HYDRATED

- Drink 1 to 2 cups of warm water when you first wake up.
- Hydrate between meals.
- Stop drinking water 20 to 30 minutes before your meal.
- Wait 90 minutes after your meal to drink again.

As with all the other strategies in this book, it's important to be consistent. You can't make up for lost time by drinking a lot of water in one sitting. Follow a schedule and soon it will become a habit. As you become better hydrated, you will notice improvements in your energy level and mood.

OBEY YOUR PLAN—NOT YOUR THIRST

While training for my first competitive triathlon, I wanted to plan ahead to stay well hydrated. The race consisted of running 10 miles, biking 50 miles, and swimming 1 mile. I mentioned my concern about hydration to my doctor. I knew that he was familiar with exercise physiology and that he would have good advice. "Wes," he said, "if you get thirsty out there, you've already lost the race."

My doctor knew that thirst isn't a reliable guide for determining how much water to drink. Thirst only occurs when the cells have already been dehydrated for quite some time. If I waited to drink until I got thirsty, I would significantly decrease my performance.

This doesn't happen only during vigorous exercise. It happens every day. Thirst is a delayed response to dehydration. Instead of waiting to drink *until* you get thirsty, drink to *prevent* getting thirsty. That's why it's important to plan ahead and to stay on schedule when it comes to drinking water.

WHY WATER IS BEST

A trip to your local grocery store reveals that the beverage industry is booming. A wide variety of juices, sodas, coffees, teas, energy drinks, milks, and alcoholic beverages are readily available. With so many different options, plain old water can seem, well...boring. But from a nutritional standpoint, water is the best choice. Let's take a look at a few different types of beverages and see how they compare to water.

COFFEE

In Chapter 17, I told the story of my caffeine-fueled finals week and the lesson I learned about avoiding drinks that contain caffeine. Not only is coffee high in caffeine, which stresses your system and robs your body of future vitality, but it also causes dehydration[11] and can contribute to blood sugar problems.[12]

Some diabetics, including my former patient Luke, find that coffee causes significant and unexpected blood sugar changes. Luke, the ex-navy seal from Chapter 9, made tremendous progress toward reversing his diabetes. After going through our lifestyle program, Luke continued to follow the strategies he'd learned. A year after our program ended, Luke still had his blood sugars under excellent control. In fact, he no longer fit the diagnosable criteria for diabetes. However, Luke continued to monitor his blood sugars regularly to make sure he was aware of what was happening in his body.

One day, Luke was shocked when his blood sugar level was 200 one hour after breakfast. It was typically under 140. He exercised regularly, ate healthy foods, and consistently balanced his meals. Why would his blood sugar suddenly spike? Luke was alarmed when the high blood sugars continued for the next several days. He didn't understand how they could be so high when he was still following the program. Feeling defeated, he set up an appointment with his physician to see if he needed to start taking insulin again.

But Luke solved the mystery for himself. The next morning while eating breakfast, he noticed the gourmet coffee jar sitting on the counter. *That's what I've been doing differently,* he thought. *It must be the coffee!*

Luke had given up caffeine and coffee when he'd gone through our lifestyle program. For the past year, he had replaced his usual morning coffee with a mug of warm water instead. But a few days earlier, Luke's wife had been cleaning out some cupboards and had found a jar of gourmet coffee—an old gift from a family friend. They had decided to enjoy the coffee for old time's sake. Every morning that week, Luke drank a mug of coffee instead of his usual water.

Luke immediately stopped drinking the coffee and went back to his warm water routine. His blood sugars stabilized right away. Luke happily called the doctor's office to cancel his appointment.

Not everyone responds to coffee the same way, but many diabetics have reported coffee-induced blood sugar changes. It's important to carefully monitor your blood sugar levels to identify and eliminate those things that negatively impact you.

DEBUNKING THE COFFEE MYTH

Coffee-lovers rejoiced when they heard about a Harvard-affiliated study concluding that women who drank four or more cups of coffee each day were less likely to develop diabetes than those who did not drink coffee.[13] That means that drinking coffee must decrease the risk of diabetes, right?

Before jumping to that conclusion, it is important to take a closer look at the study. The patients I see who drink four or more cups of coffee a day generally have adrenal fatigue and hypoglycemia issues. They use coffee as a crutch to solve their low blood sugar and low energy problems. They may not develop diabetes, but they often have other serious health problems. And the study doesn't prove that you decrease your risk for diabetes by drinking *more* coffee.

SODA

Kentucky Fried Chicken® (KFC) recently started a fundraising campaign to help fight diabetes. It challenged customers to purchase a half-gallon "mega jug" of soda with their meals for $2.99, and KFC would donate $1.00 to the Juvenile Diabetes Foundation to aid in finding a cure for diabetes.

Unfortunately, KFC's mega jug of soda does more to contribute to diabetes than it does to help find a cure. Soda is full of empty calories that fuel the metabolic mess and wreak havoc on blood sugar levels. Regular soda consumption increases the risk of obesity, diabetes, heart disease, and stroke.

DIET SODA

Once the soda industry realized that health-conscious consumers weren't excited about empty soda calories, they decided to come up with a new strategy—diet soda. Diet soda is calorie free, which means no weight gain and no negative health consequences, right? Wrong! Believe it or not, diet soda is actually worse for your health than regular soda.[14] It causes weight gain and increases risk of heart disease.[15, 16] Artificial sweeteners in diet soda also have been associated with increased risk of cancer.[17]

Many find this difficult to understand. If it doesn't have calories, how could it promote weight gain and disease? Artificial sweeteners are like toxic chemicals or drugs. Certain drugs promote weight gain and have other side effects. The drug itself doesn't contain any calories, but it causes changes in the body that promote weight gain and disease. I encourage everyone to avoid diet sodas as well as any other artificially sweetened foods. In fact, while neither beverage is ideal, I believe that regular soda is actually preferable to diet soda. The good news is that you don't have to choose between the two. You can choose the best option—pure, clean water!

JUICE

Fruit juice that is 100 percent juice is a better option than soda or diet soda. It contains healthy vitamins and minerals found in the original fruit. It doesn't, however, contain the healthy roughage and fiber found in whole fruit. This makes it easy to consume excess calories by drinking too much juice. In addition, juice contains highly concentrated fruit sugars that can cause rapid spikes in blood sugar levels.

If you have any tendency toward blood sugar spikes or other metabolic problems, be especially careful to limit the amount of juice you drink. It's okay to occasionally drink a small amount of fruit juice with a well-balanced meal (maybe 1/2 cup). Make sure that you don't drink juice between meals though, as this can spike your blood sugars.

ALCOHOL

Alcohol is bad news for diabetes and for your health in general. Not only does alcohol contain empty calories your body doesn't need, but it also contributes to the "metabolic mess" and promotes obesity (see Chapter 3). In addition, we learned in Chapter 17 that alcohol has a negative impact on sleep and contributes to poor blood sugar management.

Perhaps the most damaging effect of alcohol is its impact on the mind. Alcohol lowers inhibition and increases the tendency to make poor choices. To be in control of your health, you need to be in control of your mind.

DEBUNKING THE ALCOHOL MYTH

You've probably heard that drinking alcohol, particularly red wine, will improve cardiovascular health. This popular myth has been embraced by the public and touted by the alcohol industry. However, it's not supported by science.

Studies used in defense of this theory have been misrepresented and misunderstood. When comparing the heart health of "drinkers" versus "nondrinkers," the researchers did not take into account that many of the "nondrinkers" were former alcoholics or people who had serious health problems that kept them from drinking. Because ex-problem drinkers have high rates of heart disease and many other diseases, the results were significantly skewed.

More recent studies have disproved this theory by showing that people who drink alcohol do not have any cardiovascular advantage over people who have never drunk alcohol.[18]

Let's take a look at the official position of the American Heart Association on the connection between alcohol and cardiovascular health:

> "Over the past several decades many studies have been published in science journals about how drinking alcohol may be associated with reduced mortality due to heart disease in some populations.... The linkage reported in many of these studies may be due to other lifestyle factors rather than alcohol. Such factors may include increased physical activity, and a diet high in fruits and vegetables and lower in saturated fats. No direct comparison trials have been done to determine the specific effect of wine or other alcohol on the risk of developing heart disease or stroke.... The American Heart Association does not recommend drinking wine or any other form of alcohol."[19]

CHOOSING THE BEST

Other beverages simply can't compete with the health benefits of pure, clean water. It's what we were designed to drink. By making regular water drinking a habit, you can increase your energy and improve your health.

CHAPTER SUMMARY

- Water is the most important nutrient.
- Adequate hydration is essential for good health.
- Adequate hydration:
  - Cleanses the body and removes wastes
  - Optimizes circulation
  - Lowers inflammation
  - Carries nutrients and oxygen to cells
  - Improves digestion
  - Helps with weight management
  - Increases alertness and memory
  - Aids in immunity and prevents sickness
  - Helps regulate body temperature
  - Lubricates and cushions the joints
- 75 percent of Americans suffer from chronic, mild dehydration.
- Dehydration increases risk for all diabetes-related complications, including heart attack and stroke.
- High blood sugar levels cause dehydration, and dehydration contributes to high blood sugar levels.
- Most adults need 8 to 10 cups of water per day.
- Your urine color can indicate your hydration status.
- The best times to drink are when you first wake up, and between meals.
- Thirst isn't an adequate guide. Follow your plan, not your thirst.

—NINETEEN—

Soak up the Sun

Truly the light is sweet, and it is a pleasant thing
for the eyes to behold the sun.
—King Solomon

TRADITIONAL JAPANESE WOMEN ARE AFRAID OF GETTING a tan. Pale skin is seen as a symbol of status, while freckles, sunspots, and tan skin are considered unattractive. UV-blocking umbrellas, SPF 50+ sunscreen, and colorful hats and scarves are used to protect the skin from the sun.

Aya was no exception. This middle-aged woman had left Japan years before, and now owned a successful consulting firm on Guam. Every morning she would slather herself with sunscreen, put on a hat and sunglasses, and make a mad dash from her front door to her car to commute to work. Afraid of the effect the tropical sun would have on her skin and health, Aya wanted to completely avoid all direct exposure. She stayed indoors as much as possible and made elaborate plans to protect her skin when she did have to go outdoors. Whenever she felt the sun's warmth on her skin, Aya felt like she was in a microwave oven. She imagined all the damage the sun was causing to her skin and body.

Aya came to me for help with digestive issues. She also shared that she was suffering from significant anxiety despite the fact that her business was going well. Her lab tests revealed that she had multiple hormonal imbalances and an extremely low vitamin D level.

I immediately started Aya on a vitamin D supplement. I also encouraged her to come to a lecture I was giving on the benefits of vitamin D and sunlight. Aya was resistant to the idea at first, but was so desperate to improve her health that she decided to come. I noticed that Aya had a bewildered and perplexed look on her face as she listened to my lecture. After it was over, I greeted her and asked if she had any questions.

"I'm very confused," she said. "I've always been told to avoid the sun for cosmetic reasons as well as for my health. My entire life I've avoided the sun as much as possible. And now you're saying that I have to get sun exposure to be healthy?"

I explained to Aya that, while it is important to use moderation and to avoid overexposure, sunlight can help decrease anxiety, improve digestion, lower risk for disease, and further boost vitamin D levels. I encouraged her to begin exercising outdoors in the fresh air. Although the advice seemed counterintuitive, Aya was eager to feel better, so she began going outside in the sun.

We met several times during the next few months, and Aya's health and outlook improved dramatically. Her vitamin D level rose from 12 to 53, her digestive problems subsided, and a sense of peace and well-being replaced her usual anxiety.

At one of her follow-up visits, Aya told me what she had initially thought of my advice. "I have to admit, Dr. Youngberg," she said, "the first time you mentioned the importance of regular sun exposure I thought to myself, *How could someone so well-educated and apparently credible be so foolish as to think that it's a good thing to be in the sun? Everyone knows that you're supposed to stay away from the sun!* But I'm so glad I gave your advice a chance. I feel much better! I can't believe that it took 50 years for someone to finally tell me the truth!"

MY WATERSHED MOMENT

Like Aya, I learned about the benefits of sunlight and vitamin D late in life—I actually had the same problem. It wasn't that I had avoided the sun like Aya, but I hadn't understood until just a few years before what a powerful impact sunlight and vitamin D could have on a person's health.

About ten years ago, I stumbled upon an article in the health section of my local newspaper. I have always read a lot to keep up-to-date on the latest research, looking for new approaches to help my patients. In the wellness field, there are a wide variety of lab tests available to evaluate patients. At that time, I believed that I had developed a comprehensive and thorough testing system. But I was in for a surprise.

That day, I read an article interviewing a Harvard physician who described the connection between vitamin D and cancer. He had conducted a meta-analysis (i.e., combining and analyzing the results of numerous previous studies) to determine whether low vitamin D levels were associated with increased rates of cancer. After explaining the results of his study, he made a statement that completely shocked me: "This evidence shows that inadequate levels of vitamin D are more strongly associated with increased cancer risk than smoking is."

I could hardly believe what I had read. I read the statement again, and then a third time to make sure I understood it correctly. I had been involved in numerous community health programs to help people stop smoking. I was well aware of the significant connection between tobacco and cancer. But this well-documented, scientifically sound article was showing that low vitamin D levels were more strongly associated with increased cancer than smoking!

I had never heard such powerful evidence about the importance of vitamin D. *Where have I been all of these years?* I thought to myself. *I'm supposed to keep up with all this stuff!* All throughout my professional career, I heard that it was important to avoid too much sun exposure because it would cause cancer. Now I was reading that *inadequate* sun exposure increased the risk of cancer more than smoking!

As I began to further research its health benefits, I discovered that vitamin D plays an enormous role—not only in cancer prevention, but in essentially every facet of our health. Excited about this new information, I wanted to put it into practice. That same week, I began ordering vitamin D tests for my patients. I soon started testing the vitamin D levels of every single patient and have done so ever since.

I was surprised by the test results of my patients. I had assumed that, on the sunny, tropical island of Guam, everyone would have an optimal vitamin D level, but the tests showed differently. The vast majority of my patients had inadequate levels of vitamin D. I was no exception. I certainly thought I would be in a healthy range. I lived right next to the beach and spent a lot of time exposed to bright sunlight, but my vitamin D level was only 25—about half of what it should have been. I now live and practice in sunny Southern California. Despite the weather, the vast majority of my patients are vitamin D deficient when they are first tested.

Between 1988 and 2004, the rates of vitamin D deficiency in the United States skyrocketed from 55 to 77 percent.[1] At least 90 percent of the patients I test have vitamin D levels that I consider less than ideal.

I believe that testing and optimizing your vitamin D level is one of the most valuable contributions you can make to your health. It's a simple, painless, and inexpensive thing to do—yet the reward can be profound. In this chapter, I'll outline some of the many health benefits of vitamin D and describe how you can evaluate and optimize your level.

WHAT MAKES VITAMIN D SO IMPORTANT?

Vitamin D impacts nearly every aspect of your health. Research shows that people with adequate vitamin D levels are less likely to suffer from a variety of different diseases, including:[2]

- **Diabetes –** both type 1 and type 2
- **Cancer –** including breast, colon, prostate, lung, and many other forms
- **Cardiovascular Disease –** heart attacks, strokes, high blood pressure, and atherosclerosis
- **Kidney Disease**
- **Obesity –** especially abdominal fat
- **Common Sicknesses –** colds, flus, and upper respiratory infections
- **Bacterial Infections –** pneumonia, tuberculosis, MRSA
- **Musculoskeletal Disorders –** osteoporosis, weakened muscles, fractures
- **Autoimmune Disorders –** rheumatoid arthritis, lupus, multiple sclerosis, thyroid dysfunction
- **Mental Health Disorders –** depression, anxiety, bipolar disorder, hostility

How could one single nutrient be involved in so many different aspects of our health, reducing the risk for such a wide variety of diseases? It may seem too good to be true, but the weight of evidence shows that *it is*. Understanding the role vitamin D plays in the body will help us understand why its impact is so far-reaching.

HOW VITAMIN D WORKS

From gestation throughout the entire lifespan, vitamin D helps to facilitate proper growth, development, and maintenance of the human body. Vitamin D plays a major roll in the way our genes express information.

You may recall from Chapter 4 that each person has about 20,000 genes. These genes contain the information cells need to complete all bodily functions. Your heart beats because your body has followed a genetic code designed to develop cardiac tissue and blood vessels. The code also gives those tissues information on how to function. It influences every aspect of your health, from the way your body grows and develops to how it responds to disease.

A study in 2005 showed that more than 900 of the body's 20,000 genes are directly regulated by vitamin D. These genes contain valuable information to help the body enhance health and respond to disease. If vitamin D levels are adequate, genes function properly and the information is released. If levels are inadequate, the gene regulation is diminished, and the body misses out on valuable information. Vitamin D expert Dr. Robert Heaney describes vitamin D as "the key that unlocks the genetic library."[3] It provides the body with information it needs to fight disease.

Vitamin D doesn't force the body to do anything. It simply unlocks the genetic code that enables the body to do many of the things it needs to do for itself. That explains why such a wide variety of health conditions and diseases are so powerfully influenced by vitamin D. Let's take a closer look at a few of those conditions.

TYPE 1 DIABETES

Vitamin D deficiency significantly increases the risk of developing type 1 diabetes. A study from Finland, which evaluated 12,000 children for 20 years, revealed that those who were given 2,000 units of vitamin D every day from birth through adolescence were 80 percent less likely to develop type 1 diabetes than those who took less.[4]

Each year in the United States, roughly 30,000 people are newly diagnosed with type 1 diabetes. Imagine the public health impact of preventing 80 percent of new cases.[5] Adequate vitamin D levels could theoretically prevent 24,000 of these cases. If this information had been understood and followed in the past, instead of 3 million Americans currently suffering from type 1 diabetes, there might only be 600,000.[6]

Type 1 diabetes fits the profile of a disease caused by vitamin D deficiency. Rates of this disease are greatest in high latitude locations with diminished sun exposure.[7] Sunny countries with higher measurements of UVB (ultraviolet) radiance have lower rates of type 1 diabetes. New cases of this disease also appear more frequently in the winter months than in the summer.

Vitamin D fights infection and enhances the immune system.[8] This may be the main reason why it helps prevent type 1 diabetes, which is an autoimmune condition usually triggered by a virus or infection. As the immune system attempts to respond to the infection, it accidentally attacks the insulin-producing cells of the pancreas. Because vitamin D so powerfully protects and enhances the immune system, it decreases the chance that a virus or infection could ever become powerful enough to trigger an autoimmune response. This also explains why vitamin D has a powerful impact on many other autoimmune conditions.[9, 10]

TYPE 2 DIABETES

Vitamin D may also help in the prevention of type 2 diabetes. A Harvard study revealed that people taking more than 800 units of vitamin D per day, along with 1200 mg of calcium, were 33 percent less likely to develop type 2 diabetes than those supplementing with less than 400 units of vitamin D and less than 1200 mg of calcium.[11]

Another Finnish study revealed that men who had optimal vitamin D levels were 72 percent less likely to develop type 2 diabetes by age 50.[12] Additional studies have shown similar findings.[13]

Vitamin D decreases inflammation,[14] which is one of the main drivers of diabetes. Research suggests that vitamin D may also increase insulin production and insulin sensitivity.[15, 16, 17]

Not only can vitamin D help prevent both types of diabetes, it can also help improve the conditions if they already exist. By optimizing vitamin D levels, people with blood sugar problems can greatly reduce their risk for diabetes-related complications, including heart and kidney disease.[18]

While most people believe that only type 1 diabetes has an autoimmune component, many people who struggle with type 2 diabetes also have underlying autoimmune problems. For this reason, the immune-boosting benefit of vitamin D can help to prevent or improve both types of diabetes. I will discuss autoimmunity more fully in Chapter 22.

Sickness or infection can dramatically increase blood sugar levels for anyone with prediabetes or diabetes. Something as simple as having a cold or flu can cause dramatic changes in blood sugar levels. Vitamin D helps to prevent those spikes by stopping sickness in its tracks.

COLDS AND FLUS

"If you ask anybody who takes 5,000 units of vitamin D a day, they'll tell you they just don't get sick anymore. Colds and flus just don't happen." This is what Dr. John Cannell said in a video interview on the many benefits of vitamin D.[19] Dr. Cannell is the founder of the Vitamin D Council, and one of the top experts in his field.

He went on to explain why vitamin D protects against colds and flus. The immune system produces hundreds of natural antibiotics called antimicrobial peptides—"secret weapons" that fight infection and disease. For several decades, researchers have been looking for natural ways to increase the production of these immune-boosting substances. Research now shows that vitamin D significantly increases the production of these natural antibiotics.[20, 21]

This explains why people with adequate vitamin D levels are so much less likely to suffer from colds and flus than those with low levels of vitamin D.[22, 23]

CANCER

Cancer is the second leading cause of death in the United States.[24] Nearly 12 million Americans have or have had cancer.[25] Nearly 600,000 of these people are expected to die in 2012.[26] Cancer is a cruel, insidious disease that causes untold pain and suffering.

Imagine a drug that would prevent more than a third of all cancer cases in the United States. This drug would dominate the pharmaceutical industry, saving the lives of millions of Americans. While researchers continue to search for a cure, few people are aware that vitamin D, while not a drug, could actually have this kind of impact.

Dr. Cedric Garland, a vitamin D expert from the University of California, San Diego, estimates that increasing the average American's vitamin D level from 25 to 40 ng/mL could prevent at least 35 percent of all cases of cancer.[27, 28]

Dr. Garland has been studying the connection between cancer and vitamin D for more than 30 years. After learning that colon cancer is 3 times more prevalent in New York than it is in New Mexico, Garland, and his brother, Dr. Frank Garland, were curious to know why. The Garland brothers set out to discover whether it had anything to do with sunlight and vitamin D. They published their hypothesis in 1980 in the *International Journal of Epidemiology*.[29]

More than three decades later, a wealth of information continues to support this claim. Between 15 to 20 types of cancer have been found to be less prevalent in areas with increased sun exposure.[30] People with adequate levels of vitamin D are much less likely to develop cancer than those who are vitamin D deficient.[31]

Vitamin D causes epigenetic changes, turning off cancer-promoting genes and turning on cancer-fighting genes. In the quest to find a cure for cancer, vitamin D is certainly a step in the right direction.

BUT WHAT ABOUT SKIN CANCER?

One of the main reasons people avoid the sun or lather on sunscreen before going outside is their fear of developing skin cancer. Since the sunscreen movement started in the 1980s, many people have become afraid of direct sun exposure. In spite of the increased use of sunscreen, however, skin cancer rates have dramatically increased in the last 30 years.[32] If sun avoidance and sunscreen effectively solved the skin cancer problem, the opposite would have happened.

The risks of sunlight have been greatly exaggerated, and the benefits of sunlight have been minimized. It's important to understand the facts. While some forms of skin cancer can be caused by excessive sun exposure (sunburn), these are primarily the less serious forms of skin cancer—squamous cell and basal cell carcinomas.[33, 34] These forms of cancer are slow growing, can usually be easily removed, and have a very low death rate.[35]

Melanoma is the most dangerous type of skin cancer and has a much higher mortality rate than squamous cell and basal cell carcinomas.[36] Many people blame the sun for melanoma, but emerging evidence suggests that this is not the case.[37] Many melanomas actually occur in areas of the body that aren't even exposed to sunlight. Multiple studies have shown that *proper* sunlight exposure actually *decreases* risk of developing melanoma.[38, 39]

In one study of United States Navy workers, researchers found that those who worked exclusively indoors were almost twice as likely to develop melanoma as those who worked outdoors in the sunlight.[40] Not only does sunlight protect against melanoma, but it also can also help in treating it. People diagnosed with melanoma have better survival rates if they get regular sun exposure.[41, 42]

The benefits of sunlight clearly outweigh the risks. While you should avoid sunburn and should gradually work up your tolerance to the sun, prudent sun exposure can work wonders to improve your health. Proper nutrition and hydration can also minimize sun-associated skin cancer risk.[43]

But if the sun isn't to blame for most melanoma cases, what is? My own hypothesis is that some melanoma cases develop because of the consumption of meat that contains melanoma. When animals are killed for food, any visible areas of cancer are removed from their bodies. It's not economically feasible, however, to detect all skin cancers or to remove all of the tentacles of the cancer, which may have metastasized to areas where they are not visible.

HEART DISEASE

Vitamin D deficiency has also been linked to heart disease.[44] One Harvard study that followed over 18,000 men showed that those who were vitamin D deficient were twice as likely to have a heart attack as those with adequate levels of vitamin D.[45] Other studies have shown that vitamin D may help in controlling blood pressure[46] and preventing atherosclerosis.[47]

THE LIST GOES ON

I've described only a few of the many health conditions affected by vitamin D deficiency. This list is by no means exhaustive. As research continues, I believe more and more evidence will emerge regarding the countless positive benefits of vitamin D in disease prevention and treatment. Vitamin D doesn't just treat a specific disease. Instead, it treats the body as a whole, allowing it to optimize its healing potential. That's why vitamin D has such a wide variety of positive effects.

TAKING ADVANTAGE OF VITAMIN D

Now that you know about the amazing benefits of vitamin D, it's time to evaluate your vitamin D level and set up a plan to optimize it! The first thing to do is get tested.

You might be tempted to avoid testing and just begin taking vitamin D supplements or getting more sunlight. If you don't get tested, however, you won't know what your baseline level is—and you won't know when (or whether) you've optimized it. Some people naturally have lower vitamin D levels than others, and some need higher amounts of vitamin D to achieve the same blood levels. That's why testing is so important. Testing one of the most practical things you can do to improve your health.

When you visit your doctor, ask him or her to order the "25 Hydroxy Vitamin D Test" (25(OH)D Test). This measures the storage form of vitamin D in your blood. Make sure your doctor does not confuse this with the "1,25 Dihydroxy Vitamin D Test," which is something very different. Depending on your insurance coverage, you may prefer to order an in-home test kit. To do this, take a small blood sample from your finger (similar to checking your blood sugar levels) and mail it to the laboratory. The results will be mailed back to you.

Once you know your vitamin D level, you'll be able to determine whether it places you at risk. Current laboratory guidelines state that any level between 30 and 100 ng/mL is "normal." However, vitamin D experts worldwide believe that the higher end of this range is much healthier than the lower end. The 30 ng/mL value may protect you against developing rickets or osteoporosis; however, higher levels are needed for the prevention of many other diseases previously discussed.[48]

A much safer guideline is to make sure your levels are between 50 and 100 ng/mL.[49] This will lower your overall disease risk.[50] Robert Heaney, MD, one of the world's leading vitamin D researchers, recommends maintaining a minimum vitamin D level between 40 and 60 ng/mL.[51] I currently recommend 50 to 80, but levels up to 100 are still in the normal range. Don't be discouraged if your level is low. Bringing it up is simple and inexpensive.

How can you bring your vitamin D level into the optimal range? Is it simply a matter of spending more time in the sun? Is supplementation necessary? Let's take a look at the different options.

SUNLIGHT[52, 53, 54]

Skin manufactures vitamin D when it is exposed to the sun. That's only one of the benefits of sun exposure. However, many people find it challenging—even impossible—to optimize their vitamin D levels through sun exposure alone. Let me explain why.

While it's true that you can produce 15,000 units of vitamin D in 15 to 20 minutes of direct sun exposure, there are several qualifications. First, you need to be outside in the middle of the day—as near to solar noon as possible. The sun has to reach at least a 45-degree angle for vitamin D synthesis to occur. This is generally between 10 a.m. to 3 p.m. when the sun is at its highest. Ultra-violet light from the sun comes in two different forms: UVA and UVB. UVB rays stimulate the skin to produce vitamin D; UVA rays do not. While UVA rays are present throughout the entire day, UVB rays are *only* present in the middle of the day.

Second, you need to live in the right place during the right season. North Americans who live farther north than Atlanta, Georgia, essentially can't produce any vitamin D except in the summer months. Vitamin D levels can dramatically drop in the winter and spring.

Third, to optimize vitamin D production, it's best to expose a large portion of your body to the sun. Getting a little sun on your face and hands is not sufficient. Also, sunscreen blocks UVB rays and vitamin D production. You may want to apply sunscreen after the first 15 minutes (the time necessary to stimulate vitamin D production) to avoid getting sunburned. Remember to build your sun tolerance up gradually. If you want to get your vitamin D from the sun, however, you can't let sunscreen sabotage that process.

Fourth, be careful in the shower or bath.[55] Because vitamin D is fat soluable, if you take a soapy shower right after being in the sun, you may wash off most of the vitamin D you just produced. It can take up to 48 hours for vitamin D to fully absorb into the bloodstream and actually raise blood levels.

Historically, when people did not bathe as frequently as we do today, they were able to absorb more of the vitamin D they produced from the sun. However, in our hygiene-conscious society, vitamin D absorption is more challenging. Since we tend to wash our hands and face frequently, simply getting sun exposure to these areas is not likely to optimize vitamin D levels.

If you do take a shower or bath after being in the sun, you can minimize the amount of vitamin D loss by only using soap to wash your underarms and groin area. The rest of your skin will lose some vitamin D from the water, but not as much as it would lose if you used soap everywhere.

People with dark skin have an even more difficult time producing vitamin D from the sun. The melanin in dark skin partially blocks the UVB rays, preventing vitamin D synthesis from occurring. This explains why vitamin D deficiency is even more prevalent in blacks.[56]

Even though it's possible to produce vitamin D from the sun, after testing patient's vitamin D levels for the past 10 years, I've found that nearly everyone needs supplementation. Unless you can verify with a blood test that your vitamin D level is sufficient (year-round) with regular sun exposure, you are highly likely to be deficient. Remember, your goal should be to keep your vitamin D level between 50 and 100 ng/mL.

SUPPLEMENTATION

Most people need to take vitamin D supplements in order to optimize their levels. Vitamin D supplements are a safe, inexpensive, and effective option that may be one of the wisest investments you make to improve your health.

How much vitamin D do you need? However much it takes for you to get your blood level up to between 50 and 100 ng/mL! This can vary by individual. Current guidelines are much lower than many researchers and clinicians believe they should be. The official recommended dietary reference intake (DRI) is that people ages 1 to 70 should take 600 units per day, and people over 70 should take 800 units per day.[57] Vitamin D researchers worldwide know these levels are woefully inadequate. They are based on the amount of vitamin D necessary to prevent rickets, but are not high enough to prevent many other diseases!

Some researchers who are more aware of the benefits of vitamin D suggest that everyone, from birth to death, should take at least 2,000 units of vitamin D a day.[58] That's a *minimum*. These guidelines are better than the RDI, but in reality, after years of testing vitamin D levels I have only seen a few people who could maintain optimal vitamin D levels with only 2,000 units of vitamin D a day.

After blood tests are obtained, I typically start my adult vitamin D-deficient patients at 10,000 units per day. After two to three months, I test my patients again. If their level is above 80, I may suggest cutting back to a maintenance dose of 6,000 units a day for men and 5,000 units a day for women. Most patients need about four or five months to bring their levels to between 50 to 100 ng/mL. After that, it's important to test vitamin D levels at least two to three times per year. The best times to test are in the fall (when levels are highest due to summer sun exposure) and in the spring (when levels are lowest due to winter sunlight deprivation.) The important thing is to find out how much you need to take in order to keep your blood levels stable year-round.

CAN I GET VITAMIN D IN MY DIET?

Obtaining sufficient vitamin D in your diet is virtually impossible. Most people think they get enough vitamin D because they drink milk every day. Vitamin D isn't in milk naturally—it's added. The amount added is so low that it doesn't make much difference. This applies to most vitamin D-fortified foods. There is some vitamin D found in fatty fish (salmon, trout and sardines), liver, and shiitake mushrooms. I discourage people from eating liver because it is generally full of toxins. Fish contain toxins as well. Unless you frequently eat large amounts of these foods, they will not provide you with enough Vitamin D.

WHAT ABOUT TOXICITY?

That's a lot of vitamin D! you may be thinking. *Isn't there a chance that I might develop vitamin D toxicity?* It's only natural to be concerned about getting too much of a good thing. However, you can be assured that vitamin D toxicity is extremely rare. Research has shown that, unless you're taking at least 30,000 units a day consistently for many months, there's no toxic effect.[59]

Vitamin D toxicity does not occur until your serum level reaches 200 to 250 ng/mL.[60] The doses I've listed will not result in toxicity. I am not aware of any health benefit for having serum levels higher than 100 ng/mL, so maintaining your levels between 50 and 100 is both safe and effective. If you fall below 50 ng/mL, it's time to take more vitamin D. If your levels are over 100, you can cut back slightly. There's no need to be alarmed if your levels are around 100 because there is a big safety gap between 100 and the toxic 200 to 250 ng/mL.

In one account, a man consumed powdered supplements that had inadvertently been tainted with millions of units of vitamin D.[61] He consumed up to 2.6 million units per day, for many months before showing signs of toxicity. After the problem was identified and resolved, his symptoms quickly reversed. According to the Poison Control Center, medically relevant cases of vitamin D toxicity are extremely rare, with zero reported deaths.[62] Deficiency of this nutrient is of much greater concern than toxicity from it.

THE OCCASIONAL MEGA DOSE

Let me share with you a powerful secret that my family and friends use to keep from getting sick. If you are exposed to a bug or virus, taking a temporary mega-dose of vitamin D can help to stop it in its tracks. Studies show that it's safe to take up to 1,000 units for every pound of body weight for two to three days.[63] This boosts the immune system and fights off sickness. For example, a person weighing 150 pounds could take 150,000 units, three days in a row. However, I don't think this much is necessary, especially for people who carry a lot of weight.

If you feel that you are coming down with a cold or flu, I recommend taking 50,000 units per day for two to three days. This should be sufficient to powerfully boost your immunity. In fact, I've never seen anything work better. I could tell you story after story of patients and family members who used vitamin D to stop a cold or flu before it could get the best of them.

Several years ago, I flew to Geneva, Switzerland, to speak at a wellness conference. My parents joined me, and we planned to travel through Europe for a few weeks after the meetings. By the time we arrived in Geneva, we were exhausted. We had flown overnight and had also lost sleep preparing for the trip. My then 84-year-old mother could tell she was getting sick.

"I think I'm coming down with the flu," she said. "When I feel this way, I'm usually out for a week." It was the worst time to get sick, and it threatened to ruin our entire trip. I had come prepared. I pulled out a bottle of high-potency liquid vitamin D3 and squirted an entire dropper (50,000 units) into her mouth. Mom woke up the next morning feeling great.

Even if you have already come down with a cold or flu, taking a large dose is a good idea. It will help your immune system fight the bug, resulting in a quicker recovery.

BEYOND VITAMIN D—OTHER BENEFITS OF THE SUN

Vitamin D isn't the only benefit of getting regular sun exposure. Sunlight has a wide variety of health benefits unrelated to vitamin D. Just because you're taking a vitamin D supplement doesn't mean that you don't need to get good old-fashioned sunshine!

OTHER BENEFITS OF SUNLIGHT

- Improves sleep
- Synchronizes hormones
- Reduces stress
- Boosts serotonin/enhances mood
- Improves digestion
- Increases metabolism
- Lowers heart rate
- Reduces pain

TWO PIECES IN THE PUZZLE

Vitamin D and sunlight can work wonders to improve our health. However, it's important to remember that they are only two pieces in the puzzle. If you truly want to optimize wellness and prevent disease, you need to take a comprehensive approach. Your body is also designed to need optimal nutrition, adequate exercise, sufficient sleep, and pure water. It's okay to get excited about vitamin D. After all, it's such a simple and inexpensive way to improve your health. But don't let that be the only thing you do. As you take advantage of all the various strategies available, they will unite to produce tremendous results.

CHAPTER SUMMARY

- Vitamin D is an important component of an optimal wellness program.
- The vast majority of Americans are vitamin D deficient.
- Adequate vitamin D intake can improve health and prevent many kinds of diseases: diabetes, heart disease, cancer, and many others.
- Vitamin D levels can be increased through sunlight exposure and supplementation.
- Very little vitamin D is found in food.
- Vitamin D blood levels should be between 50 and 100 ng/mL.
- Test your vitamin D level before starting a supplement, and then every fall and spring.
- You can initially take 10,000 units of vitamin D per day to bring your level up.
- To maintain a healthy level, most men need 6,000 units per day and women need 5,000 units.
- Vitamin D toxicity is very rare.
- For a temporary boost to your immune system, take a mega dose of vitamin D for two to three days. This can help prevent sickness, or help you to recover more quickly if you are sick.

—TWENTY—

Ten Super Supplements

All illness is caused by a deficiency or an excess.
—Anonymous

I FIRST MET AMIL WHILE EXERCISING AT MY LOCAL GYM. He was the coach of an Olympic judo team, and a former competitive judo wrestler. In his late 30s, he was still a gifted wrestler, but had become more sedentary than he had been in college. His diet wasn't optimal, and he'd gained some belly fat. About a year before, Amil had been diagnosed with diabetes. He'd started coming to the gym more frequently to try to regain his health.

One day, I saw Amil standing in the waiting room of the clinic where I worked. He was waiting to see one of the physicians. I greeted him and asked how he was doing. "Well, my feet are really bothering me," he said. "They hurt and tingle. I can't relax. If I sit down, it hurts even worse. If I lay down, it's *horrible!*"

Amil's complaints sounded familiar. He was describing typical symptoms caused by diabetic neuropathy, an often painful and irritating complication of diabetes. Neuropathy occurs when high blood sugar levels damage nerve fibers throughout the body. An estimated 60 to 70 percent of diabetics have some form of neuropathy.[1] I explained to Amil what neuropathy was, and then gave him a few suggestions.

"It's good that you're here to get some help," I said. "I'm sure your doctor will have good advice, but let me share two suggestions with you. First, make sure you're managing your blood sugars well. This will go a long way toward halting nerve damage. Second, a supplement called "alpha lipoic acid" can help heal and protect your nerve fibers. It can greatly reduce symptoms associated with diabetic neuropathy. Start taking about 300 milligrams twice daily. Chances are, you'll feel an improvement."

Just two days later, Amil spotted me at the gym and approached me with exciting news. "I just wanted to thank you for your recommendation," he said. "Right after my visit to the clinic, I bought some alpha lipoic acid. That same evening I could already tell that the nerve pain was a lot better. The next day it was completely gone. I'm so glad I can get back to exercising!"

I was excited for Amil, but not surprised by the results. I've had many diabetic patients who have experienced similar results from using alpha lipoic acid as a supplement. For some, it takes several weeks, or even several months, to heal damaged nerves. Others, like Amil, have seen results very quickly. Alpha lipoic acid also has multiple other health benefits. I don't have diabetes or prediabetes, but I've been taking it for the past 20 years. It's just one of a variety of nutritional supplements that can powerfully enhance health, especially for people with diabetes.

My friend, Eric Madrid, is a family physician in Southern California. A few years ago, he attended a medical lecture on strategies for treating peripheral neuropathy. After introducing his topic, the lecturing physician said something that surprised Dr. Madrid.

"I just want you all to be aware that alpha lipoic acid is a great supplement to help treat, and even cure, diabetic neuropathy," the physician said. "Few physicians are aware of this, but it can be very effective. However, that really isn't within the scope of this lecture. Instead, we're going to look at medications that will help to relieve the symptoms of neuropathy."

Dr. Madrid was shocked. An affordable supplement was available that could effectively treat—and even *cure*—neuropathy, but the focus was still placed on medications that would alleviate symptoms?

His story didn't surprise me. In our healthcare system today, few physicians are trained to understand the benefits of nutritional supplements. In this chapter, I will outline 10 nutritional supplements that may be beneficial for people with diabetes or prediabetes. Since everyone has differing needs, it is important to have a qualified health professional guide this process.

PILLS AND POTIONS

When it comes to healthcare products, it's hard to know who to trust. Many consumers are confused about the vast selection of drugs, herbs, and nutritional supplements. Television commercials promise magic pills that will solve every healthcare concern. Health food stores carry a wide variety of difficult-to-pronounce pills and potions. With so many products making competing claims, it's difficult to know how to make the right choices.

Most people look only to their doctor for help, allowing him or her to make all their healthcare decisions. Few patients understand the drugs they are taking, the way they work, the long-term side effects, or other treatment options.

I believe it's important for all adults to take personal responsibility for their own health. Think of yourself as the chairman of the board for your health concerns. Your board of directors includes your doctor, your diabetes educator, your dietitian, and other healthcare professionals. They can provide you with valuable information. You can also glean more information from other credible sources. But at the end of the day you have to make your own healthcare choices, including choices about drugs and supplements. You need to understand the options available to you.

Some drugs and nutritional supplements are appropriate and beneficial. Others do more harm than good. The only way to know for sure is to examine the evidence. Throughout my career, I have done my best to recommend products to people based on scientific evidence that shows the products are both beneficial and safe. In this chapter, we'll take a look at a variety of different nutritional supplements. My goal is to help you become as well-informed as possible so you can make responsible decisions about your health.

When I sit down with new patients, I outline wellness plans that are specific to their needs. I talk to them about nutrition, meal balancing, exercise, sleep, and all the basic lifestyle strategies that can dramatically improve their health. These strategies should be your primary focus, as well, when it comes to combating degenerative diseases like obesity, diabetes, and heart disease.

After outlining these fundamental principles, I take it one step further by suggesting nutritional supplements that can further help heal the body and restore normal function.

The dictionary defines the word supplement as, "Something that completes or enhances something else when added to it."[2] Supplements cannot replace lifestyle measures, but they *can* enhance them. Nutritional supplements should be used *in addition to,* not *instead of* lifestyle strategies. Remember, it's a supplement, not a substitute!

Because each person is unique, supplemental needs can substantially vary based on lab results and individual health status. However, I highly recommend several core supplements to my patients—especially those suffering from diabetes.

TOP 10 SUPPLEMENTS FOR DIABETES

1. High Potency Multivitamin
2. Vitamin D
3. Omega-3 Fatty Acids
4. Magnesium
5. Alpha Lipoic Acid
6. Vitamin C
7. Chromium
8. Biotin
9. Berberine
10. Tocotrienols

Let's take a closer look at each supplement and at the powerful ways in which they can improve your health.

1. HIGH POTENCY MULTIVITAMIN

Choose a high-quality multivitamin that contains all the basic vitamins and minerals. The best multivitamins have higher amounts of vitamins and minerals than the typical RDA recommendations. Make sure your multivitamin includes B vitamins. Most multivitamins require that you take one to two tablets per day for optimal benefit. Be sure to check the directions on your multivitamin packaging. I encourage you to use a multivitamin that uses natural forms of nutrients instead of the cheaper, synthetic forms.

2. VITAMIN D

In the previous chapter, I discussed at length the benefits of vitamin D. Optimizing your vitamin D level may significantly lower your risk of heart disease, cancer, diabetes, and high blood pressure as well as improve your overall immune health. Ask your doctor for the 25 Hydroxy Vitamin D Test. Your goal should be to keep your level within the range of 50 and 100 nanograms per milliliter (ng/mL). If you need to raise your level, start by taking 10,000 International Units of vitamin D per day. Check again after two to three months of supplementation. Once optimal levels are reached, most men can maintain those levels with 6,000 units per day, and women with 5,000 units per day. However, testing is the only way to know how much your body needs. Recheck levels every fall and spring. The amount of vitamin D you need may vary, depending on the season.

3. OMEGA-3 FATTY ACIDS[3]

Omega-3 fatty acids have a wide range of health benefits and are especially helpful for people with diabetes. These fatty acids can lower elevated triglycerides, reduce inflammation, protect the heart and blood vessels, improve insulin sensitivity, boost thyroid and adrenal function,[4] and improve mental functioning and emotional well-being. Omega-3 fatty acids also help protect the body from diabetes-related complications, including neuropathy.[5]

I recommend taking purified forms of arctic cod liver or fish oil, which are high in Omega-3s. The goal is to get 4,000 milligrams of combined EPA and DHA (two specific types of fatty acids) every day. Almost all fish oils and cod liver oils contain both types and their packaging tells the measurements of each. Remember, 4,000 milligrams of EPA and DHA is not the same as 4,000 milligrams of fish oil. DHA and EPA make up only a portion of the oil (usually ¼ to ⅓ of the total). Keep your oil refrigerated and take it during any meal of the day. Avoid taking between meals, as this can cause fishy-smelling breath.

Omega-3s are also available in capsules, but you have to take a larger number of the capsules to get the same dose as you can easily get in a small amount of oil. Be sure to buy a molecularly distilled oil free from toxins or impurities that may have originally been in the fish. Vegan omega-3 formulas are available as well, but they're usually more expensive than other forms.

4. MAGNESIUM[6, 7, 8]

Magnesium is a secret weapon against heart disease. It helps prevent cholesterol and plaque buildup in the arteries.[9] People with adequate magnesium levels are less likely to suffer heart attack or stroke.

Magnesium also lowers inflammation, blood pressure, and blood sugars, and helps to prevent headaches, cramps, restless leg syndrome, constipation, insomnia, and depression. In addition, magnesium helps improve bone health.

Most people in the industrialized world are magnesium-deficient.[10] Processed, nutrient-depleted foods do not contain magnesium. Most first-class foods do contain magnesium, but these foods need to be eaten in high volumes to keep levels adequate.

Diabetics are at even higher risk for magnesium deficiency, as the kidneys release more magnesium into the urine when blood sugars are high. Magnesium supplementation is beneficial for almost everyone, and especially for diabetics.

Take 250 milligrams of magnesium citrate at bedtime and the same amount when you wake up in the morning. Avoid magnesium oxide, the cheapest form of magnesium available. It is not as well absorbed. Magnesium citrate and other chelated forms work best. One tablet usually contains 250 milligrams. You can build up to 500 milligrams per day (250 milligrams in the morning and 250 milligrams at bedtime). Decrease the amount you're taking if your stools become watery. If you have a problem with constipation, it may help to increase your bedtime magnesium dose until you have regular bowel movements.

5. ALPHA LIPOIC ACID[11, 12, 13]

I already mentioned the benefits of alpha lipoic acid for healing the nerves and preventing diabetic neuropathy. Many of my patients have found relief from neuropathy by using this supplement. Alpha lipoic acid is also a powerful antioxidant. It's especially helpful for people with liver problems. Alpha lipoic acid can boost cellular energy and is sometimes used to enhance athletic performance. I recommend that diabetics take 300 milligrams of alpha lipoic acid two times per day. Taking vitamin C at the same time will increase the benefit of this supplement.

6. VITAMIN C

Vitamin C is a powerful immune booster and antioxidant.[14, 15, 16] Countless studies have documented the wide range of health benefits that vitamin C brings to the table. Vitamin C is a cheap, effective way to protect against the common cold,[17, 18] help wounds to heal,[19, 20] lower blood pressure,[21, 22] and reduce the risk of heart disease[23] and cancer.[24]

Vitamin C is especially important for people with diabetes.[25] For example, 1,000 milligrams of vitamin C per day for three months can lower hemoglobin A1c by roughly 18 percent.[26] One study showed that vitamin C added to drinking water actually neutralized a genetic mutation in mice that was causing diabetes, heart disease, cancer, and accelerated aging.[27] Correcting the relative insufficiency of vitamin C in the mice led to improved fat burning, decreased inflammation, and reduced oxidative stress. After treatment, the mutant mice were as healthy—and lived as long—as the non-mutant mice.

To obtain the maximum benefit from vitamin C, I usually recommend that patients take 1,000 mg three times per day.

7. CHROMIUM

Chromium is a key nutrient that improves insulin sensitivity.[28] It can actually increase the number of insulin receptors on muscle and liver cells.[29] Taking chromium is a natural and healthy way to optimize blood sugars.

I generally recommend taking 200 to 1,000 micrograms of chromium per day. To optimize blood sugar levels, take 1,000 micrograms per day.

Once blood sugars are consistently controlled, the dose of chromium can be decreased. Chromium is even more effective when paired with biotin.[30, 31]

8. BIOTIN

Biotin helps increase insulin sensitivity and control blood sugars.[32] Biotin and chromium are often given together, because they work synergistically and increase each other's effects. Biotin can be dosed up to 5,000 micrograms per day. One nutraceutical company combines 600 micrograms of chromium with 2,000 micrograms of biotin to double the increase in insulin sensitivity.

9. BERBERINE

Berberine is a powerful herb shown to be more effective in improving insulin sensitivity than metformin—the most popular diabetes drug on the market. In one study, berberine improved insulin sensitivity by 45 percent, reducing the need for insulin production by 28 percent.[33] Diabetics can take up to 1,500 milligrams of berberine per day, but it's best to start with 500 milligrams once per day and work up (if necessary) to three times per day.

10. TOCOTRIENOLS

Because diabetics are just as likely to have a heart attack as people who have already had a heart attack, medical protocol requires that diabetics be treated as if they have already had a heart attack. That's why so many diabetics are put on a statin or other cholesterol lowering medication, whether or not their cholesterol is elevated. While I prefer to use more natural strategies, I believe in being every bit as aggressive in preventing heart disease. All the supplements outlined in this chapter can help improve cardiovascular health. Tocotrienols are especially valuable for preventing toxic plaque buildup in the arteries.[34]

Tocotrienols are a special form of vitamin E. They can significantly lower the tendency of cholesterol to become oxidized. Oxidized cholesterol is the sticky, toxic goo that promotes plaque formation. Tocotrienols are powerful antioxidants that lower the oxidation of LDL as well as total cholesterol.[35] I typically recommend taking 100 milligrams of tocotrienols in the evening or at least six hours after taking any vitamin E supplement, as they can compete for absorption.

DON'T OVERMEDICATE!

Following the information outlined in this book can quickly and dramatically lower your blood sugar levels. That's why it's so important to work with your healthcare provider to adjust medications accordingly. You don't want to end up in an emergency room in a severe hypoglycemic crisis. Anytime you do something different—whether it's changing your diet, increasing your exercise, or taking advantage of nutritional supplements—you need to frequently check your blood sugar levels and adjust your medications as necessary.

ADDITIONAL INSTRUCTIONS

Most supplements are best absorbed if you take them with food, unless instructed otherwise. Your urine may appear bright yellow when you start taking certain supplements. Don't be alarmed. This is normal.

DON'T JUST POP PILLS

Far too many people depend on medications alone to solve their health problems. A false sense of security is gained from popping pills, while basic lifestyle interventions are neglected. Whether you're taking prescription drugs or nutritional supplements, this is a dangerous mindset.

Remember, supplements are designed to be used *in addition to*, not instead of, lifestyle strategies like nutrition, exercise, sunshine, sleep, etc. There are no magic shortcuts. If you want comprehensive health results, you need to take a comprehensive approach.

CHAPTER SUMMARY

- You are personally responsible for your own health.
- Choices about supplements (or drugs) should be based on scientific evidence that demonstrates their safety and effectiveness.
- The primary focus in combating diabetes should be to follow basic lifestyle strategies.
- Nutritional supplements can enhance your wellness plan.

- » The top ten supplements I recommend for diabetics are:
    1. High Potency Multivitamin
    2. Vitamin D
    3. Omega-3 Fatty Acids
    4. Magnesium
    5. Alpha Lipoic Acid
    6. Vitamin C
    7. Chromium
    8. Biotin
    9. Berberine
    10. Tocotrienols
- » Making lifestyle changes and taking supplements can quickly and dramatically lower blood sugar levels. Work with your doctor to appropriately adjust medications and supplements.
- » Supplements are just one part of a comprehensive lifestyle approach.

—TWENTY-ONE—

Drugs and Diabetes

Medicine sometimes snatches away health, sometimes gives it.
—Ovid

LET ME TELL YOU THE *TALE OF THREE PATIENTS*. All three had diabetes. Each one nearly died. One, because she took too much insulin—the other two, because they wouldn't take any. Their stories reveal valuable lessons about the relationship between diabetes and drugs.

LISA

Lisa was in her 60s and had finally reached a point where she was motivated to take charge of her health. She had been taking insulin for ten years. After watching several relatives develop diabetes-related complications, Lisa knew she was at risk. But she hadn't been controlling her type 2 diabetes very well. Her blood sugars were constantly running high, and her doctor frequently had to increase her insulin dose.

Lisa finally got sick and tired of being sick and tired. Her doctor referred her to a diabetes specialist, who then referred her to the diabetes-reversal program offered at our clinic. At first, Lisa was apprehensive about trying something new, but after our initial consultation, I could tell she was excited. She realized there was hope for improving her condition and preventing the devastating complications her family members had experienced. She joined our six-month outpatient wellness program, which began with two weeks of intensive lifestyle therapy.

Lisa had been taking insulin multiple times per day—a total of 80 units. Our clinical team knew that her insulin needs would decrease as a result of the dramatic lifestyle changes she was making. And that's exactly what happened. After just three days of eating first-class foods and participating in after-meal exercise and group support, Lisa's insulin needs dropped to 40 units per day—a 50 percent decrease!

This scenario is typical for people who adopt new lifestyle programs. Results can be rapid and dramatic. That's why it's so important to carefully monitor blood sugars during this time and to adjust insulin and other medications accordingly. Lifestyle interventions dramatically lower blood sugar levels. Unless medications are adjusted, patients may be at risk for hypoglycemia.

By Wednesday of the second week, Lisa's blood sugars had improved even more. Her insulin dose dropped to 20 units daily. An hour after supper, we rechecked the participants' blood sugar levels before sending them home for the night. Lisa's level was 150—very close to the one-hour blood sugar target for a diabetic. Lisa was ecstatic about the dramatic improvements she was experiencing. We were excited too.

The next morning, I got a disturbing phone call that didn't seem to make sense. Lisa was in the hospital after suffering a severe hypoglycemic reaction. *How could that have happened?* I wondered. We had already cut her insulin by 75 percent!

After a few more phone calls the story seemed even stranger. Apparently Lisa had returned home that night and checked her blood sugar on her personal glucose meter.

Lisa then called her diabetes nurse educator and reported that her blood sugar was 300. The nurse educator was alarmed after learning that Lisa had cut her insulin so dramatically and called the primary care doctor to request an order for an increased dose. The doctor ordered Lisa to immediately take 40 units of insulin, and also to increase her regular daily dose. Lisa took 40 units and hoped for the best.

Soon, she started to feel confused, anxious, and shaky. Within a few hours, she was unconscious. Lisa's husband rushed her to the emergency room. She was admitted to the hospital and treated for severe hypoglycemia.

Well, of course she bottomed out with 40 units of insulin, I thought to myself. *There's no way her blood sugar was 300. We had just checked it right before she went home.* I called Lisa to express my concern and asked her to bring her home glucose meter to the clinic next time she attended class.

Lisa was released from the hospital late that afternoon and showed up for our evening group session. She brought her glucose meter with her. When it came time to check blood sugars, we first tested with our equipment. Her level was 105 before dinner. Lisa then checked her blood sugar level using her own meter, which gave a reading of 258. Lisa almost lost her life because of a faulty, uncalibrated glucose meter.

While Lisa's story is sobering, it proves an exciting point. Lifestyle strategies can dramatically lower blood sugars! While it's important to carefully decrease medication accordingly, it's also exciting to no longer need as much medication! Lisa represents millions of people who could decrease their need for insulin (and other diabetes medications) simply by optimizing their lifestyle.

SISTER MARY

Sister Mary was a different story. Mary was a 57-year-old nun. Like Lisa, she had been battling type 2 diabetes for many years. Her blood sugars were out of control, running 200 to 250 before meals, and 400 to 450 after meals. Every three months, Sister Mary had a check-up with her physician. For years, he had tried to convince her that she needed to take insulin.

Mary was very opposed to the idea. She begged her doctor not to prescribe insulin. She wanted to try every other option available. He would concede, prescribing multiple forms of oral medications and encouraging her to exercise and eat healthfully.

But Sister Mary's blood sugars remained dangerously high. Her doctor informed her that she was at imminent risk for complications and that he didn't see any safe option other than insulin. But Mary would not comply. She actually experienced several panic attacks when thinking about taking insulin. After running out of options, Mary's physician referred her to see me.

Before sitting down with Mary, I reviewed her medical history. Mary's chronically high blood sugars had caused serious damage to her pancreas. It was no longer capable of producing the amount of insulin her body required. Lifestyle strategies could definitely help, but all the evidence pointed to the fact that she would also need insulin to control her blood sugars. Mary's diabetes had essentially become more like type 1 than type 2.

"Sister Mary," I said. "I know you're hesitant to take insulin. But your lab results show that this is the best option for you. I agree with your doctor's concerns." Mary looked terrified, avoiding eye contact. She sank down in her chair. Several moments passed, but Mary remained silent.

I knew there had to be a reason why she was so terrified of insulin. There had to be an explanation for her anxiety. "Sister Mary," I said. "I can tell that the thought of taking insulin is very frightening to you. What do you think will happen if you start taking it?"

Mary braced herself, looked at me with a very sad expression, and said, "Dr. Youngberg, I don't want to die."

She thinks she's going to die if she takes insulin, I thought to myself. *I wonder where that thought came from?*

"You believe that if you start taking insulin, you will die?" I asked quietly.

"Well, yes," she responded.

"Why do you think that?"

Mary became very thoughtful, waited a few moments, then replied, "Because that's what happened to my sister when she started taking insulin. For years, the doctors had told her she should take it, but she didn't want to. Finally, she gave in, but within two weeks she was dead."

Finally understanding the source of Mary's fear, I gently explained to her that it wasn't the insulin that caused her sister's death—it was the damage done to her organ systems because of her chronically high blood sugars. For her sister—and for Mary—insulin wasn't the problem. It could have been part of the solution.

I still remember the look on Mary's face when things clicked and the information finally made sense. She had assumed that giving insulin was a measure taken during the final stages of life. She didn't want to die. Due to a lack of information, she had spent years living in fear of something that could have helped her. By the time she left my office, she was completely willing to start taking insulin as well as to begin improving her diet and exercise program.

RUDY

Personality-wise, Rudy was the complete opposite of Sister Mary. While Mary was quiet and gentle, Rudy was loud and obnoxious. Health-wise, they suffered from the same problem. Rudy was just as afraid to take insulin as Mary. He was a Vietnam veteran who had suffered from severe post-traumatic stress disorder (PTSD) for many years. He had a variety of health problems, including out-of-control diabetes.

Rudy's blood sugar levels were sky-high. His doctor had repeatedly advised him that he needed to take insulin. Rudy came to me because he wanted to address his diabetes without insulin. During our first visit, Rudy laid down the rules.

"I just want to make one thing clear," he said. "I want you to understand that I don't want to hear anything about going on insulin. I refuse to take insulin. I would rather cut my [blankety-blank] foot off than take [blankety-blank] insulin."

I assured Rudy that I would do my best to help him improve his health without insulin. We designed a program to help him reach his goals. He made a commitment to exercise after meals, check his blood sugar more frequently, and eat first-class foods.

A few months later, Rudy still hadn't experienced the results he wanted. Although he'd made changes in his lifestyle, his blood sugars were still very high and his hemoglobin A1c was above 10. I suspected that Rudy's pancreas had been damaged after years of high blood sugars and that he did need insulin—at least for the time being.

I had a responsibility to be honest with Rudy about his risk. I carefully suggested that he consider taking insulin. As soon as I mentioned it, Rudy's temper exploded: "I told you I don't want to take [blankety-blank] insulin! I'll do anything else, really. I'll try harder. Just give me two more weeks, I'll try really hard."

"All right, Rudy," I said. "I believe that your pancreas is damaged and that we won't see a big improvement in two weeks, but let's give it a shot."

Two weeks later, Rudy's labs showed no improvements. "Rudy, " I said. "We really need to talk about how valuable insulin can be for you." Rudy exploded again—yelling, screaming, and calling me names.

There's always a reason people react the way they do. In Sister Mary's case, a misconception about insulin had prevented her from taking it. In contrast, Rudy seemed to be aware that insulin would help his health, but he was terrified to take it.

I suspected it might have something to do with needles. Sometimes, people with PTSD have a difficult time dealing with needles and blood. But Rudy was willing to have his blood drawn for lab tests. They require a much bigger needle than insulin. Still, I had a sneaking suspicion that the real cause of Rudy's fear of insulin was a fear of needles.

As we sat in my office, I gave Rudy time to vent his frustration. When he finally stopped talking, I did something that surprised him.

"Look Rudy, I'm gonna show you how it's done," I said, pulling out an insulin syringe and a vial of water from my desk drawer. "See how tiny this is?" I drew up 15 units of water, and squirted the air out of the top while Rudy was watching in horror.

"I've never done this before," I said. "But I bet I'm not even going to feel it." I lifted up my shirt a few inches, pinched an inch of my abdomen, plunged the needle in, and injected the water. "See Rudy, it's that simple!"

"Well, if you can [blankety-blank] do that, I sure can [blankety-blank] do that, too. Give me one of those [blankety-blank] needles."

Rudy walked out of my office that day completely fine with the idea of giving himself insulin injections. His blood sugars improved significantly, and he continued to incorporate healthy lifestyle habits to increase his sensitivity to insulin. I believe Rudy's decision to begin taking insulin probably added an extra ten years to his life.

"I WANT TO GET OFF OF MY MEDICATION!"

When I sit down with new patients, I always ask them what their goals are. One response I frequently hear is, "I want to get off of my medication!" These patients are aware of the side effects of most prescription drugs and are interested in finding an alternative.

But "getting off medication" isn't the best goal. There are plenty of people not taking medication who still aren't healthy. Perhaps a better goal would be, "I want to *improve my health* so that I no longer need medication," or, "I want *to improve my health* so that I'm able to decrease the amount of medication I need."

Lisa improved her health so much that she decreased her need for insulin. If she had stopped taking insulin without making lifestyle changes, however, her blood sugars would have run dangerously high. Sister Mary and Rudy both tried to improve their health without taking insulin, but they were fighting an uphill battle. Because they both had pancreatic damage, the healthiest option for them was to start taking insulin. However, they still had the opportunity to decrease the amount of insulin they needed by eating healthy foods, exercising, and following other natural strategies to increase their bodies' sensitivity to insulin. Not only do these habits improve health as it relates to diabetes, but they also improve health overall.

Most diabetics and prediabetics are like Lisa. They can experience dramatic blood sugar improvements through simple lifestyle choices alone. If they are on medication, they can significantly reduce or eliminate their need for that medication. Because high insulin levels increase risk for many diseases including heart disease,[1] obesity,[2] and cancer,[3] overcoming insulin resistance and reducing the amount of insulin needed can dramatically improve health.

However, all type 1 diabetics and some type 2 diabetics who have sustained pancreatic damage need the aid of insulin to keep their blood sugars under control. Oral diabetes medications are sometimes necessary as well. Lifestyle strategies are certainly still important as they help the body to become more responsive to insulin, thereby decreasing the amount of insulin needed.

I am a big proponent of "getting off medication" when you can accomplish what the medication was designed to accomplish, but in a more healthy way. However, for some people medication is appropriate and essential.

One way to help determine whether you need to be on insulin is to take the stimulated C-peptide test, which measures your pancreatic function. This test was described in Chapter 9.

WHY NOT JUST DEPEND ON INSULIN INJECTIONS?

The most common form of injectable insulin is bio-identical to the insulin produced by the pancreas. So what's the harm in depending on insulin injections to control your blood sugars? Remember that the main problem associated with prediabetes and type 2 diabetes is not a lack of insulin production; rather, it's a lack of *sensitivity* to insulin. Unless you address the cause of insulin resistance, you will require more and more insulin to lower your blood sugars. Extra insulin means weight gain, which increases insulin resistance even more which requires an increase in the insulin dose—and the cycle continues. Further, excess insulin can cause hypoglycemia and high blood pressure and can increase the risk of heart disease, cancer, and many other diseases.

Type 2 diabetics generally require far more insulin than type 1 diabetics. While there's nothing wrong with taking insulin when your body is unable to produce an appropriate amount, the main goal of therapy for type 2 diabetes should be to address insulin resistance, which will then lower—or completely eliminate—the need for insulin injections.

DIABETES AND DRUGS

Besides insulin, diabetics are prescribed a variety of other medications. Despite uncertain economic times, the global diabetes market is booming. Currently, diabetes drugs and devices alone cost the world $41 billion annually. That's expected to rise to over $114 billion by 2018.[4]

Numerous types of diabetes medications are available. Some slow the absorption of sugar during digestion, others increase insulin sensitivity, others stimulate the pancreas to produce more insulin, and still others prevent the liver from releasing too much glucose into the bloodstream.

Numerous studies have shown that even the best of these medications are not as effective as simple lifestyle changes in fighting diabetes. Metformin is one of the most popularly prescribed oral diabetes medications. It causes the muscles and the liver to be more sensitive to insulin, preventing blood sugars from going up in the first place. Metformin can be effective in controlling blood sugars, but a landmark study by the Diabetes Prevention Program Research Group found that prediabetics who walked at least 150 minutes per week and followed a healthy diet plan were much more successful in decreasing their risk for developing diabetes than patients who took metformin but did not follow lifestyle strategies.[5, 6]

Many diabetes medications have side effects. Weight gain, hypoglycemia, nausea, infection, stomach pain, kidney and liver damage, increased risk of heart attack and stroke, and increased risk of sudden death are a few of the potential side effects of these medications.

LEARNING TO PRIORITIZE

One of the best things you can do to improve your health is to learn how to prioritize your approach in making healthy decisions. I call this first-line, second-line, and third-line therapy.

First-line therapy involves implementing basic lifestyle strategies your body was designed to thrive on. This is where you should start. Eat first-class foods. Get regular exercise. Drink enough water. Get some sunshine. Get adequate sleep. Take advantage of the information you have to optimize your habits in all these areas. These changes are simple, inexpensive, and extremely effective. Putting these principles into practice will greatly decrease your risk for developing disease and will dramatically improve your health if you already are suffering from disease.

Second-line therapy involves adding appropriate nutritional supplements to enhance your approach. First-class foods provide a wide variety of vitamins and minerals, but even people who eat healthfully are often deficient in certain nutrients. Vitamin D, vitamin C, omega-3 fatty acids, magnesium, and the other top 10 supplements mentioned in the previous chapter are naturally occurring nutrients that can improve your health without dangerous side effects.

Third-line therapy involves taking pharmaceutical drugs. If you have type 2 diabetes and have tried your very best to improve your health by using first- and second-line therapy, but are still struggling with poorly controlled blood sugars (consistently greater than 100 fasting and frequently greater than 140 two hours after a meal), you may need to consider medication. Remember that first- and second-line therapies are still extremely important, and should be your priority. Health is not just about blood sugars. Without question, anyone can benefit from lifestyle changes and most people can benefit from supplements. Those who find that they cannot control their blood sugars effectively without medication will benefit from adding third-line therapy to their approach.

I hope this system helps you prioritize the decisions you make about your health. My goal as a clinician is to educate my patients about all the tools available to them as they seek to experience optimal wellness. Henry Ward Beecher once said, "To array a man's will against his sickness is the supreme art of medicine." I couldn't agree more. You can experience dramatic results by taking personal responsibility for your health and combatting disease to the best of your ability.

CHAPTER SUMMARY

- Many diabetics have the potential to significantly decrease and eventually eliminate their need for insulin and other diabetes medications.
- For some diabetics, medication is appropriate and essential.
- All type 1 diabetics and some type 2 diabetics need to take insulin.
- The C-peptide test can help you determine whether you need insulin long-term.
- A variety of other diabetes medications are also available. These come with potential side effects and are usually not as effective as basic lifestyle interventions.
- You can make better health decisions by prioritizing your approach.
- First-line therapy involves nutrition, exercise, water, sunshine, and sleep. This is where you should start.
- Second-line therapy involves taking nutritional supplements that can further enhance your health.
- Third-line therapy involves taking pharmaceutical drugs. This is necessary for some people, but should always be combined with first- and second-line therapy as well.

—TWENTY TWO—

Fight Hidden Culprits

What you don't know can kill you.
—Anonymous

"MOST OF YOU ARE THINKING THIS, SO I'M JUST GONNA say it. People are just fat and lazy, and that's what causes diabetes!" You could have heard a pin drop.

I was attending a medical conference on diabetes. A well-respected psychologist had just made this claim during one of the main lectures. The audience was shocked. His assertion seemed insensitive and inappropriate. But as I've talked with many healthcare professionals over the years, I've come to realize that generally they hold the opinion that if type 2 diabetics would just lose weight and exercise more, their problem would be solved.

There's no question that losing excess weight and getting regular exercise can have a profound impact on preventing, controlling, and even reversing diabetes. But are excess weight and inactivity the only factors to blame? I've had many type 1 and type 2 diabetic patients who maintain a healthy weight and exercise more than I do, but they still struggle with diabetes. I've also had numerous overweight patients who can't seem to lose weight despite the fact that they exercise regularly and eat sensibly. What is going on?

Sometimes "hidden culprits" contribute to diabetes and other degenerative diseases. These factors are usually overlooked, rarely discussed, and seldom screened for, even though they play a significant role in the development and progression of diabetes. In this chapter, we'll examine three hidden diabetes culprits: autoimmunity, toxins, and low-grade infections.

THE AUTOIMMUNE EPIDEMIC

It's common knowledge that type 1 diabetes is an autoimmune disorder. But what exactly does that mean? Autoimmune disease occurs when the body's immune system mistakenly attacks itself ("auto" means self). Examples of autoimmune disease include rheumatoid arthritis, multiple sclerosis, Chrohn's disease, type 1 diabetes, latent autoimmune diabetes, asthma, and many others.

Autoimmune disease has increased dramatically in the past few decades. One in twelve Americans (about 23.5 million people) suffer from an autoimmune disorder.[1] This is how the National Institutes of Health defines autoimmune disease:

> "Normally the immune system's army of white blood cells helps protect the body from harmful substances, called antigens. Examples of antigens include bacteria, viruses [and] toxins.... But in patients with an autoimmune disorder, the immune system can't tell the difference between healthy body tissue and antigens. The result is an immune response that destroys normal body tissues."[2]

In the case of type 1 diabetes, the immune system attacks and destroys the insulin-producing cells of the pancreas, mistakenly identifying them as foreign invaders (i.e., antigens). This halts insulin production and makes it necessary for type 1 diabetics to take insulin injections.

While type 1 diabetes is accepted as an autoimmune problem, however, few people are aware that all forms of diabetes can actually have an autoimmune component. Type 1, type 2, gestational, and latent autoimmune diabetes in adults (LADA) can all be triggered—or worsened—by underlying autoimmune issues.

WHAT IS LADA?

Becky was 28 weeks pregnant with her second child when she was diagnosed with gestational diabetes. The picture of health, Becky ate a largely plant-based diet, worked out at the gym at least five times per week, and cycled competitively. Becky was shocked by the diagnosis and concerned for her baby.

"I was really surprised to be diagnosed with diabetes. It was unexpected for sure. I was really active. I was very healthy. I was cycling with a women's team, and I just didn't think of myself as someone who would have diabetes. I felt very healthy, and it just wasn't consistent with the way that I felt and with the way I thought of myself as an athlete," she said.

She found a physician who specialized in gestational diabetes and did her very best to control her blood sugars throughout the rest of her pregnancy. Becky expected that the diabetes would resolve itself after her daughter was born.

But in the days following her daughter's birth, Becky's blood sugars remained high. Her doctors worked to identify the problem. They soon discovered that Becky had been misdiagnosed. Instead of gestational diabetes, Becky had latent autoimmune diabetes in adults (LADA).

LADA is sometimes referred to as slow-onset type 1 diabetes or type 1.5 diabetes. It combines certain characteristics of type 1 and type 2. LADA occurs when the body slowly attacks and destroys the insulin-producing cells of the pancreas. The process is more gradual than it is in type 1 diabetes. It can progress over months or even years.

In the beginning stages, people with LADA are still producing some insulin, but their insulin production gradually decreases as more and more insulin-producing cells die off. Patients with LADA are frequently misdiagnosed with type 2 diabetes, while their underlying autoimmune problem is not addressed. Overall, 10 percent of people who have been diagnosed with type 2 diabetes have LADA.[3] This increases to 20 percent in type 2 diabetics who are not overweight.[4]

MOST PEOPLE WHO SUFFER FROM LADA[5]

- have the classic symptoms of diabetes.
- are diagnosed with diabetes in adulthood, but before age 50.
- are not overweight.
- may have a family history of autoimmune disease.
- may have another autoimmune condition.

In an Australian study, 90 percent of diabetics who had two or more of the above traits had LADA.[6] If you suspect that you have this form of diabetes, you should talk to your doctor about getting tested for the antibodies associated with autoimmune-related diabetes.

Remember that any form of diabetes can include or be aggravated by an autoimmune process. That's why it's important to protect your immune system from harmful substances that could trigger an autoimmune response. Let's take a look at some of those substances.

TREATING THE CAUSE

What actually causes autoimmune disease? Can anything be done to prevent or improve it? Part of the answer is found in the National Institutes of Health definition of autoimmune disease, stated earlier. An autoimmune response doesn't happen unless the body is trying to protect itself from a foreign invader, or antigen. These antigens—viruses, bacteria, or toxins—are what start the war. In an attempt to fight against them, the body mistakenly attacks itself. The pancreatic cells are killed under "friendly fire."

But where do these antigens come from? Can anything be done to prevent them from starting the war in the first place?

There is still much to discover about treatment for autoimmune disease. It's a complex process that warrants further investigation. However, research has identified some of the specific viruses and toxins that can initiate autoimmune disease. Sometimes these triggers are out of our control. Other times they are not.

In her groundbreaking book *The Autoimmune Epidemic*, Donna Jackson Nakazawa tackles the often-overlooked topic of the role that environmental toxins play in the development of autoimmune disease.[7] Nakazawa presents a compelling case to support her claim that the recent marked increased in autoimmune disease can largely be attributed to the body's response to environmental triggers.

ENVIRONMENTAL TOXINS

The United States produces or imports roughly 42 billion pounds of industrial chemicals every day.[8] These chemicals are used in a wide variety of different products, but have a sneaky way of seeping into the environment and then into our bodies. A study by the CDC found that the average American has traces of 212 environmental chemicals in his or her bloodstream.[9] These traces include toxic substances like pesticides, arsenic, flame-retardants, cadmium, mercury, lead, and perchlorate (an ingredient found in rocket fuel).

Even trace amounts of toxic chemicals can have a negative impact on health. BPA (bisphenol A) is a dangerous chemical found in many forms of plastic. This chemical is easily absorbed by the human body. BPA has been associated with an increased risk for several diseases including diabetes, cardiovascular disease, breast and prostate cancer, and neurological and behavioral disorders.[10] A CDC study revealed that 93 percent of Americans surveyed had detectable levels of BPA in their bloodstreams.[11]

Mercury is another toxic substance commonly found in the bloodstream.[12] One in three American women have detectable mercury levels in their blood.[13, 14] Research suggests that mercury increases the risk of heart disease,[15] promotes autoimmune changes, and causes neurological damage.[16]

Noel Rose, MD, PhD, director of the Autoimmune Disease Research Center at Johns Hopkins Medical Institute, strongly believes that the increased prevalence of autoimmune disease can be explained by an increase in environmental toxicity. He says, "We have no other good explanation as to why there should be an increase in autoimmune diseases, except for the things to which we are exposed in the environment. Autoimmunity is our immune system's effort to adapt to all the new environmental agents and shifts that we're being bombarded with. It's an unsuccessful adaptation, but it's our body's way of trying to fight back."[17]

WHAT CAN WE DO ABOUT IT?

Twelve-step programs like Alcoholics Anonymous have adopted a prayer that contains a lot of wisdom. It says: "God grant me serenity to accept the things I cannot change, courage to change the things I can, and wisdom to know the difference." When it comes to taking care of our health and avoiding toxin exposure, some factors are out of our control. There are things you cannot change. The air pollution of your city, the paint that your next-door neighbor uses, or the chemical cleaners you breathe in at work—these are things you may not have any say in.

However, there are other choices you have control over. You can do a few simple things to reduce your exposure to toxins. Let's take a look at some practical tips for safeguarding yourself against many food and environmental toxins.

AVOID FOOD TOXINS

Most of the toxins in our bodies come from what we eat. In the past 100 years, the Western diet has changed dramatically. Healthy, minimally-processed foods have been replaced with chemically- and genetically-modified, nutrient-depleted foods. In *The Autoimmune Epidemic,* Nakazawa aptly describes the problem with artificially-preserved foods:

> Centuries ago, salt, sugar, and vinegar were among the first food preservatives. Today, industrial food manufacturers have at their disposal an endless variety of chemical ways to preserve food....In an ironic sense, food processing might be defined thus: taking a food from nature, removing everything natural from it, then adding preservatives, dyes, bleaches, flavors, emulsifiers, and stabilizers to make it taste, look, feel, and smell like what it was originally supposed to be, but no longer is. The resemblance is there, but little else remains.[18]

Mounting research shows that many additives, chemicals, and dyes in commonly processed foods are not safe for human consumption. Nakazawa and other autoimmune specialists believe that these changes in our food may help to explain the growing prevalence of autoimmune disease.

One of the best things you can do to prevent or improve autoimmune disease is to eat a first-class diet. Whole, first-class foods are much less likely to be contaminated with toxic chemicals and preservatives. The powerful nutrients in these foods can actually help detoxify your body and rid it of substances that shouldn't be there.

Improving digestion will also help guard against autoimmune disease. Nakazawa writes about this in her book as well:

> An essential first step for anyone suffering from autoimmune disease is to ensure that his or her gastrointestinal tract is thriving.... A healthy intestine allows only digested nutrients to pass into the bloodstream. In patients with immune and inflammatory-based illnesses, the body's intestinal lining often becomes impaired, thus permitting larger molecules, such as bacteria and undigested foods, to slip through. In the bloodstream, these foreign items can trigger an immune reaction, making the body think that it's under attack and prompting the body's immune system to lash out to battle those foreign pathogens.[19]

By following the strategies in Chapter 14, you can improve your digestion and minimize your risk for autoimmune complications.

AVOIDING ENVIRONMENTAL TOXINS

In addition to food-related toxins, a variety of harmful toxins are found in the environment and in common household items used every day. People with a tendency toward autoimmune disease should especially be careful to limit their exposure to these toxins as far as possible.

Manufacturers of household cleaning supplies are not required to list the toxins those supplies contain. The safest bet is to purchase toxin-free cleaners that are now available at most grocery stores (for example, Seventh Generation®, Earth Friendly®, Biokleen®, etc.).

Because the government doesn't regulate personal hygiene products or cosmetics, these are another avenue for toxins to be introduced into your body. For example, women who use dark hair dyes have a three times greater risk for developing lupus than those who do not. For more information about safe personal products, visit www.safecosmetics.org.

USE COMMON SENSE

A little common sense goes a long way in reducing your personal toxin exposure as well as your environmental footprint. Wash your hands frequently. Carpool. Eat whole, plant-based foods. Choose organic when possible. Optimize your immune-enhancing vitamin D level. Avoid foods and substances that you know are unhealthy. The overall success or failure of your health and the health of your planet can be powerfully influenced by these small choices.

LOW-GRADE INFECTIONS

Another hidden culprit that can contribute to diabetes is the presence of a chronic, low-grade infection. If you've had diabetes for any length of time, you know that coming down with a cold, flu, or other sickness can cause your blood sugars to immediately shoot up. It's common for blood sugars to run at least 50 to 100 points higher as the result of an acute infection. These levels will remain high until the infection is effectively eradicated from the body. For this reason, diabetics are taught to monitor their blood sugars closely during bouts of acute infection.

But chronic, low-grade infections can also contribute to chronically high blood sugars. Gum or periodontal infections, yeast infections, stomach infections, sinus infections, and other infections that are sometimes accepted as "normal" can contribute to a chronic elevation in blood sugars. These infections cause a continual, low-grade form of inflammation in the body.

People who have periodontal disease are almost twice as likely to have a heart attack or stroke as people who do not have periodontal disease.[20] We usually don't think of our oral hygiene as being important to our overall health, but even the infection and inflammation that exists in our mouths can profoundly influence our risk. Infection in any part of the body will impact the health of the entire body. I frequently encourage my patients to go to the dentist to undergo routine cleanings and any necessary procedures.

It's critical that you pay attention to all forms of low-grade infection. If you have an infection, talk to your physician about aggressive ways to get rid of it for good.

Some infections are not as easy to detect as others. Studies show that seventy percent of elderly people[21] and 50 percent of the worldwide population[22] have an H. pylori bacterial infection in the stomach. This infection is often asymptomatic and can remain undetected for decades. You may want to talk to your doctor about being tested and treated for *H. pylori*.

In Chapter 20, I mentioned the benefit of the supplement berberine for blood sugar control. This supplement is also a powerful antimicrobial agent and may be beneficial for treating chronic, low-grade infections.[23]

PUTTING IT ALL TOGETHER

I hope this chapter encourages you to pay attention to health factors you may not have previously considered. You live in an imperfect world and are exposed to health hazards on a regular basis. However, you can take simple steps to reduce your risk by avoiding exposure to toxins and eliminating infections that increase risk of diabetes and other autoimmune disorders.

CHAPTER SUMMARY

- Diabetes is influenced by a variety of factors, some of which are not commonly understood.
- Diabetes can be caused or worsened by autoimmune problems.
- The worldwide prevalence of autoimmune conditions is increasing rapidly.
- At least 1 in 12 Americans has an autoimmune disorder.
- Type 1 diabetes is caused by an autoimmune reaction.
- Latent autoimmune diabetes in adults (LADA) is an autoimmune disorder.
- Many people with LADA are misdiagnosed with type 2 diabetes.
- If you suspect you have LADA, talk to your doctor about being tested for the antibodies associated with diabetes.
- There are practical things you can do to reduce your risk for autoimmune disease.

- The marked rise in environmental and food toxins may be contributing to the increase in autoimmune disorders.
- To avoid food toxins, eat whole, unprocessed, first-class foods.
- Choose toxin-free household supplies and personal care products.
- Chronic, low-grade infections can cause chronic blood sugar elevation.
- It is important to aggressively address and eradicate all forms of infection.

—TWENTY-THREE—

Reach Out for Help

Alone we can do so little. Together we can do so much.
—Helen Keller

I USED TO HAVE A PET *CONEJO*. THAT'S THE SPANISH WORD for rabbit. I was seven years old and living in Argentina with my missionary parents, my older brother, and of course my little rabbit, Peter. Peter's name came from the children's story, *The Tale of Peter Rabbit,* by Beatrix Potter.[1]

In this popular children's book, Peter Rabbit disobeys his mother and sneaks into Mr. McGregor's garden to snatch some vegetables: "First he ate some lettuces and some French beans; and then he ate some radishes; and then...he went to look for some parsley."

Mr. McGregor, who chased after Peter with a rake, scaring him almost to death, cut short Peter's first-class feast. Eventually, Peter escaped and made it back home. Shaken by the ordeal, Peter had a short bout with post-traumatic stress disorder. His mother gave him chamomile tea and put him to bed.

I recently heard another story about rabbits that I found absolutely fascinating. It wasn't from a children's book, but instead was from a study performed by researchers at the University of Texas.[2]

The researchers wanted to examine the correlation between diet and heart disease in rabbits. Instead of feeding them lettuce, French beans, radishes, and parsley, they fed them extra fatty, artery-clogging rabbit food.

But there was a twist to the study. Some of the rabbits were frequently held, petted, talked to, and played with, while others were not given extra attention.

As you might expect, the high-fat, high-cholesterol diet contributed to plaque formation and heart disease in many of the rabbits. But amazingly, the rabbits that had been loved and petted actually had 60 percent less plaque buildup in their arteries than the other rabbits!

SAY WHAT?

Wait a second! you might be thinking. *Do you mean to tell me that diet really isn't as important as I thought?* Before you throw in the towel and head to your nearest fast-food restaurant, let me explain. Diet is *extremely* important, as are all of the health strategies we've talked about. Most likely, none of the rabbits would have developed heart disease if they hadn't been placed on such an unhealthy diet. Even the rabbits that developed 60 percent less plaque still developed more plaque than they would have if they had been eating Peter Rabbit's kind of food.

This study shouldn't cause us to minimize the importance of diet. Instead, it should pique our interest in a health strategy that is often overlooked—the importance of love and positive support.

Rabbits aren't the only ones to experience health benefits from being loved. People do too. Multiple studies have shown that people who live isolated, lonely lives are more likely to suffer from heart disease, obesity, and diabetes than those who have strong support systems.[3, 4, 5]

LOVE AND SURVIVAL

In Chapter 4, I mentioned the success of Dr. Ornish who proved for the first time to the medical community that heart disease can be reversed by adopting a healthy lifestyle, including diet changes, regular exercise, stress-management, and group therapy and support.[6]

When the medical community learned of Dr. Ornish's success, they attributed it to changes in diet and exercise. The group support seemed like an adjunct and possibly unnecessary component of the program. That would seem to be logical. A tremendous amount of research supports the conclusion that simple changes in diet and exercise can reverse chronic diseases like heart disease and diabetes. But love? Support? What does all that touchy-feely stuff have to do with it?

Dr. Ornish believes that social support is an integral part of the healing process. In 1998, he published the national bestseller *Love and Survival,* which documents the scientific evidence that love and intimacy profoundly influence health and risk for disease. In the first chapter of the book, Dr. Ornish makes this bold statement, "I am not aware of any other factor in medicine that has a greater impact on our survival than the healing power of love and intimacy. Not diet, not smoking, not exercise, not stress, not genetics, not drugs, not surgery."[7]

Dr. Ornish then presents a compelling and scientifically sound case as to why love and support are important for our health. He outlines many studies that prove the same conclusion.

For instance, a Yale University study of 159 people undergoing coronary angiography found that the people who said that they felt loved and supported had significantly less arterial blockage than the people who did not. These results were independent of lifestyle habits and other risk factors such as diet, exercise, smoking, cholesterol, and genetics.[8]

A similar study in Sweden also showed decreased arterial blockage in women who reported close, supportive relationships—even when other lifestyle factors and risks were taken into consideration.[9]

Men who do not feel loved or supported by their wives are two to three times more likely to develop stomach ulcers than those who do feel loved and supported.[10]

In one Harvard University study, young, healthy students were asked to rate their relationship with their parents as: 1) very close, 2) warm and friendly, 3) tolerant, or 4) strained and cold. Thirty-five years later, 91 percent of those who had described that relationship negatively had developed a serious disease in mid-life, while only 45 percent of those who had rated it positively had developed a serious disease.[11]

Numerous studies indicate a powerful correlation between the health of our relationships and the health of our bodies. The good news is that we can take advantage of this information to reduce risk and promote wellness.

LEARN TO LOVE AND BE LOVED

Psychiatrist David Viscott insightfully stated, "To love and be loved is to feel the sun from both sides."[12] We were designed both to give and to receive love. One of the most powerful things you can do to improve your health is to learn to love and to be loved. If you have a strong spiritual, social, and family background, you may already be experiencing the health benefits of love. But in our fast-paced, individualized society, many people feel isolated and unconnected. Let's look at a few practical tips for building and maintaining loving relationships.

1. GET INVOLVED.

The ancient king Solomon wrote, "A man that has friends must show himself friendly."[13] It's just common sense. If you want to meet people and build quality friendships, you need to get involved with them and show that you care.

You can meet people in countless ways. Join a diabetes support group, a craft or hobby club, or an exercise team at your local gym. Volunteer at a community service organization, get involved in your local church, or invite your neighbors over for dinner. Don't wait for someone else to ask you—take the initiative to get involved.

One of the healthiest ways to get involved is to reach out to someone else. Focusing on improving the happiness of others will profoundly influence your own health. In the Old Testament, Isaiah wrote about the health benefits that could come from ministering to others: "Then your light will break forth like the dawn, and your healing will quickly appear."[14]

2. FIND SUPPORT.

It's important to have a strong support system. This may include your doctor and healthcare team as well as your spouse, family, and friends. Tell your loved ones how they can help encourage you to be healthy. Have a plan in place that includes someone you can talk to when you're feeling discouraged or overwhelmed. Then, share the favor with others.

3. MAKE PEOPLE A PRIORITY.

In our fast-paced, deadline-oriented society, it's easy to push relationships to the back burner. Far too many people sacrifice quality relationships while heavily investing in their career and other pursuits. But relationships are what make life worth living. If you have a hectic schedule, you may need to intentionally schedule time to spend with people. This is a necessity, not a luxury. You can experience lasting health benefits by making family and friends a priority.

4. FIND A HEALTH BUDDY.

Find someone in your life who wants to follow the same health strategies you do, then team up and do it together! You can find an exercise buddy, a nutrition buddy, or someone who wants to start drinking more water. Share your goals with each other, and then hold one another accountable. You can share with your buddy the things you've learned in this book. Not only will this benefit him or her, but it will also reinforce the information in your own mind.

You're more likely to be successful if you have the support of someone else who is moving in a similar direction. King Solomon described this well when he wrote, "Two are better than one.…If one falls down, his friend can help him up. But pity the man who falls and has no one to help him up!"[15]

5. PRACTICE FORGIVENESS.

Failing to give or receive forgiveness is one of the most destructive factors that affects overall health. Lack of forgiveness causes hostility, resentment, and regret. Redford Williams, MD, is the head of behavioral medicine at Duke University Medical Center and the coauthor of *Anger Kills: 17 Strategies for Controlling the Hostility that Can Harm Your Health.*[16] His numerous studies have shown that people with hostile personalities are at an increased risk for obesity, high cholesterol, high blood pressure, heart disease, and premature death. Hostility and stress lead to elevated levels of the stress hormone cortisol and increase arterial inflammation.

Often, people who are unwilling to receive forgiveness or to forgive others shut themselves off from healing and rewarding relationships. One example of this is my former patient, Nancy, who was in her early sixties when she participated in my six-month outpatient lifestyle program. Nancy wanted to stop her prediabetes in its tracks and reduce her risk of heart disease. She was serious about improving her health. She quickly began incorporating all the information she was learning. Soon, she dramatically lowered her blood sugar levels, inflammation levels, and cholesterol. Excited about her progress, Nancy remained consistent in making good health decisions.

About three months into the program, I lectured on the healing benefits of love and forgiveness. I shared that hostility and resentment are some of the most *dangerous* risk factors for disease. I had the participants fill out a questionnaire to determine their level of hostility, anger, and depression. They were not required to share the score with me or anyone else, but could use it confidentially to asses their risk. I noticed that Nancy looked very troubled as she answered the questions and scored her results.

After the questionnaire, I encouraged the patients to do what they could to improve their results. "If you're concerned with your score, there's good news," I said. "There are simple things you can do to reduce your level of hostility."

I shared a story about an interpersonal conflict I had recently had with a colleague. After the argument, we avoided one another. This continued for several weeks and was negatively impacting our professional relationship and friendship. I realized that the isolation and ill feelings were eating away at me and negatively impacting my health. I was embarrassed to deal with the situation, but decided it must be done. I picked up the phone, called, and apologized. I immediately felt a tremendous sense of relief, like a weight had been lifted from my shoulders.

"You may have unresolved conflicts in your life that are negatively impacting you," I said. "Sometimes we are hesitant and embarrassed to try to resolve these things because we don't know how the other person will respond. But we don't have to worry about their response. The important thing is to take the first step to initiate resolution." I finished my talk and left them with a challenge, "What can you do in the next 24 hours to deal with unresolved conflicts that are impacting your health?"

After the lecture, Nancy approached me with tears in her eyes. She shared with me that the test results had shown that she was experiencing a high level of anger and hostility. Nancy knew this was terrible for her health. She wanted to resolve it once and for all, but didn't know if she could.

Nancy then shared with me a story about an event that had happened 20 years before when her children were teenagers. Nancy's best friend was her next-door neighbor, Lisa. She and Lisa had connected when Nancy's family had moved into the neighborhood. For years their families had done fun activities together. The women shared a special bond. Nancy knew that Lisa was someone she could trust.

Then something unexpected happened. Lisa made a critical comment about Nancy's teenage son that deeply offended Nancy. Nancy was so upset that she told Lisa she never wanted to talk to her again. Lisa was surprised by Nancy's harsh reaction and also became offended. Despite the fact that they still lived next door to each other, they hadn't spoken during the past 20 years.

If they both went to take the trash to the curb at the same time, they would turn their backs and totally ignore each other. If they were walking toward each other on the sidewalk, one of them would cross over and walk on the other side of the street.

"What Lisa said made me so upset that I completely shut her out of my life," Nancy said. "But now I've realized that this anger I have toward her is actually hurting me. It's an even worse risk factor than my high cholesterol and blood sugars are." Nancy wanted to resolve the issue, but the thought of approaching Lisa seemed too embarrassing: "How can I talk to her now? I've let this go so long." I prayed with Nancy and encouraged her to keep praying and thinking about the best way to resolve this situation that was causing her so much grief.

Nancy went home burdened with her concern. As part of the program, we had encouraged participants to find exercise buddies. Nancy had chosen another neighbor whom she now walked with two times per day. The next morning, Nancy met with her walking partner and shared what was on her heart. She was honest about what had happened. She confided in her friend that she didn't know how to deal with the embarrassment of the situation, but wanted to make things right. Her friend listened patiently and then prayed again with Nancy. They agreed to meet again later to walk after dinner.

That evening, Nancy heard the usual knock and opened her front door, expecting to see her walking buddy. Her walking buddy was there, but so was someone else—Lisa. Overwhelmed with emotion, Nancy stepped out the door and looked Lisa in the face for the first time in 20 years. Both of them had tears in their eyes. Knowing that this was her chance, Nancy mustered the courage to say, "Lisa, I just want to tell you that I'm really sorry for what happened." Nancy held her breath, not knowing what to expect.

"No," Lisa said. "I'm so sorry for what I said. I hope we can be friends again." They both reached out, gave each other a big hug, and then went for a walk.

Later that evening, Nancy came to our group lecture and told us her story. A heavy burden had lifted from her shoulders. For 20 years, this stress and hostility had been eating at her, but now she realized that resolving the issue was the best thing she could have done. "I was excited when my cholesterol and blood sugar levels came down," Nancy said. "But I can tell that resolving this issue has improved my health and sense of well-being more than any other aspect of this program."

Dealing with past or present conflicts can be difficult and embarrassing. "I'm sorry" is a simple phrase, but those two words can be very difficult to say. Reconciliation begins with uncertainty and a willingness to feel vulnerable.

Often we are tempted to avoid the pain and leave issues unresolved. In his book *The Road Less Traveled*, Scott Peck, MD, defines mental health as "the willingness to deal with pain at all cost."[17] Our willingness to deal with painful situations (regardless of how other people respond) profoundly influences both mental and physical health.

Forgiveness is a cornerstone of the healing process. We are imperfect people living in an imperfect world. We make mistakes, and other people do too. Learning to love and forgive unconditionally can profoundly improve our health and reduce our risk for disease. It can also improve the lives of the people around us. If you want to learn more about how forgiveness can transform your physical and emotional health, I recommend the book, *Forgive to Live* by Dr. Dick Tibbits.[18]

RECEIVING FORGIVENESS

It is just as important to receive forgiveness as to give forgiveness. In fact, we may be unable to forgive others if we haven't first experienced forgiveness ourselves. We can't give what we don't have. I've experienced this firsthand. I can remember numerous times in my life when I've said or done things that were unkind. The guilt and remorse I experienced as a result started to change the way I felt about myself and others.

What has really helped me is the realization that God offers me unconditional love and forgiveness, regardless of what I have done. Accepting His forgiveness has motivated me to be more forgiving and to ask for forgiveness from others.

I now make it a personal goal to forgive quickly when I have been wronged and to ask for forgiveness quickly when I have been in the wrong. Forgiveness is the *only* solution in the universe that is powerful enough to unlock the chemical bonds of hostility, resentment, and bitterness. It is a medicine of the greatest importance.

CHAPTER SUMMARY

- Love and support are key components of the healing process.
- People who feel isolated and alone are much more likely to suffer from disease than those who have adequate support.
- There are several things you can do to improve the relational aspect of your health:
    - Get involved in your community and in the lives of people around you.
    - Reach out to help people in need.
    - Build a strong support system, including your family, friends, and healthcare team.
    - Find a health buddy. Encourage and support each other on the journey toward optimal health.
    - Be willing to give and receive forgiveness—from others, yourself, and God.

—APPENDIX—

Food Lists for Meal Balancing

THE FOLLOWING LISTS WILL HELP YOU DETERMINE serving sizes of different carbohydrate, protein, and fat foods. Remember, in order to experience optimal health, you need to eat the right *quantity* of the best possible *quality* of foods. The lists below are designed to help you understand serving sizes (quantity). Refer to the first-class foods lists in Chapter 13 to review the best *quality* of foods.

CARBOHYDRATE

Starchy Grains and Starchy Vegetables

1 serving = 15 grams of carbohydrate

Goal: 1–3 servings/meal

Starchy Grains

(Choose first-class whole grains.)

- 1 slice bread (1 ounce)
- 1 tortilla (6-inch size)
- ¼ large bagel (1 ounce)
- 2 taco shells (5-inch size)
- ½ hamburger bun or hot dog bun (1 ounce)
- ¾ cup ready-to-eat cereal
- ½ cup cooked cereal
- 4–6 small crackers
- ⅓ cup pasta or rice (cooked)
- ¾ ounce pretzels, potato, or tortilla chips
- 3 cups popcorn (popped)

STARCHY VEGETABLES

½ cup corn, sweet potatoes, winter squash, or mashed or boiled potatoes
¼ large baked potato (3 ounces)
½ cup beans, peas, or lentils (These are also protein foods. If you count this as a protein serving, you do not need to count it as a carb serving.)

FRUIT

1 serving = 15 grams of carbohydrate
Goal: 3–5 servings per day (roughly 1–2 servings per meal)

1 small fresh fruit (4 ounces)
½ cup canned fruit (in its own juice)
¼ cup dried fruit (2 tablespoons)
17 small grapes (3 ounces)
1 cup melon or berries
2 tablespoons raisins or dried fruit
½ cup fruit juice (4 ounces)

MILK AND MILK SUBSTITUTES

I strongly recommend avoiding dairy. Non-dairy substitutes are a better alternative. If you do choose to use dairy, be sure to use organic, fat-free products. Depending on the products you choose, you may need to count these as carbohydrate servings.

1 cup soy milk—check the label, as sugar content varies (unsweetened soymilk is free since it has less than 5 grams carb per serving)
1 cup almond milk – check the label, as sugar content varies (unsweetened almond milk is free since it has less than 5 grams carb per serving)
1 cup fat-free milk
⅔ cup plain, fat-free yogurt (6 ounces) – check the label, as sweetened yogurts have more sugar

NON-STARCHY VEGETABLES (CARBOHYDRATES THAT DON'T COUNT.)

1 serving = about 5 grams of carbohydrate = 1 cup raw vegetables or ½ cup cooked vegetables

Fill half your plate with 3 or more servings.
No need to count them in your carb servings.

Artichoke
Asparagus
Bamboo shoots
Broccoli
Brussel sprouts
Cabbage (green, bok choy, Chinese)
Carrots
Cauliflower
Celery
Chayote
Cucumber
Daikon
Eggplant
Gourds (bitter, bottle, luffa, bitter melon)
Green Onions or Scallions
Greens (collard, kale, mustard, turnip)
Hearts of Palm
Jicama
Kohlrabi
Leeks
Mung bean sprouts
Mushrooms
Okra
Onions
Pea Pods
Peppers

Radishes
Rutabaga
Salad Greens (chicory, endive, escarole, lettuce, romaine,
arugala, radicchio, watercress)
Spinach
Squash (summer, crookneck, zucchini)
Sugar Snap Peas
Swiss Chard
Tomato (raw)
Turnips
Water chestnuts

PROTEIN

1 serving = 7 grams of protein
Goal: 2 servings per meal

As discussed in Chapter 12, plant-based proteins are the best protein option for blood sugar management and overall health. When you choose plant-based proteins, such as those listed below, you don't have to count their carbohydrate content into your carb servings.

½ cup beans (black, garbanzo, kidney, lima, navy, pinto, white, edamame)
½ cup peas (green, black-eyed and split peas)
½ cup lentils (brown, green, or yellow)
1/3 cup hummus
½ cup tofu (4 ounces)
¾ cup tempeh
3 patties falafel (2 inches across—Mediterranean chick pea and wheat patties)
3 ounces meatless burger (soy-based)
1 patty meatless burger (2½ ounces)
1 meatless hot dog (soy-based)
1 tablespoon nut spreads (almond, cashew, peanut, and soy nut butters)

Keep in mind that many animal protein foods are high in fat and cholesterol. Avoid third-class animal foods altogether, and minimize second-class animal foods as much as possible.

1 egg
2 egg whites
¼ cup egg substitutes
¼ cup fat-free cottage cheese
1 ounce meat (chicken, turkey, fish)

FAT

1 serving = 5 grams of fat
Goal: 2-4 servings per meal

The healthiest way to eat fats is in whole, unrefined plant foods such as olives, nuts, seeds, coconut, and avocado.

HEALTHY FATS

2 tablespoons (1/8) avocado
2 teaspoons nut spreads (almond butter, cashew butter, peanut butter)
8 large olives
6 almonds
2 brazil nuts
6 cashews
5 filberts (hazelnuts)
3 macadamia nuts
10 peanuts
4 pecan halves
16 pistachios
4 walnut halves
1 tablespoon pine nuts
1 tablespoon flaxseed, pumpkin, sunflower, or sesame seeds
2 teaspoons tahini or sesame paste
2 tablespoons coconut, shredded
1/3 cup light coconut milk
1½ tablespoons regular coconut milk
1 teaspoon olive or coconut oil (use sparingly)

Endnotes

CHAPTER 1: THE DIABEDEMIC

1 Centers for Disease Control and Prevention, "National Diabetes Fact Sheet: National Estimates and General Information on Diabetes and Prediabetes in the United States," US Department of Health and Human Services, Centers for Disease Control and Prevention, Atlanta, GA, 2011.

2 Centers for Disease Control and Prevention, Crude and Age-Adjusted Percentage of Civilian, Noninstitutionalized Population with Diagnosed Diabetes, Atlanta, GA, 1980-2010. Last modified 12/9/2011, http://www.cdc.gov/diabetes/statistics/prev/national/figage.htm.

3 World Health Organization, Diabetes Fact Sheet, August 2011, http://www.who.int/mediacentre/factsheets/fs312/en/.

4 Cowie, Catherine, et al, "Full Accounting of Diabetes and Pre-Diabetes in the U.S. Population in 1988-1994 and 2005-2006" *Diabetes Care*. 32.2 (2009): 287–294.

5 American Diabetes Association, "Prediabetes FAQ's," Accessed July 2012, http://www.diabetes.org/diabetes-basics/prevention/pre-diabetes/pre-diabetes-faqs.html.

6 See Endnote 1.

7 See Endnote 4.

8 See Endnote 1.

9 National Institutes of Health News, "One Third of Adults with Diabetes Still Don't Know They Have It," Accessed July 2012, http://www.nih.gov/news/pr/may2006/niddk-26.htm.

10 See Endnote 1.

11 See Endnote 1.

12 Centers for Disease Control and Prevention, "Leading Causes of Death," Atlanta, GA, 2011, http://www.cdc.gov/nchs/fastats/lcod.htm.

13 See Endnote 3

14 Hu, Frank, et al, "Diet, Lifestyle, and the Risk of Type 2 Diabetes Mellitus in Women," *New England Journal of Medicine*, 345.11, (2001): 790-797.

15 See Endnote 1.

CHAPTER 2: DIABETES FOR DUMMIES

1 American Heart Association, "Cardiovascular Disease and Diabetes," Accessed July 2012, http://www.heart.org/HEARTORG/Conditions/Diabetes/WhyDiabetesMatters/Cardiovascular-Disease-Diabetes_UCM_313865_Article.jsp#.T3yR3lGsf_Z.

2 See Endnotes 1 and 4, Chapter 1.

3 See Endnote 1, Chapter 1.

4 National Diabetes Information Clearinghouse, "Diabetes Overview," National Institutes of Health, Bethesda, MD, 2008, http://diabetes.niddk.nih.gov/dm/pubs/overview/#types.

5 See Endnote 1, Chapter 1.

6 Jean-Pierre Després, et al, "Hyperinsulinemia as an Independent Risk Factor for Ischemic Heart Disease," The New England Journal of Medicine, 334 (1996): 952-958.

7 American Diabetes Association, "What is Gestational Diabetes," Accessed July 2012, http://www.diabetes.org/diabetes-basics/gestational/what-is-gestational-diabetes.html.

CHAPTER 3: A METABOLIC MESS

1 Random House Dictionary, "Metabolism," Accessed July 2012, http://dictionary.reference.com/browse/metabolism.

2 See Endnote 12, Chapter 1.

3 National Heart, Lung, and Blood Institute, "What is diabetic heart disease?," National Institutes of Health, Bethesda, MD, 2011, http://www.nhlbi.nih.gov/health/health-topics/topics/dhd/.

4 American Heart Association, "Cardiovascular Disease & Diabetes," Accessed July 2012, http://www.heart.org/HEARTORG/Conditions/Diabetes/WhyDiabetesMatters/Cardiovascular-Disease-Diabetes_UCM_313865_Article.jsp.

5 Bowie, A, et al, "Glycosylated Low Density Lipoprotein is More Sensitive to Oxidation: Implications for the Diabetic Patient?," Atherosclerosis, 102.1(1993): 63-67.

6 American Diabetes Association, "Standards of Medical Care in Diabetes—2011," *Diabetes Care,* 34.1(2011):S11–S61, table 9.

7 Stratton, Irene, et al, "Association of Glycaemia with Macrovascular and Microvascular Complications of Type 2 Diabetes (UKPDS 35): Prospective Observational Study," BMJ, 321.7258 (2000): 405-412.

8 Pitsavos, Christos, et al, "Association Between Low-Grade Systemic Inflammation and Type 2 Diabetes Mellitus Among Men and Women from the ATTICA Study," The Review of Diabetic Studies, 4.2 (2007): 98-104.

9 Libby, P. and Ridker, P.M., "Inflammation and Atherosclerosis: Role of C-reactive Protein in Risk Assessment," The American Journal of Medicine, 116.6A (2004): 9S-16S.

10 Gorman, Christine, et al, "Health: The Fires Within," Time, Accessed July 2012, http://www.time.com/time/magazine/article/0,9171,993419,00.html.

11 Kotz, Deborah, "Chronic Inflammation: Reduce It to Protect Your Health," U.S. News, Accessed July 2012, http://health.usnews.com/health-news/family-health/articles/2009/11/02/chronic-inflammation-reduce-it-to-protect-your-health.

12 Hyman, Mark "Is Your Body Burning Up With Hidden Inflammation?," Huffington Post, Accessed July 2012, http://www.huffingtonpost.com/dr-mark-hyman/is-your-body-burning-up-w_b_269717.html.

13 See Endnote 8.

14 Baker, SM, *Detoxification and Healing*, Revised 2nd Edition, (Chicago, IL, McGraw Hill, 2003).

15 Centers for Disease Control and Prevention, "Vital Signs: Prevalence, Treatment, and Control of Hypertension—United States, 1999-2002 and 2005-2008," Morbidity and Mortality Weekly Report, 60.4 (2011):103-108.

16 Centers for Disease Control and Prevention, "High Blood Pressure Facts," Atlanta, GA, Accessed July 2012, http://www.cdc.gov/bloodpressure/facts.htm.

17 World Heart Federation, "Diabetes," Geneva, Switzerland, Accessed July 2012, http://www.world-heart-federation.org/cardiovascular-health/cardiovascular-disease-risk-factors/diabetes/.

18 Personal phone call with Gerald Reaven, July 9, 2012.

19 Reaven, Gerald M., *Syndrome X: The Silent Killer* (New York: Simon and Schuster, 2000).

20 Doron Aronson and Elliot J. Rayfield, "How Hyperglycemia Promotes Atherosclerosis: Molecular Mechanisms," Cardiovascular Diabetology, 1.1 (2002).

CHAPTER 4: THE DIABETIC'S GENETICS

1 National Human Genome Research Institute, "The Human Genome Project," Accessed July 2012, http://www.genome.gov/10001772/.

2 National Human Genome Research Institute, "The Human Genome Project," Accessed July 2012, http://www.genome.gov/12011238.

3 Waterland, R.A. and Jirtle, RL, "Transposable Elements: Targets for Early Nutritional Effects on Epigenetic Gene Regulation," Molecular Cell Biology, 23 (2003): 5293-5300.

4 PBS. "Nova Science Now," Epigenetics Video (2007), http://www.pbs.org/wgbh/nova/body/epigenetics.html.

5 Watters, Ethan, "DNA is Not Destiny," Discover Magazine, 11 (2006), http://discovermagazine.com/2006/nov/cover.

6 See Endnote 5.

7 Ornish, Dean, "Dr. Dean Ornish's Program for Reversing Heart Disease," (New York, Ballantine Books, 1996).

8 Ornish, Dean, "Changes in Prostate Gene Expression in Men Undergoing an Intensive Nutrition and Lifestyle Intervention," National Academy of Sciences. 105. 24 (2008): 8369-8374.

9 "Change in diet, exercise may change your genes," Reuters: June 16, 2008

10 American Cancer Society, "Breast Cancer," Accessed July 2012, http://documents.cancer.org/acs/groups/cid/documents/webcontent/003090-pdf.pdf.

11 National Breast Cancer Foundation, "What Is Breast Cancer?," Accessed July 2012, http://www.nationalbreastcancer.org/about-breast-cancer/what-is-breast-cancer.aspx.

12 Narod, Steven, "BRCA1 and BRCA2 in 2005," Discovery Medicine, 74 (2012), http://www.discoverymedicine.com/Steven-A-Narod/2009/07/16/brca1-and-brca2-in-2005/.

CHAPTER 5: THERE'S A CURE FOR SURE!

1 Howe, Rebekah and Harrison, Alex, "Google SWOT Analysis," Google News Online, 2011, Accessed July 2012, http://www.googlenewsonline.com/google-swot-analysis.html.

2 The American Heritage Dictionary of the English Language, "Cure," (New York: Houghton Mifflin Company, Fourth Edition, 2000).

3 American Diabetes Association, "Standards of Medical Care in Diabetes—2010," Diabetes Care, 33 (2010): S11-S61.

4 World Health Organization, Obesity and Overweight Fact Sheet, May 2012, http://www.who.int/mediacentre/factsheets/fs311/en/.

5 See Endnote 4.

6 Buettner, Dan, "The Secrets of Living Longer," National Geographic. 11 (2005).

7 Anderson, James, "High Fiber Diets for Diabetic and Hypertriglyceridemic Patients," CMA Journal, 123 (1980): 977-979.

8 "Supersize Me," directed by Morgan Spurlock (United States: Samuel Goldwyn Films, 2004), DVD.

9 Buchwald, Henry, et al, "Bariatric Surgery: A Systematic Review and Meta-analysis," The Journal of the American Medical Association, 292.14 (2004): 1724-1737.

10 Associated Press, "Beating Diabetes: Some do, but are they cured?," MSNBC, April 2009. Accessed July 2012, http://www.msnbc.msn.com/id/30294089/ns/health-diabetes/t/beating-diabetes-some-do-are-they-cured/#.T_s_gFGsf_Y.

11 Hellmich, Nanci, "Bill Clinton Declares Vegan Victory," USA Today Online, August 2011. Accessed July 2012, http://yourlife.usatoday.com/fitness-food/diet-nutrition/story/2011-08-23/Bill-Clinton-declares-vegan-victory/50111212/1.

12 Hicks, J. Morris and Hicks, J. Stanfield, "Healthy Eating. Healthy World. Unleashing the Power of Plant-Based Nutrition," (Dallas, Texas: Benbella Books, Inc., 2011).

13 Wyrick, Jason. "Cured Type 2 Diabetes. No Cost." Dr. McDougall's Health and Medical Center, Accessed July 2012, http://www.drmcdougall.com/stars/jason_wyrick.html.

14 Physicians Committee for Responsible Medicine Diabetes Success Story, "Jason Wyrick," YouTube, 2008, Accessed July 2012, http://www.youtube.com/watch?v=6jRMrkR9ROU.

15 Barnard, Neal, "Dr. Neal Barnard's Program for Reversing Diabetes," (Emmaus, PA: Rodale Inc. Books, 2007).

16 Barnard, Neal, et al, "A Low-fat Vegan Diet Improves Glycemic Control and Cardiovascular Risk Factors in a Randomized Clinical Trial in Individuals with Type 2 Diabetes," Diabetes Care, 29.8 (2006): 1777-1783.

17 See Endnote 15.

18 Physicians Committee for Responsible Medicine Diabetes Success Story, "Nancy Boughn," YouTube, 2008, Accessed July 2012, http://www.youtube.com/watch?v=ljlCrAiDgVk.

19 Fuhrman, Joel, "Eat to Live," (New York: Little, Brown and Company, 2003) 185-190.

20 Fuhrman, Joel, "American Diabetes Alert Day," DrFuhrman.com, March 2010, Accessed July 2012, http://www.drfuhrman.com/library/american_diabetes_association_alert.aspx.

21 Romans 8:24 (New International Version).

CHAPTER 6: WARNING SIGNS

1 American Diabetes Association, "Who is at a Greater Risk for Type 2 Diabetes," Accessed July 2012, http://www.diabetes.org/diabetes-basics/prevention/risk-factors/.

2 See Endnote 4, Chapter 1.

3 Manson, Joann, "Nurses' Health Study," (paper presented at the American College of Nutrition Annual Meetings, 1994).

4 National Diabetes Prevention Program, "About the Program," Centers for Disease Control and Prevention, Accessed July 2012, http://www.cdc.gov/diabetes/prevention/about.htm.

5 Biggs, Mary L., et al, "Association Between Adiposity in Midlife and Older Age and Risk of Diabetes in Older Adults," *The Journal of the American Medical Association,* 303.24 (2010):2504-2512.

6 Haffner, Steven, "Abdominal Obesity, Insulin Resistance, and Cardiovascular Risk in Prediabetes and Type 2 Diabetes," European Heart Journal Supplements, 8.B (2006): 20-25.

7 Harvard Medical School, "Abdominal Fat and What to do About it,", 2006, Accessed July 2012, http://www.health.harvard.edu/newsweek/Abdominal-fat-and-what-to-do-about-it.htm.

8 Havard Public Health School, "The Obesity Prevention Source: Waist Size Matters," Accessed July 2012, http://www.hsph.harvard.edu/obesity-prevention-source/obesity-definition/abdominal-obesity/index.html.

9 National Center for Health Statistics, "Most Americans Don't Exercise Regularly," CNN Health Online, April 2002, Accessed July 2012, http://articles.cnn.com/2002-04-07/health/americans.exercise_1_vigorous-activity-leisure-time-exercise-activity-at-least-three?_s=PM:HEALTH.

10 Mokdad AH, et al, "Actual Causes of Death in the United States, 2000," *Journal of American Medical Association*, 291.10 (2004):1238-1245.

11 Spelsberg, Angela and Manson, Joann, "Physical Activity in the Treatment and Prevention of Diabetes," *Comprehensive Therapy*, 21.10, (1995): 559-564.

12 Bruce, CR and Hawley JA, "Improvements in Insulin Resistance with Aerobic Exercise Training: a Lipocentric Approach," Medical Science Sports Exercise, 36.7, (2004): 1196-201.

13 Rose, Adam and Richter, Erik, "Skeletal Muscle Glucose Uptake During Exercise: How is it Regulated?," Physiology. 20.4 (2005): 260-270.

14 Centers for Disease Control and Prevention, "High Blood Pressure Facts," Accessed July 2012, http://www.cdc.gov/bloodpressure/facts.htm.

15 World Heart Federation, "Diabetes," Accessed July 2012, http://www.world-heart-federation.org/cardiovascular-health/cardiovascular-disease-risk-factors/diabetes/.

16 Discovery Fit and Health. "What's the Difference Between LDL and HDL Cholestrol?," Accessed July 2012, http://health.howstuffworks.com/diseases-conditions/cardiovascular/cholesterol/difference-between-ldl-and-hdl-cholesterol1.htm.

17 Staprans, I, et al, "Oxidized Cholesterol in the Diet Accelerates the Development of Atherosclerosis in LDL Receptor and Apolipoprotein E-deficient Mice," *Arteriosclerosis, Thrombosis, and Vascular Biology*, 20.3 (2000): 708-714.

18 CHIP, "The Good and Bad Kinds of Cholestrol," Accessed July 2012, http://www.chiphealth.com/health_topics/topics/kinds_of_cholesterol.php.

19 Harvard Public Health School, "The Nutrition Source," Accessed July 2012, http://www.hsph.harvard.edu/nutritionsource/what-should-you-eat/fats-full-story/#cholesterol.

20 Kratz, M, "Dietary Cholesterol, Atherosclerosis, and Coronary Heart Disease," *Handbook of Experimental Pharmacology*, 170 (2005): 195-213.

21 American Heart Association, "About Cholesterol," Accessed August 2012, http://www.heart.org/HEARTORG/Conditions/Cholesterol/AboutCholesterol/About-Cholesterol_UCM_001220_Article.jsp.

22 Mayo Clinic, "Cholestrol Levels: What Numbers Should you Aim For?," Accessed August 2012, http://www.mayoclinic.com/health/cholesterol-levels/CL00001.

23 CNN Health. "One Third of Americans Have High Triglycerides," March 2009, Accessed August 2012, http://articles.cnn.com/2009-03-24/health/hm.cholesterol.heart_1_triglyceride-levels-bad-cholesterol-deciliter?_s=PM:HEALTH.

24 Harvard Medical School, "How to Improve Tryglyceride Levels," October 2007, Accessed August 2012, http://www.health.harvard.edu/newsletters/Harvard_Womens_Health_Watch/2007/October/how_to_improve_triglyceride_levels_.

25 Stannard, SR and Johnson, NA, "Insulin Resistance and Elevated Triglyceride in Muscle," *Journal of Physiology*, 554 (2004): 595-607.

26 American Diabetes Association, "Prediabetes FAQs," Accessed August 2012, http://www.diabetes.org/diabetes-basics/prevention/pre-diabetes/pre-diabetes-faqs.html#QA-4.

27 Tirosh, Amir, et al, "Changes in Triglyceride Levels Over Time and Risk of Type 2 Diabetes in Young Men," *Diabetes Care*, 31.10 (2008): 2032–2037.

28 BBC News, "China Faces Diabetes Epidemic', Research Suggests,"' March 2010, Accessed August 2012, http://news.bbc.co.uk/2/hi/8587032.stm.

29 See Endnote 2.

30 Central Intelligence Agency, "The World Fact Book: Nauru," Accessed August 2012, https://www.cia.gov/library/publications/the-world-factbook/geos/nr.html.

31 Marks, Kathy, "Fat of the Land: Nauru Tops Obesity League," The Independent, December 2010, Accessed August 2012, http://www.independent.co.uk/life-style/health-and-families/health-news/fat-of-the-land-nauru-tops-obesity-league-2169418.html.

32 "King, H. and Rewers M., "Diabetes in Adults is Now a Third World Problem," *Ethnicity & Disease* 3 (1993): 67–74.

33 World Health Organization, "Nauru," Accessed August 2012, http://www.who.int/countries/nru/en/index.html.

34 ABC News Online, "The Fattest Place on Earth," Frontline, Accessed August 2012, http://abcnews.go.com/Nightline/video/fattest-place-earth-12533987.

35 Wikipedia, "Young Naurun People.jpg," Accessed July 2012, http://upload.wikimedia.org/wikipedia/commons/thumb/1/12/Young_nauruan_people.jpg/543px-Young_nauruan_people.jpg).

36 See Endnote 34.

37 Manner, HI, et al, "Plant succession after phosphate mining on Nauru," *Australian Geographer, 26.3 (1985): 185-195.*

38 BBC News, "Nauru Profile," Accessed August 2012, http://www.bbc.co.uk/news/world-asia-pacific-15433616.

39 See Endnote 34.

40 Centers for Disease Control and Prevention, "Diabetes Complications," Accessed August 2012, http://www.cdc.gov/diabetes/statistics/complications_national.htm.

CHAPTER 7: HOW ARE YOUR SUGARS

1 Guthrie, Diana and Humphreys, Selbys, "Diabetes Urine Testing: An Historical Perspective," *The Diabetes Educator*, 14.6 (1988): 521-525.

2 American Diabetes Association, "Screening for Type 2 Diabetes," *Diabetes Care*, 27.1 (2004): 511-514.

3 American Diabetes Association, "Who is at a Greater Risk for Type 2 Diabetes," Accessed July 2012, http://www.diabetes.org/diabetes-basics/prevention/risk-factors/.

4 National Diabetes Information, "Am I at Risk for Type 2 Diabetes? Taking Steps to Lower Your Risk of Getting Diabetes," National Institutes of Health, Accessed July 2012, http://diabetes.niddk.nih.gov/dm/pubs/riskfortype2/#6.

5 See Endnote 4, Chapter 1.

6 American Diabetes Association, "Screening for Diabetes," *Diabetes Care*, 25.1 (2002): 521-524.

7 National Diabetes Information Clearninghouse, "Diagnosis of Diabetes," National Institutes of Health, Accessed July 2012, http://diabetes.niddk.nih.gov/dm/pubs/diagnosis/#what.

8 Buysschaert, Martin and Bergman, Michael, "Definition of Prediabetes," Accessed July 2012, http://info.theclinics.com/mdconsult/pdf/Medical_Clinics_sample_article.pdf.

9 Simon, K, "Tests for Diagnosing Diabetes Mellitus. Glucose Tolerance Test is Most Sensitive," *BMJ*, 309.6953 (1994): 537-538.

10 National Library of Medicine, "Glucose Tolerance Test," Accessed July 2012, http://www.nlm.nih.gov/cgi/mesh/2011/MB_cgi?mode=&term=Glucose+Tolerance+Test.

11 American Diabetes Association, "Standards of Medical Care in Diabetes-2010," *Diabetes Care*, 33.1 (2010): 511-561.

12 See Endnote 7.

13 See Endnote 11.

14 Sciacqua, A, et al, "One-hour Postload Plasma Glucose Levels and Left Ventricular Mass in Hypertensive Patients," *Diabetes Care*, 34.6 (2011): 1406-1411.

15 Lamar, M.E., et al, "Jelly Beans as an Alternative to a Fifty-Gram Glucose Beverage for Gestational Diabetes Screening," *American Journal or Obstetrics and Gynecology*, 181.5 (1999): 1154-1157.

16 See Endnote 4, Chapter 1.

17 See Endnote 7.

18 Medical Dictionary, "Glycosylated Hemoglobin Test," The Free Dictionary, Accessed July 2012, http://medical-dictionary.thefreedictionary.com/glycosylated+hemoglobin+test.

19 Nathan, D.M., Genuth, S, Lachin, J, et al, "The Effect of Intensive Treatment of Diabetes on the Development and Progression of Long-Term Complications in Insulin-Dependent Diabetes Mellitus," *The New England Journal of Medicine*, 329.14 (1993): 977–986.

20 American Diabetes Association , "ADA's New Clinical Practice Recommendations Promote A1c as Diagnostic Test for Diabetes," Accessed July 2012, http://www.diabetes.org.

21 Bayer Diabetes Care, "How Does A1c Relate to Glucose Control?," Accessed July 2012, http://www.A1cnow.com/Professionals/About-A1c/How-Does-A1c-Relate-to-Glucose-Control#ref2.

22 Stratton, Irene, et al, "Association of Glycaemia with Macrovascular and Microvascular Complications of Type 2 Diabetes (UKPDS 35): Prospective Observational Study," *BMJ*, 321.7258 (2000): 405-412.

23 Vlassara, H, "Chronic Diabetic Complications and Tissue Glycosylation. Relevant Concern for Diabetes-Prone Black Population," *Diabetes Care*, 13.11 (1990): 1180-1185.

CHAPTER 8: THE FIVE STAGES OF HIGH BLOOD SUGAR

1 Guam Diabetes Prevention & Control Program, "Island of Guam," Department of Public Health and Social Services, Accessed August 2012, http://www.guamdiabetes.org/pdf/Prevalence%20of%20Diabetes%20from%202001%20-%202010.pdf.

2 Buysschaert, Martin, et al, "Definition of Prediabetes," Accessed July 2012, http://info.theclinics.com/mdconsult/pdf/Medical_Clinics_sample_article.pdf.

3 National Institutes of Health, "What is Prediabetes?," Accessed July 2012, http://diabetes.niddk.nih.gov/dm/pubs/stroke/#what-pre.

4 Youngberg, Wes, et al, "Diabetes Care on Guam: Guidelines for Prevention, Early Detection, and Treatment," Governor's Vision 2001 Task Force on Health Care, Guam Department of Public Health and Social Services, July 1997.

CHAPTER 9: HOW'S YOUR PANCREAS?

1 Lab Tests Online, "Insulin," Accessed July 2012, http://labtestsonline.org/understanding/analytes/insulin/tab/test.

2 Mayo Clinic, "Type 2 Diabetes," Accessed July 2012, https://www.mayoclinic.com/health/hyperinsulinemia/HQ00896.

3 Reaven, Gerald, "Insulin Resistance/Compensatory Hyperinsulinemia, Essential Hypertension, and Cardiovascular Disease," *The Journal of Clinical Endocrinology and Metabolism*, 88.6 (2003): 2399-2403.

4 Despres, Jean-Pierre, et al, "Hyperinsulinemia as an Independent Risk Factor for Ischemic Heart Disease," *The New England Journal of Medicine*, 334 (1996): 952-958.

5 Modan, Michaela, et al, "Hyperinsulinemia: A Link Between Hypertension Obesity and Glucose Intolerance". *Journal of Clinical Investigation, 75* (1985): 809-817.

6 Barnard, R. James, "Prostate Cancer Prevention by Nutritional Means to Alleviate Metabolic Syndrome," *The American Journal of Clinical Nutrition*, 86.3, (2007): 8895-8935.

7 Giovannucci, Edward, "Insulin and Colon Cancer," *Cancer Causes and Control*, 6.2 (1995): 164-179.

8 Novosyadlyy, Ruslan and LeRoith, Derek, "Hyperinsulinemia and Type 2 Diabetes," *Cell Cycle*. 9.8 (2010): 1449-1450.

9 Sakumoto, Tetsurou, et al, "Insulin Resistance/Hyperinsulinemia and Reproductive Disorders in Infertile Women," *Reproductive Medicine and Biology*, 9.4 (2010): 185.

10 Osterweil, Neil, "Elevated Insulin Increases Alzheimer's Disease Risk," MedPage Today. August 2005, Accessed August 2012, http://www.medpagetoday.com/Neurology/AlzheimersDisease/1506.

11 Bohanon, Nancy, Family Practice Audio Digest. 1991-1992.

12 Hyman, Mark, *The Blood Sugar Solution* (New York: Little, Brown and Company, 2012),180.

13 See Endnote 12.

14 Lab Tests Online, "C-Peptide," Accessed July 2012, http://labtestsonline.org/understanding/analytes/c-peptide/tab/test.

15 WebMD, "Diabetes Health Center: C-peptide," Accessed August 2012, http://diabetes.webmd.com/c-peptide.

16 Weinstock, Ruth and Zygmont, Steven, "Pancreatic Islet Function Tests," EndoText.org, January 201o, Accessed August 2012, http://www.endotext.org/protocols/protocols5/protocols5.htm.

17 Personal interview, George Guthrie and Charles Zeno Marcell, American College of Lifestyle Medicine Meeting, September 2006.

CHAPTER 10: LOOKING AT THE BIG PICTURE

1 World Health Organization, "The Top 10 Causes of Death," Updated June 2011, Accessed July 2012, http://www.who.int/mediacentre/factsheets/fs310/en/index.html.

2 Lloyd-Jones, Donald, et al, "Heart Disease and Stroke Statistics- 2009 Update. A Report From the American Heart Association Statistics Committee and Stroke Statistics Subcommittee," Circulation Online, December 2008, http://circ.ahajournals.org/citmgr?gca=circulationaha;CIRCULATIONAHA.108.191261v1.

3 American Heart Association, "Cardiovascular Disease & Diabetes," Updated February 2012, Accessed August 2012, http://www.heart.org/HEARTORG/Conditions/Diabetes/WhyDiabetesMatters/Cardiovascular-Disease-Diabetes_UCM_313865_Article.jsp.

4 See Endnote 5, Chapter 1.

5 Stanton, Robert, "Diabetic Kidney Disease," Joslin Diabetes Center, YouTube, Accessed July 2012, http://www.youtube.com/watch?v=w2TdxGZjg7Y.

6 See Endnote 1, Chapter 1.

7 Collazo-Clavell, Maria, "Expert Answers. Diabetes: How Do I Help Protect My Liver?," Mayo Clinic, Accessed http://www.mayoclinic.com/health/diabetes/AN00193.

8 ABC News Online, "FDA: New Warning Labels for Statins," February 2012, Accessed August 2012, http://abcnews.go.com/Health/Wellness/warning-labels-highlight-statin-dangers/story?id=15810244#.T_3jqlGsdZk.

9 Blackwell, J, "Evaluation and Treatment of Hyperthyroidism and Hypothyroidism," *Journal of the American Academy of Nurse Practioners*, 16.10 (2004): 422-425.

10 Wu, Patricia, "Practical Pointers: Thyroid Disease and Diabetes, *Clinical Diabetes*, 18 (2000), Accessed July 2012, http://journal.diabetes.org/clinicaldiabetes/v18n12000/pg38.htm.

11 Klein, Irwin and Danzi, Sara, "Cardiovascular Involvement in General Medical Conditions," *Circulation*, 116 (2007): 1725-1735.

12 Ginde, Adit, et al, "Demographic Differences and Trends of Vitamin D Insufficiency in the US Population, 1988-2004" Archives of Internal Medicine, 169.6 (2009): 626-632.

13 Coyne, Daniel, "Vitamin D and the Diabetic Patient," MedScape.org. Accessed August 2012, http://www.medscape.org/viewarticle/573383.

14 Hypponen, Elina, et al, "Intake of Vitamin D and Risk of Type 1 Diabetes: A Birth Cohort Study" *The Lancet*. 358.9292 (2001) 1500-1503.

15 Knekt, P, et al, "Serum Vitamin D and Subsequent Occurrence of Type 2 Diabetes," Epidemiology, 19 (2008):666-671.

16 Vitamin D Council, "Vitamin D News," Accessed July 2012, http://www.vitamindcouncil.org/.

CHAPTER 11: THINK GOOD THOUGHTS

1 Meyer, Paul, "What would you do if you knew you couldn't fail? Creating S.M.A.R.T. Goals," *Attitude Is Everything: If You Want to Succeed Above and Beyond*, (Waco, Texas: Meyer Resource Group, 2003).

2 Marketing Campaign Case Studies, "Obey Your Thirst Campaign (2004)," Accessed July 2012, http://marketing-case-studies.blogspot.com/2008/05/obey-your-thirst-campaign-2004.html.

3 Behavioral Diabetes Institute, "Breaking Free from Depression and Diabetes," San Diego, CA, Accessed July 2012, http://behavioraldiabetesinstitute.org/downloads/Breaking-Free-from-Depression-and-Diabetes.pdf.

4 Shryock, Harold. *Family Medical Guide to Health and Fitness Volume 1*. (Washington DC: Review & Herald + Pacific Press, 1991), 114-135.

CHAPTER 12: EAT TO LIVE

1 Fuhrman, Joel, *Eat to Live* (New York: Little Brown and Company, 2003), 7.

2 Joslin Diabetes Center, "How Does Fiber Affect Blood Glucose Levels?," Accessed July 2012, https://www.joslin.org/info/how_does_fiber_affect_blood_glucose_levels.html.

3 Brown, Lisa, et al, "Cholesterol-lowering effects of dietary fiber: a Meta-analysis," *The American Journal of Clinical Nutrition*, 69.1 (1999): 30-42.

4 Slavin, JL, "Dietary Fiber and Body Weight," *Nutrition*, 21.3 (2005): 411-418.

5 American Institute for Cancer Research, "Major New Analysis: Fiber May Prevent Breast Cancer," January 2012, Accessed August 2012, http://blog.aicr.org/2012/01/11/major-new-analysis-fiber-may-prevent-breast-cancer/.

6 American Heart Association, "Whole Grains and Fiber," Updated January 2011, Accessed July 2012, http://www.heart.org/HEARTORG/GettingHealthy/NutritionCenter/HealthyDietGoals/Whole-Grains-and-Fiber_UCM_303249_Article.jsp.

7 Tabatabai, A and Li, S, "Dietary Fiber and Type 2 Diabetes," Clinical Excellence for Nurse Practioners, 4.5 (2000): 272-276.

8 Burkitt, DP, et al, "Dietary Fiber and Disease," *The Journal of the American Medical Association*, 229.8 (1974): 1068-1074.

9 Park, J and Flock, M.H., "Prebiotics, Probiotics, and Dietary Fiber in Gastrointestinal Disease," *Gastroenterology Clinics of North America*, 36.1 (2007): 46-63.

10 Kokke, F, et al, "A Dietary Fiber Mixture Versus Lactulose in the Treatment of childhood Constipation: A Double-Blind Randomized Controlled Trial," *Journal of Pediatric Gastroenterology and Nutrition*," 47.5 (2008): 592-597.

11 "Trends in Dietary Fiber Intake in the US, 1999-2008," *Journal* of *the Academy ofNutrition and Dietetics*, 112 (2012):642-648.

12 Anderson, James, et al, "Carbohydrate and Fiber Recommendations for Individuals with Diabetes: A Quantitative Assessment and Meta-Analysis of the Evidence," *Journal of the American College of Nutrition*, 23.1 (2004): 5-17.

13 Chandalia, Manisha, et al, "Beneficial Effects of High Dietary Fiber Intake in Patients with Type 2 Diabetes Mellitus," *The New England Journal of Medicine*, 342.19 (2000): 1392-1398.

14 Higgins, Janine A., "Whole Grains, Legumes, and the Subsequent Meal Effect: Implications for Blood Glucose Control and the Role of Fermentation," *Journal of Nutrition and Metabolism*, Accessed September2012, http://www.hindawi.com/journals/jnume/2012/829238/.

15 Mates, JM, et al, "Anticancer Antioxidant Regulatory Functions of Phytochemicals," *Current Medicinal Chemistry*, 18.15 (2011): 2315-2338.

16 American Heart Association, "Phytochemicals and Cardiovascular Disease," Accessed July 2012, http://www.heart.org/HEARTORG/GettingHealthy/NutritionCenter/Phytochemicals-and-Cardiovascular-Disease_UCM_306020_Article.jsp.

17 Dembinska-Kiec, Aldona, et al, "Antioxidant Phytochemicals Against Type 2 Diabetes," *British Journal of Nutrition*, 99.1 (2008): 109-117.

18 Nascimento, Gislene G.F., et al, "Antibacterial Activity of Plant Extracts and Phytochemicals on Antibiotic-Resistant Bacteria," *Brazilian Journal of Microbiology*, 31.4 (2000): 247-256.

19 Fulgoni, III, L.V., "Current Protein Intake in America: Analysis of the National Health and Nutrition Examination Survey, 2003–2004," *American Journal of Clinical Nutrition*, 87.5 (2008): 1554S-1557S.

20 Physicians Committee for Responsible Medicine, "How Can I Get Enough Protein? The Protein Myth," Accessed July 2012, http://www.pcrm.org/search/?cid=251.

21 Campbell, T. Colin, "Animal vs. Plant Protein," T. Colin Campbell Foundation, Accessed July 2012, http://www.tcolincampbell.org/courses-resources/article/animal-vs-plant-protein/?tx_ttnews[backPid]=76&cHash=d5607d1968.

22 Campbell, T. Colin and Campbell II, Thomas M., *The China Study* (Dallas, TX: Ben Bella Books, 2005).

23 Curry, Andrew, "The Gladiator Diet," Archaeology, 61.6 (2008), http://www.archaeology.org/0811/abstracts/gladiator.html.

24 British Broadcasting Corporation, "Gladiator Graveyard," Accessed July 2012, http://www.youtube.com/watch?v=nMpf_XYXEJk&feature=gv.

25 McDougall, John," What do Bill Clinton, Steve Wynn, John Mackey, and Mike Tyson Have in Common?," McDougall Newsletter, Accessed July 2012, http://www.drmcdougall.com/misc/2010nl/sep/powerful.htm.

26 Collier, G., McLean, A., and O'Dea, K., "Effect of Co-Ingestion of Fat on the Metabolic Responses to Slowly and Rapidly Absorbed Carbohydrates," *Diabetologia*, 26.1 (1984): 50-54.

27 Functional Medicine Research Center, "The Use of Coconut Oil, a Healthy Medium-Chain Fatty Acid, as part of the FirstLine Therapy® Program," Accessed July 2012, http://www.metadocs.com/pdf/position_papers/MET1621_coconut_oil.pdf.

28 Freeman, Mason W., Junge, Christine, *The Harvard Medical School Guide to Lowering Your Cholesterol* (New York, NY: McGraw-Hill, 2005).

29 Johns Hopkins Medicine, "High Cholesterol and Triglyceride Levels," Health alerts, Accessed July 2012, http://www.johnshopkinshealthalerts.com/symptoms_remedies/hyperlipidemia/91-1.html.

30 Nature, "Immunology: Saturated Fats Up Inflammation," *Nature*, 472.139 (2011), Accessed July 2012, http://www.nature.com/nature/journal/v472/n7342/full/472139b.html.

31 Jakobsen, Marianne U., et al, "Major Types of Dietary Fat and Risk of Coronary Heart Disease: A Pooled Analysis of 11 Cohort Studies," *The American Journal of Clinical Nutrition*, 89.5 (2009): 1425-1432.

32 Cho, E., Spiegelman, D., Hunter, D., et al, "Premenopausal Fat Intake and Risk of Breast Cancer," *Journal of the National Cancer Institute* , 95.14 (2003): 1079-1085.

33 Meyer, Katie A., et al, "Dietary Fat and Incidence of Type 2 Diabetes in Older Iowa Women," *Diabetes Care*, 24.9 (2001): 1528-1535.

34 Mozaffarian, Dariush, et al, "Trans Fatty Acids and Cardiovascular Disease," *The New England Journal of Medicine*, 354 (2006): 1601-1613.

35 Harvard School of Public Health, "The Bottom Line: Choose Foods with Healthy Fats, Limit Foods High in Saturated Fat, and Avoid Foods with Trans Fat," The Nutrition Source, Accessed July 2012, http://www.hsph.harvard.edu/nutritionsource/what-should-you-eat/fats-and-cholesterol/.

36 Public Health Law Center, "Trans Fat Bans: Policy Options for Eliminating the Use of

Artificial Trans Fats in Restaurants," Tobacco Law Center, Accessed July 2012, http://publichealthlawcenter.org/sites/default/files/resources/phlc-policy-trans-fat.pdf.

37 U.S. Food and Drug Administration, "Trans Fat Now Listed With Saturated Fat and Cholesterol," Accessed July 2012, http://www.fda.gov/Food/ResourcesForYou/Consumers/NFLPM/ucm274590.htm#after.

CHAPTER 13: BE A FIRST-CLASS FOODIE

1 Newscorp Australian Papers, "Hospital-Themed Restaurant Serves 'Patients' Quadruple Bypass Burgers, Flatliner Fries," Foxnews.com, Accessed July 2012, http://www.foxnews.com/story/0,2933,528069,00.html.

2 ABC News Nightline, "The Heart Attack Grill," Youtube, March 2011, Accessed July 2012, https://www.youtube.com/watch?v=hqf_SIQ3JAk.

3 Memmott, Mark, "Diners Not Fazed By Second Collapse At 'Heart Attack Grill'; Would You Be?," NPR.org, April 2012, Accessed July 2012, http://www.npr.org/blogs/thetwo-way/2012/04/24/151274493/diners-not-fazed-by-second-collapse-at-heart-attack-grill-would-you-be.

4 CBS, "A Meal To Die For," Youtube, November 2008, Accessed August 2012, http://www.youtube.com/watch?v=zbKRSYAuSNg&feature=player_embedded#!.

5 See Endnote 4

6 Craig, W.J and Mangels, A.R., "Position of the American Dietetic Association: Vegetarian Diets," *Journal of the American Dietetic Association*, 109.7 (2009): 1266-1282.

7 Craig, W.J., "Nutrition Concerns and Health Effects of Vegetarian Diets," *Nutrition in Clinical Practice*, 25.6 (2010): 613-620.

8 Craig, W.J., "Health Effects of Vegan Diets," *The American Journal of Clinical Nutrition*," 89.5 (2009): 1627S-1633S.

9 Hung, H.C., et al, "Fruit and Vegetable Intake and Risk of Major Chronic Disease," *Journal of the National Cancer Institute*, 96.21 (2004): 1577-1584.

10 Fuhrman, Joel, *Eat to Live* (New York, NY: Little Brown and Company, 2011) 118-120.

11 American Institute for Cancer Research, "Foods That Fight Cancer: Dark Green Leafy Vegetables," Accessed July 2012, http://preventcancer.aicr.org/site/PageServer?pagename=foodsthatfightcancer_leafy_vegetables.

12 Joshipura, K.J., et al, "The Effect of Fruit and Vegetable Intake on Risk for Coronary Heart Disease," *Annals of Internal Medicine*, 134.12 (2001): 1106-1114.

13 Manning, Anita, "If You Eat a Lot of Fish, You May Run Health Risk," USA Today, November 2002, Accessed July 2012, http://www.usatoday.com/news/health/2002-11-04-fish-1acover_x.htm.

14 Hoffman, Matthew, "Safer Food For a Healthier You," Webmd.com, Accessed July 2012, http://www.webmd.com/diet/features/safer-food-healthier-you.

15 Fuhrman, Joel, *Eat to Live* (New York, NY: Little Brown and Company, 2011) 165.

16 Masters, Rachel C., et al, "Whole and Refined Grain Intakes Are Related to Inflammatory

Protein Concentrations in Human Plasma," *The Journal of Nutrition*, 140.3 (2010): 587-594.

17 Liu, Simin, "Intake of Refined Carbohydrates and Whole Grain Foods in Relation to Risk of Type 2 Diabetes Mellitus and Coronary Heart Disease," *Journal of the American College of Nutrition*, 21.4 (2002): 298-306.

18 Pan, An, et al, "Red Meat Consumption and Mortality: Results from Two Prospective Cohort Studies," *Archives of Internal Medicine*, 172.7 (2012): 555-563.

19 Pan, An, et al, "Red Meat Consumption and Risk of Type 2 Diabetes: Three Cohorts of US Adults and an Updated Meta-Analysis," *The American Journal of Clinical Nutrition*, August 2011, Accessed July 2012, http://www.ajcn.org/content/early/2011/08/10/ajcn.111.018978.abstract.

20 See Endnote 19.

21 Davis, Brenda and Barnard, Tom, (Summertown: Healthy Living Publications, 2003) Visit: www.brendadavisrd.com

22 See Endnote 1, Chapter 12.

23 Houghton, Karen, *Naturally Gourmet* (Fallbrook: Hart Books, 2010) Visit: www.naturallygourmet.com

---

CHAPTER 14: OPTIMIZE DIGESTION

1 Williams, Tennessee. *The Glass Menagerie*, (New York: New Directions Books, 1945).

2 Hashimoto, T, et al, "Serum Magnesium, Ambulatory Blood Pressure, and Carotid Artery Alteration: the Ohasama Study," *American Journal of Hypertension*, 23.12 (2010):1292-1298.

3 Rosanoff, A, "Magnesium and Hypertension," *Clinical Calcium*, 12.2 (2005): 255-260.

4 Bo, S and Pisu, E, "Role of Dietary Magnesium in Cardiovascular Disease Prevention, Insulin Sensitivity, and Diabetes," Current Opinion in Lipidology, 19.1 (2008):50-56.

5 Sales, CH and Pedrosa, LF, "Magnesium and Diabetes Mellitus: Their Relation," 25.4 (2006):554-562.

6 Shaheen, Nicholas, and Ransohoff, David, "Gatroesophageal Reflux, Barrett Esophagus, and Esophageal Cancer," *The Journal of the American Medical Association*, 287.15 (2002):1972-1981.

7 Hyman, Mark, "Three Simple Steps to Eliminate Heartburn and Acid Reflux," July 2010, Accessed August 2012, http://www.huffingtonpost.com/dr-mark-hyman/3-simple-steps-to-elimina_b_649609.html.

8 Watson, Brenda, "Is That Antacid Killing You?," Accessed August 2012, http://www.brendawatson.com/in-the-news/brenda's-news/is-that-antacid-killing-you-/.

9 ProHealth.com, "Acid Stomach—or Not Enough Stomach Acid?," September 2006, Accessed August 2012, http://www.prohealth.com/library/showarticle.cfm?libid=12108.

10 RefluxDefense.com, "Side Effects of Antacids and Acid Blockers," Accessed August 2012, http://refluxdefense.com/heartburn_GERD_articles/side-effects-antacids-and-acid-blockers.html.

11 Food and Drug Administration, "Low Magnesium Levels Can Be Associated With Long-term Use of Proton Pump Inhibitor Drugs," March 2011, Accessed August 2012, http://www.fda.gov/drugs/drugsafety/ucm245011.htm.

12 Walling, Elizabeth, "Drinking Water With Meals Can Impair Digestion," September 2011, Accessed August 2012, http://www.naturalnews.com/033731_digestion_drinking_water.html.

13 Colbert, Donald, *Eat This and Live*, (Lake Mary, Florida, Siloam, 2008)

14 Bond, Owen, "Why Drink Warm Water?," July 2011, Accessed August 2012, http://www.livestrong.com/article/477337-why-drink-warm-water/?utm_source=popslideshow&utm_medium=a1.

15 Ewe, Klaus, et al, "Gastric Emptying of Indigestible Tablets in Relation to Composition and Time of Ingestion of Meals Studied by Metal Detector," *Digestive Diseases and Sciences*, 36.2 (1991):146-152.

16 Abbott, George Knapp, *The Witness of Science,* (Mountain View, CA: Pacific Press, 1948) 36.

17 Bolondi, L, et al, "Measurement of Gastric Emptying Time by Real-Time Ultrasonography," *Gastroenterology*, 89.4 (1985):752-759.

18 O'Sullivan, Therese A., et al, "A Good-Quality Breakfast is Associated with Better Mental Health in Adolescence," *Public Health Nutrition*, 12.2 (2008):752-759.

19 Kivisto, K.T., et al, "Inhibition of Norfloxacin Absorption by Dairy Products," *Antimicrobial Agents and Chemotherapy*, 36.2 (1992):489-491.

20 Kiefer, Dale, "Promoting Optimal Nutrition with Digestive Enzymes," *Life Extension Magazine*, January 2008, Accessed July 2012, http://www.lef.org/magazine/mag2008/jan2008_report_digestiveEnzymes_01.htm.

21 The Harvard Medical School Family Health Guide, "Health Benefits of Taking Probiotics," September 2005, Accessed July 2012, http://www.health.harvard.edu/fhg/updates/update0905c.shtml.

22 Kennedy, Ron, "Hypochlorhydia," The Doctors' Medical Library, Accessed July 2012, http://www.medical-library.net/hypochlorhydria.html

23 Thrash, Agatha, and Thrash, Calvin, *RX: Charcoal* (Seale, AL: New Lifestyle Books, 1988).

24 Acts 2:46 (NASB)

CHAPTER 15: GET A MOVE-ON

1 Spelsberg, A., and Manson, J.E., "Physical Activity in the Treatment and Prevention of Diabetes," *Comprehensive Therapy*, 21.10 (1995):559-562.

2 Borghouts, L.B., and Keizer, H.A., "Exercise and Insulin Sensitivity: A Review," *International Journal of Sports Medicine*, 21.1 (2000):1-12.

3 Duncan, Glen E., et al, "Exercise Training, Without Weight Loss, Increases Insulin Sensitivity and Postheparin Plasma Lipase Activity in Previously Sedentary Adults," *Diabetes Care*, 26.3 (2003):557-562.

4 Colberg, Sheri R., et al, "Postprandial Walking is Better for Lowering the Glycemic Effect of Dinner than Pre-Dinner Exercise in Type 2 Diabetic Individuals," *Journal of the American Medical Directors Association*," 10.6 (2009):394-397.

5 American Diabetes Association, "Postprandial Blood Glucose," *Diabetes Care*, 24.4 (2001):775-778.

6 Ceriello, A., "Mechanisms of Tissue Damage in the Postprandial State," *International Journal of Clinical Practice, Supplement*, 123 (2001):7-12.

7 Aadland, Eivind, and Hostmark, Arne T., "Very Light Physical Activity after a Meal Blunts the Rise in Blood Glucose and Insulin," *The Open Nutrition Journal*, 2 (2008):94-99.

8 Knab, A.M., et al, "A 45-Minute Vigorous Exercise Bout Increases Metabolic Rate for 14 Hours," *Medicine and Science in Sports and Exercise*, 43.9 (2011):1643-1648.

9 Herzberg, G.R., "Aerobic Exercise, Lipoproteins, and Cardiovascular Disease: Benefits and Possible Risks," *Canadian Journal of Applied Physiology*, 29.6 (2004):800-807.

10 Sessim H.D., et al, "Physical Activity and Coronary Heart Disease in Men: The Harvard Alumni Health Study," *Circulation*, 102.9 (2000):975-980.

11 Nelson, Valerie J., "Ralph S. Paffenbarger Jr., 84; His Key Study Confirmed that Exercise Boosts Longevity," Los Angeles Times, July 15, 2007, Accessed July 2012, http://articles.latimes.com/2007/jul/15/local/me-paffenbarger15.

12 Church, T.S., et al, "Effects of Aerobic and Resistance Training on Hemoglobin A1c Levels in Patients with Type 2 Diabetes: a Randomized Controlled Trial," *The Journal of the American Medical Association*, 304.20 (2010):2253-2262.

13 Ibanez, Javier, et al, "Twice-Weekly Progressive Resistance Training Decreases Abdominal Fat and Improves Insulin Sensitivity in Older Men With Type 2 Diabetes," *Diabetes Care*, 28.3 (2005):662-667.

14 Mayo Clinic Staff, "Weight Training: Improve Your Muscular Fitness," February 12, 2011, Accessed July 2012, http://www.mayoclinic.com/health/weight-training/HQ01627.

15 Perry, C.G., et al, "High-Intensity Aerobic Interval Training Increases Fat and Carbohydrate Metabolic Capacities in Human Skeletal Muscle," *Applied Physiology, Nutrition, and Metabolism*, 33.6 (2008):1112-1123.

16 Meckel, Y., et al, "The effect of Brief Sprint Interval Exercise on Growth Factors and Inflammatory Mediators," *Journal of Strength and Conditioning Research*, 23.1 (2009):225-230.

17 Hackney, Anthony C., et al, "Thyroid Hormonal Responses to Intensive Interval Versus Steady-State Endurance Exercise Sessions," *Hormones*, 11.1 (2012):54-60.

18 Tionna, A.E., et al, "Aerobic Interval Training Versus Continuous Moderate Exercise as a Treatment for the Metabolic Syndrome: a Pilot Study," *Circulation*, 118.4 (2008):346-354.

19 Powers, Scott and Howley, Edward, "Exercise Physiology," Accessed July 2012, http://www.depts.ttu.edu/hess/mccomb/documents/ess3305/ppt/chap05.pdf.

20 Ciloglu, Figen, et al, "Exercise Intensity and its Effects on Thyroid Hormones," *Neuroendocrinology Letters*, 26.6 (2005):830-834.

21 Crooks, Hulda, *Conquering life's mountains: A collection of writings* (Redlands, CA: Quiet Hour, 1996).

22 Reed, Susan, "Far from Being Over the Hill, Hulda Crooks, at 87, Is a Real Climber," *People*, 21.3 (1984):88.

23 Crooks, Hulda, *Conquering life's mountains: A collection of writings* (Redlands, CA: Quiet Hour, 1996) 1.

24 U.S. Geological Survey, "Feature Detail Report for: Crooks Peak," Accessed July 2012, http://geonames.usgs.gov/pls/gnispublic/f?p=gnispq:3:::NO::P3_FID:277451.

25 Fixx, Jim, *The Complete Book of Running* (New York, NY: Random House, 1977).

26 The Free Dictionary, "Synergy," Accessed July 2012, http://www.thefreedictionary.com/synergy.

CHAPTER 16: WHAT ABOUT WEIGHT?

1 As presented by Dr. Jo Ann Manson at the American College of Nutrition Annual Meetings, 1993-1994.

2 National Diabetes Education Program, "Diabetes Risk Factors: At-Risk Weight Charts," National Institutes of Health, Bethesda, Accessed July 2012, http://ndep.nih.gov/am-i-at-risk/DiabetesRiskFactors.aspx#weightcharts

3 Lee, Chong Do, Blair, Steven N., and Jackson, Andrew S., "Cardiorespiratory Fitness, Body Composition, and All-Cause and Cardiovascular Disease Mortality in Men," *American Journal of Clinical Nutrition*, 69.3 (1999):373-380.

4 Biggs, Mary L., et al, "Association Between Adiposity in Midlife and Older Age and Risk of Diabetes in Older Adults," *The Journal of the American Medical Association*, 303.24 (2010):2504-2512.

5 Gallagher, Dympna, et al, "Healthy Percentage Body Fat Ranges: an Approach for Developing Guidelines Based on Body Mass Index," *The American Journal of Clinical Nutrition*, 72 (2000):694-701.

6 Harvard School of Public Health, "Waist Size Matters," The Obesity Prevention Source, Accessed July 2012, http://www.hsph.harvard.edu/obesity-prevention-source/obesity-definition/abdominal-obesity/index.html.

7 See Endnote 5.

8 Hicks, Rob, "BMI," BBC Health, Accessed July 2012, http://www.bbc.co.uk/health/treatments/healthy_living/your_weight/whatis_bmi.shtml.

9 National Heart Lung and Blood Institute, "Assessing Your Weight and Health Risk," National Institutes of Health, Accessed July 2012, http://www.nhlbi.nih.gov/health/public/heart/obesity/lose_wt/risk.htm.

10 Wang, Youfa, et al, "Comparison of Abdominal Adiposity and Overall Obesity in Predicting Risk of Type 2 Diabetes Among Men," *The American Journal of Clinical Nutrition*, 81.3 (2005): 555-563.

11 Collins, Karen, "Nutrition Wise," American Institute for Cancer Research, June 6, 2008, Accessed July 2012, http://preventcancer.aicr.org/site/News2?page=NewsArticle&id=13478&news_iv_ctrl=0&abbr=pr_hf.

12 Lifelines Online, "Waist-to-Hip Ratio Measures Health Risks," Laborer's Health and Safety Fund of North America, February 2006, Accessed July 2012, http://www.lhsfna.org/index.cfm?objectID=FE2B1294-D56F-E6FA-9F62DE309AA52FCF.

13 As presented by George A. Bray, MD, Chief, Division of Clinical Obesity and Metabolism Professor, Pennington Biomedical Research Center.

14 Bray, George A., et al, "Relation of Central Adiposity and Body Mass Index to the Development of Diabetes in the Diabetes Prevention Program," *The American Journal of Clinical Nutrition*, 87.5 (2008):1212-1218.

15 Carter, J.P., Brown, J. "Dr. Cupp's simple approach to weight loss." *The Journal of Louisiana State Medical Society,* 137 (1985): 35-38.

16 Taheri, Shahrad, et al, "Short Sleep Duration Is Associated with Reduced Leptin, Elevated Ghrelin, and Increased Body Mass Index," *Plos Medicine*, 1.3 (2004), Accessed August 2012, http://www.plosmedicine.org/article/info:doi/10.1371/journal.pmed.0010062.

17 Nedley, Neil, Depression Recovery Program DVD, (2005).

18 Yoon, In-Young, et al, "Luteinizing Hormone Following Light Exposure in Healthy Young Men," *Neuroscience Letters*, 341.1 (2003):25-28.

19 Ishida, Atsushi, et al, "Light Activates the Adrenal Gland: Timing of Gene Expression and Glucocorticoid Release." *Cell Metabolism*, 2.5 (2005):297-307.

20 Holick, Michael, "Sunlight and Vitamin D," *Journal of General Internal Medicine*, 17.9 (2002):733-735.

21 University of Minnesota, "Vitamin D Levels May Predict Weight Loss Success," YouTube, December 2009, Accessed July 2012, http://www.youtube.com/watch?v=zpWuTWqWd5c.

CHAPTER 17: GET SOUND SLEEP

1 Irving, Washington, *Rip Van Winkle and The Legend of Sleepy Hollow. Harvard Classics Shelf of Fiction, Vol. X, Part 2.* (New York, NY: P.F. Collier & Son, 1917).

2 Spiegel, Karine, et al, "Sleep Loss: A Novel Risk Factor for Insulin Resistance and Type 2 Diabetes," *Journal of Applied Physiology*, 99.5 (2005):2008-2019.

3 Ayas, Najib T., et al, "A Prospective Study of Sleep Duration and Coronary Heart Disease in Women," *Archives of internal Medicine*, 163.2 (2003):205-209.

4 Cappuccio, Francesco P., et al, "Meta-Analysis of Short Sleep Duration and Obesity in Children and Adults," *Sleep*, 31.5 (2008):619-626.

5 Qureshi, Adnan I., et al, "Habitual Sleep Patterns and Risk for Stroke and Coronary Heart Disease," *Neurology*, 48.4 (1997):904-910.

6 Christos, G. A., "Is Alzheimer's Disease Related to a Deficit or Malfunction of Rapid Eye Movement (REM) Sleep?" *Medical Hypotheses*, 41.5 (1993):435-439.

7 Harvard Medical School, "Poor Sleep Habits: Heart Disease and Sleep Apnea," Harvard Health Publications, January 2007, Accessed July 2012, http://www.health.harvard.edu/press_releases/sleep-habits,

8 Park, Alice, "Lack of Sleep Linked to Heart Problems," Time Health, December 23, 2008, Accessed July 2012, http://www.time.com/time/health/article/0,8599,1868406,00.html,

9 Knutson, K.L., et al, "Association Between Sleep and Blood Pressure in Midlife: The CARDIA Sleep Study," *Archives of Internal Medicine*, 169.11 (2009):1055-1061.

10 Leproult, R., et al, "Sleep Loss Results in an Elevation of Cortisol Levels the Next Evening," *Sleep*, 20.10 (1997):865-870.

11 Donga, Esther, et al, "A Single Night of Partial Sleep Deprivation Induces Insulin Resistance in Multiple Metabolic Pathways in Healthy Subjects," *The Journal of Clinical Endocrinology & Metabolism*, 95.6 (2010):2963-2968.

12 Krystal, A.D., "Sleep and Psychiatric Disorders: Future Directions," *The Psychiatric Clinics of North America*, 29.4(2006):1115-1130.

13 Alhola, Paula, and Polo-Kantola, Paivi, "Sleep Deprivation: Impact on Cognitive Performance," *Neuropsychiatric Disease and Treatment*, 3.5 (2007):553-567.

14 Walker, Matt, "Sleep: Expert Q & A," Nova Science Now, July 2007, Accessed July 2012, http://www.pbs.org/wgbh/nova/body/walker-sleep.html,

15 Irwin, Michael, et al, "Partial Night Sleep Deprivation Reduces Natural Killer and Cellular Immune Responses in Humans," *Federation of American Societies for Experimental Biology Journal*, 10 (1996):643-653.

16 Blask, David E., "Melatonin-Depleted Blood from Premenopausal Women Exposed to Light at Night Stimulates Growth of Human Breast Cancer Xenografts in Nude Rats," *Cancer Research*, 65 (2005):11174.

17 Tillet, Tanya, "Headliners: Breast Cancer: Decreased Melatonin Production Linked to Light Exposure," *Environmental Health Perspectives*, 114.2 (2006):A99.

18 OM Buxton, et. al., "Adverse Metabolic Consequences in Humans of Prolonged Sleep Restriction Combined with Circadian Disruption," *Science Translational Medicine*, 4 (2012):1-11.

19 Shernhammer, Eva S., et al, "Rotating Night Shifts and Risk of Breast Cancer in Women Participating in the Nurses' Health Study," *Journal of the National Cancer Institute*, 93.20 (2001):1563-1568.

20 Kotz, Deborah, "Light at Night: How to Counter the Health Effects," U.S. News Health, February 2008, Accessed July 2012, http://health.usnews.com/health-news/family-health/cancer/articles/2008/02/22/light-at-night-how-to-counter-the-health-effects.

21 Griffin, R. Morgan, "Coping With Excessive Sleepiness: The Health Risks of Shift Work," WebMD, Accessed July 2012, http://www.webmd.com/sleep-disorders/excessive-sleepiness-10/shift-work

22 Onen, S.H., Onen, F., Bailly, D., and Parquet, P., "Prevention and Treatment of Sleep Disorders Through Regulation of Sleeping Habits," *Press Medicale*, 23.10 (1994):485-489.

23 Hadhazy, Adam, "iPad Could Cause Insomnia Researchers Say," NBCNews.com, April 2010, Accessed July 2012, http://www.msnbc.msn.com/id/36828043/ns/technology_and_science-tech_and_gadgets/#.UAny3lGsdZl.

24 Mayo Clinic Staff, "Can't Sleep? Try Daytime Exercise," Mayo Clinic, July 2011, Accessed July 2012, http://www.mayoclinic.com/health/health-tip/HT00072/rss=6.

25 Driver, Helen S., Taylor, Sheila R., "Exercise and Sleep," *Sleep Medicine Reviews*, 4.4 (2000):387-402.

26 Clodore, M., et al, "Psychophysiological Effects of Early Morning Bright Light Exposure in Young Adults," *Psychoneuroendocrinology*, 15.3 (1990):193-205.

27 National Sleep Foundation, "Melatonin and Sleep," Accessed July 2012, http://www.sleepfoundation.org/article/sleep-topics/melatonin-and-sleep.

28 Sin, C.W., Ho, J.S., and Chung, J.W., "Systematic Review on the Effectiveness of Caffeine Abstinence on the Quality of Sleep," *Journal of Clinical Nursing*, 18.1 (2009):13-21.

29 Kamimori, G.H., et al, "Effect of Three Caffeine Doses on Plasma Catecholamines and Alertness during Prolonged Wakefulness," *European Journal of Clinical Pharmacology*, 56.8 (2000):537-544.

30 National Institute on Alcohol Abuse and Alcoholism, "Alcohol and Sleep," *Alcohol Alert*, 41 (1998) http://pubs.niaaa.nih.gov/publications/aa41.htm.

31 National Institute on Alcohol Abuse and Alcoholism, "Alcohol's Effects on Sleep in Alcoholics," Accessed July 2012, http://pubs.niaaa.nih.gov/publications/arh25-2/110-125.htm,

32 American Diabetes Association, "Alcohol," Accessed July 2012, http://www.diabetes.org/food-and-fitness/food/what-can-i-eat/alcohol.html.

33 Emanuele, Nicholas V., Swade, Terrence F., and Emmanuele, Mary Ann, "Consequences of Alcohol Use in Diabetics," *Alcohol Health and Research World*, 22.3 (1998):211-219.

34 Zhang, Lin, et al, "Cigarette Smoking and Nocturnal Sleep Architecture," *American Journal of Epidemiology*, 164.6 (2006):529-537.

35 Willi, Carole, et al, "Active Smoking and the Risk of Type 2 Diabetes: A Systematic Review and Meta-analysis," *The Journal of the American Medical Association*, 298.22 (2007):2654-2664.

36 Centers for Disease Control and Prevention, "Health Effects of Cigarette Smoking," Accessed July 2012, http://www.cdc.gov/tobacco/data_statistics/fact_sheets/health_effects/effects_cig_smoking/

37 Centers for Disease Control and Prevention, "Heart Disease and Strokeg," Accessed July 2012, http://www.cdc.gov/tobacco/basic_information/health_effects/heart_disease/index.htm.

38 Centers for Disease Control and Prevention, "Tobacco Use in the United States," National Center for Chronic Disease Prevention and Health Promotion. Tobacco Information and Prevention Source (TIPS), January 27, 2004.

CHAPTER 18: STAY WELL HYDRATED

1 Dakss, Brian, "This Was Our Miracle," CBS News, February 2009, Accessed September 2012, http://www.cbsnews.com/2100-500202_162-692382.html.

2 O'Driscoll, Patrick, "Pulled to Sea in Minutes, Teens Survive for 6 Days," USA Today, May 2005, Accessed September 2012, http://www.usatoday.com/news/nation/2005-05-02-teens-lost-sea_x.htm.

3 U.S. Geological Survey, "The Water in You," Accessed September 2012, http://ga.water.usgs.gov/edu/propertyyou.html.

4 Mayo Clinic Staff, "Water: How Much Should You Drink Every Day?," Mayo Clinic, October 2011, Accessed September 2012, http://www.mayoclinic.com/health/water/NU00283,

5 See Endnote 3.

6 Cosgrove, William J., and Rijsberman, Frank R., *World Water Vision: Making Water Everybody's Business* (London, UK: Earthscan Publications Ltd, 2000) 6-21.

7 Chan, Jacqueline, et al, "Water, Other Fluids, and Fatal Coronary Heart Disease," *American Journal of Epidemiology*, 155.9 (2002):827-833.

8 Mukamal K.J., et al, "Increased Risk of Congestive Heart Failure Among Infarctions with Nighttime Onset," *American Heart Journal*, 140 (2000):438–442.

9 Reuters, "Drinking Less Water Tied to High Blood Sugar," Fox News, October 2011, Accessed September 2012, http://www.foxnews.com/health/2011/10/25/drinking-less-water-tied-to-high-blood-sugar/.

10 Griling, E.M.K. and Eddy, C.A., "The Hyperglycemic Effect of Vasopressin, Oxytocin and Pituitrin," *Experimental Biology and Medicine*, 26.2 (1928):146-147.

11 Marks, Diane, "Can Drinking Too Much Coffee Bring on Severe Dehydration?," Live Strong, July 2011, Accessed September 2012, http://www.livestrong.com/article/505199-can-drinking-too-much-coffee-bring-on-severe-dehydration/.

12 Adams, Mike, "Diabetics Advised to Avoid Caffeine; New Study Shows Radical Blood Sugar Effects," Natural News, July 2004, Accessed September 2012, http://www.naturalnews.com/001514.html.

13 Van Dam, R.M., et al, "Coffee, Caffeine, and Risk of Type 2 Diabetes: a Prospective Cohort Study in Younger and Middle-Aged U.S. Women," *Diabetes Care*, 29.2 (2006):398-403.

14 Fowler, Sharon, 65th Annual Scientific Sessions, American Diabetes Association, San Diego, June 10-14, 2005

15 Swithers, S.E., Martin, A.A., and Davidson T.L., "High-Intensity Sweeteners and Energy Balance," *Physiolology and Behavavior*, 100.1 (2010):55-62.

16 Gardener, H., et al, "Diet Soft Drink Consumption is Associated with an Increased Risk of Vascular Events in the Northern Manhattan Study," *Journal of General Internal Medicine*, 27.9 (2012):1120-1126.

17 Soffritti, Morando, et al, "First Experimental Demonstration of the Multipotential Carcinogenic Effects of Aspartame Administered in the Feed to Sprague-Dawley Rats," *Environmental Health Perspectives*, 114.3 (2006):379-385.

18 Fillmore, K.M., et al, "Moderate Alcohol Use and Reduced Mortality Risk: Systematic Error in Prospective Studies and New Hypotheses," *Annals of Epidemiology*, 17.5 (2007):S16-23.

19 American Heart Association, "Alcohol and Heart Disease," February 2012, Accessed September 2012, http://www.heart.org/HEARTORG/Conditions/More/MyHeartandStrokeNews/Alcohol-and-Heart-Disease_UCM_305173_Article.jsp.

CHAPTER 19: SOAK UP THE SUN

1 Ginde, Adit, et al, "Demographic Differences and Trends of Vitamin D Insufficiency in the US Population, 1988-2004," *Archives of Internal Medicine*, 169.6 (2009):626-632.

2 Vitamin D Council, "Health Conditions," Accessed July 2012, www.vitamindcouncil.org.

3 Heaney, Robert, Vitamin D Symposium, San Diego, April 9, 2008.

4 Hypponen, Elina, et al, "Intake of Vitamin D and Risk of Type 1 Diabetes: a Birth-Cohort Study," *The Lancet*, 358.9292 (2001):1500-1503.

5 National Diabetes Information Clearinghouse, "National Diabetes Statistics, 2011," National Institutes of Health, Accessed July 2012, http://diabetes.niddk.nih.gov/dm/pubs/statistics/index.aspx.

6 Journal Diabetes Research Foundation, "Type 1 Diabetes, 2010; Prime Group for JDRF," March 2011.

7 Mohr, S.B., et al, "The Association Between Ultraviolet B Irradiance, Vitamin D Status and Incidence Rates of Type 1 Diabetes in 51 Regions Worldwide," *Diabetologia*, 51.8 (2008):1391-1398.

8 Adams, John, and Hewison, Martin, "Unexpected Actions of Vitamin D: New Perspectives on the Regulation of Innate and Adaptive Immunity," *Nature Reviews Endocrinology*, 4 (2008):80-90.

9 Deluca, Hector, and Cantorna, Margherita, "Vitamin D: Its Role and Uses in Immunology," *Federation of American Societies for Experimental Biology Journal*, 15 (2001):2579-2585.

10 Guillot, Xavier, et al, "Vitamin D and Inflammation," *Joint, Bone, Spine: Revue du Rhumatisme*, 77.6 (2010):552-557.

11 Pittas, Anastassios G., et al, "Vitamin D and Calcium Intake in Relation to Type 2 Diabetes in Women," *Diabetes Care*, 29.3 (2006):650-656.

12 Knekt, P., et al, "Serum Vitamin D and Subsequent Occurrence of Type 2 Diabetes," *Epidemiology*, 19.5 (2008):666-671.

13 Rauscher, Megan, "Vitamin D May Curb Type 2 Diabetes Risk," Reuters, November 2007, Accessed August 2012, http://www.reuters.com/article/2007/11/19/us-type-idUSCOL96182020071119.

14 Zhang, Y., et al, "Vitamin D Inhibits Monocyte/Macrophage Proinflammatory Cytokine Production by Targeting MAPK Phosphatase-1," *Journal of Immunology*, 88.5 (2012):2127-2135.

15 Nikooyeh, B., et al, "Daily Consumption of Vitamin D- or Vitamin D + Calcium-Fortified Yogurt Drink Improved Glycemic Control in Patients with Type 2 Diabetes: a Randomized Clinical Trial," *The American Journal of Clinical Nutrition*, 93.4 (2011):764-771.

16 Ou, H.Y., et al, "Interaction of BMI with Vitamin D and Insulin Sensitivity," *European Journal of Clinical Investigation*, 41.11 (2011):1195-1201.

17 Chiu, Ken, et al, "Hypovitaminosis D is Associated with Insulin Resistance and *a* Cell Dysfunction," *The American Journal of Clinical Nutrition*, 79.5 (2004):820-825.

18 Cheng, S., and Coyne, D., "Vitamin D and Outcomes in Chronic Kidney Disease," *Current opinion in Nephrology and Hypertension*, 16.2 (2007):77-82.

19 Cannell, John, "Why the New Vitamin D Recommendations Spell Disaster For Your Health," Diabetic Connect, December 2011, Accessed September 2012, http://www.diabeticconnect.com/news-articles/6406-why-the-new-vitamin-d-recommendations-spell-disaster-for-your-health/portal.

20 Hata, Tissa R., et al, "Administration of Oral Vitamin D Induces Cathelicidin Production in Atopic Individuals," *The Journal of Allergy and Clinical Immunology*, 122.4 (2008):829-831.

21 Wang, Tian-Tain, et al, "Cutting Edge: 1,25-Dihydroxyvitamin D3 Is a Direct Inducer of Antimicrobial Peptide Gene Expression," *The Journal of Immunology*, 173.5 (2004):2909-2912.

22 Urashima, Mitsuyoshi, et al, "Randomized Trial of Vitamin D Supplementation to Prevent Seasonal Influenza A in Schoolchildren," *The American Journal of Clinical Nutrition*, 91.5 (2010):1255-1260.

23 Li-ng, M., et al, "A Randomized Controlled Trial of Vitamin D3 Supplementation for the Prevention of Symptomatic Upper Respiratory Tract Infections," *Epidemiology and Infection*, 137.10 (2009):1396-1414.

24 Murphy, Sherry L., et al, "Deaths: Preliminary Data for 2010," *National Vital Statistics Reports*, 60.4 (2012):1-52.

25 American Cancer Society, *Cancer Facts & Figures 2012* (Atlanta: American Cancer Society, 2012).

26 See Endnote 25.

27 Lappe, Joan M., et al," Vitamin D and Calcium Supplementation Reduces Cancer Risk: Results of a Randomized Trial," *The American Journal of Clinical Nutrition*, 85 (2007):1586-1591.

28 Grassroots Health, "Disease Incidence prevention by Serum 25(OH)D Level," March 2010, Accessed September 2012, http://grassrootshealth.net/media/download/disease_incidence_prev_chart_032310.pdf.

29 Garland, Cedric F., and Garland, Frank C., "Do Sunlight and Vitamin D Reduce the Likelihood of Colon Cancer?," *International Journal of Epidemiology*, 9.3(1980):227-231.

30 Garland, Cedric F., et al, "The Role of Vitamin D in Cancer Prevention," *American Journal of Public Health*, 96.2 (2006):252-261.

31 Holick, M.F., "Vitamin D and Sunlight: Strategies for Cancer Prevention and Other Health Benefits," *Clinical Journal of the American Society of Nephrology*, 3.5(2008):1548-1554.

32 Skin Cancer Foundation, "Skin Cancer Facts," Accessed September 2012, http://www.skincancer.org/skin-cancer-information/skin-cancer-facts.

33 Skin Cancer Foundation, "Squamous Cell Carcinoma: The Second Most Common Form of Skin Cancer," Accessed September 2012, http://www.skincancer.org/skin-cancer-information/squamous-cell-carcinoma.

34 Skin Cancer Foundation, "Basal Cell Carcinoma: The Most Frequently Occuring Form of Skin Cancer," Accessed September2012, http://www.skincancer.org/skin-cancer-information/basal-cell-carcinoma.

35 See Endnote 34.

36 Skin Cancer Foundation, "Melanoma," Accessed September 2012, http://www.skincancer.org/skin-cancer-information/melanoma.

37 British Medical Journal, "Is Sun Exposure a Major Cause of Melanoma? " Accessed September 2012, http://www.bmj.com/content/337/bmj.a764.full.

38 Egan, Kathleen, Sosman, Jeffrey, and Blot, William, "Sunlight and Reduced Risk of Cancer: Is The Real Story Vitamin D?," *Journal of the National Cancer Institute*, 97.3 (2005):161-163.

39 Levell, N.J., et al, "Melanoma Epidemic: A Midsummer Night's Dream?," *The British Journal of Dermatology*," 161.3 (2009): 630-634.

40 White, Martin R., et al, "Malignant Melanoma in U.S. Navy Personnel," Naval Health Research Center, Report 88-27 (1988), Accessed September 2012, http://www.dtic.mil/dtic/tr/fulltext/u2/a211922.pdf

41 Berwick, Marianne, et al, "Sun Exposure and Mortality from Melanoma," *Journal of the National Cancer Institute*, 97.3 (2005):195-199.

42 See Endnote 38

43 Watson, Ronald Ross, *Functional Foods and Nutraceuticals in Cancer Prevention* (Ames, Iowa: Iowa State press, 2003)105-120.

44 Wang, T.J., et al, "Vitamin D Deficiency and Risk of Cardiovascular Disease," *Circulation*, 117.4 (2008):503-511.

45 Giocannucci, E., et al, "25-Hydroxyvitamin D and Risk of Myocardial Infarction in Men: a Prospective Study," *Archives of Internal Medicine*, 168.11 (2008):1174-1180.

46 Zittermann, A., "Vitamin D and Disease Prevention with Special Reference to Cardiovascular Disease," *Progress in Biophysics and Molecular Biology*, 92.1 (2006):39-48.

47 Brewer, L.C., Michos, E.D., and Reis, J.P., "Vitamin D in Atherosclerosis, Vascular Disease, and Endothelial Function," *Current Drug Targets*, 12.1 (2011):54-60.

48 See Endnote 28.

49 Baggerly, Carole, "To All Readers," Grassroots Health, Accessed September 2012, http://www.grassrootshealth.net/recommendation.

50 Grassroots Health, "Disease Incidence prevention by Serum 25(OH)D Level," March 2010, Accessed September 2012, http://grassrootshealth.net/media/download/disease_incidence_prev_chart_032310.pdf.

51 UCSD School of Medicine, Grassroots Health, "What's a Vitamin D Deficiency," Youtube.com, February 2009, Accessed September 2012, http://www.youtube.com/watch?v=emjCzaHtSrg.

52 Hyde, Peter, *Sunlight, Vitamin D, and Prostate Cancer Risk* (Bloomington, IN: Xlibris, 2004).

53 Madrid, Eric, *Vitamin D Prescription: The Healing Power of the Sun & How It Can Save Your Life* (Charleston, SC: BookSurge Publishing, 2009).

54 Dowd, James, *The Vitamin D Cure* (Hoboken, NJ: Wiley, 2008).

55 Cannell, John, "Showering After Sunbathing," Vitamin D Council, 2009, Accessed September 2012, http://www.vitamindcouncil.org/news-archive/2009/showering-after-sunbathing/.

56 Harris, Susan S., "Vitamin D and African Americans," *The Journal of Nutrition*, 136.4 (2006):1126-1129.

57 National Research Council, *Dietary Reference Intakes for Calcium and Vitamin D* (Washington, DC: The National Academies Press, 2011).

58 See Endnote 51.

59 Hathcock, John N., et al," Risk Assessment for Vitamin D," *The American Journal of Clinical Nutrition*, 85.1 (2007):6-18.

60 See Endnote 51.

61 http Koutkia, Polyxeni, Chen, Tai C., and Holick, Michael F., "Vitamin D Intoxication Associated with an Over-the-Counter Supplement," *The New England Journal of Medicine*, 345 (2001):66 67.

62 Bronstein, Alvin C., et al, "2010 Annual Report of the American Association of Poison Control Centers ' National Poison Data System (NPDS): 28th Annual Report," *Clinical Toxicology*, 49 (2011):910-941.

63 Cannell, John, et al, "On the Epidemiology of Influenza," *Virology Journal*, 5 (2008):29.

CHAPTER 20: TEN SUPER SUPPLEMENTS

1 National Diabetes Information Clearinghouse, "Diabetic Neuropathies: The Nerve Damage of Diabetes," *National Institutes of Health*, Accessed July 2012, http://diabetes.niddk.nih.gov/dm/pubs/neuropathies/.

2 Google Dictionary, "Supplement," Accessed September 2012, http://www.google.com/search?client=safari&rls=en&q=definition+of+supplement&ie=UTF-8&oe=UTF-8#hl=en&client=safari&rls=en&q=supplement&tbs=dfn:1&tbo=u&sa=X&ei=22_bT6SJHajc2QWl8ISIBg&ved=0CGAQkQ4&bav=on.2,or.r_gc.r_pw.r_qf.,cf.osb&fp=ce0a53ad8d6bcb4b&biw=1207&bih=848.

3 Horrocks, Lloyd and Yeo, Young, "Health Benefits of Docosahexaenoic Acid (DHA)," *Pharmacological Research*, 40.3 (1999):211-225.

4 Clandinin, M. Thomas, Claerhout, Donna L., and Lien, Eric L., "Docosahexaenoic Acid Increases Thyroid-Stimulating Hormone Concentration in Male and Adrenal Corticotrophic Hormone Concentration in Female Weanling Rats," *The Journal of Nutrition*, 128.8 (1998):1257-1261.

5 Coste, T.C., et al, "Neuroprotective Effect of Docosahexaenoic Acid-Enriched Phospholipids in Experimental Diabetic Neuropathy," *Diabetes*, 52.10 (2003):2578-2585.

6 Seelig, Mildred and Rosanoff, Andrea, *The Magnesium Factor* (New York, NY: Penguin Group Inc., 2003).

7 Office of Dietary Supplements, "Dietary Supplement Fact Sheet: Magnesium," National Institutes of Health, Accessed September 2012, http://ods.od.nih.gov/factsheets/Magnesium-HealthProfessional/.

8 Pham, P.C.T., et al, "Lower Serum Magnesium Levels are Associated with More Repid Decline of Renal Function in Patients with Diabetes Mellitus Type 2," *Clinical Nephrology*, 63.6 (2005):429-436.

9 Maier, Jeanette A.M., "Low Magnesium and Atherosclerosis: an Evidence-Based Link," *Molecular Aspects of Medicine*, 24.1 (2003):137-146.

10 Nielsen, F.H., "Magnesium, Inflammation, and Obesity in Chronic Disease," *Nutrition Reviews*, 68.6 (2010):333-340.

11 Nagamatsu, Masaaki, et al, "Lipoic Acid Improves Nerve Blood Flow, Reduces Oxidative Stress, and Improves Distal Nerve Conduction in Experimental Diabetic Neuropathy," *Diabetes Care*, 18.8 (1995):1160-1167.

12 Jacob, S., et al, "Oral Administration of Rac-*a*-lipoic Acid Modulates Insulin Sensitivity in Patients with Type-2 Diabetes Mellitus: a Placebo-Controlled Pilot Trial, "*Free Radical Biology and Medicine*," 27.3 (1999):309-314.

13 Zeigler, D., et al, "Treatment of Symptomatic Diabetic Peripheral Neuropathy with the Anti-Oxidant *a*-lipoic Acid A 3-Week Multicentre Randomized Controlled Trial (ALADIN Study)," *Diabetologia*, 38.12 (1995):1425-1433.

14 Anderson, R., et al, "Vitamin C and Cellular Immune Functions. Protection Against Hypochlorous Acid-Mediated Inactivation of Glyceraldehyde-3-Phosphate Dehydrogenase and ATP Generation in Human Leukocytes as a Possible Mechanism of Ascorbate-Mediated Immunostimulation," *Annals of the New York Academy of Sciences*, 587 (1990):34-48.

15 Heitzer, Thomas, Just, Hanjorg, and Munzel, Thomas, "Antioxidant Vitamin C Improves Endothelial Dysfunction in Chronic Smokers," *Circulation*, 94 (1996):6-9.

16 Padayatty, Sabastian J., et al, "Vitamin C as an Antioxidant: Evaluation of Its Role in Disease Prevention," *Journal of the American College of Nutrition*, 22.1 (2003):18-35.

17 Anderson, T.W., Reid, D.B.W., and Beaton, G.H., "Vitamin C and the Common Cold: a Double-Blind Trial, *Canadian Medical Association Journal*, 107.6 (1972):503-508.

18 Pauling, Linus, "Vitamin C and Common Cold," *The Journal of the American Medical Association*, 216.2 (1971):332.

19 Bartlett, Marshall K., Jones, Chester M., and Ryan, Anna E., "Vitamin C and Wound Healing," *The New England Journal of Medicine*, 226 (1942): 474-481.

20 See Endnote 19.

21 Mullan, Brian A., et al, "Ascorbic Acid Reduces Blood Pressure and Arterial Stiffness in Type 2 Diabetes," *Hypertension*, 40 (2002):804-809.

22 Fotherby, Martin D., et al, "Effect of Vitamin C on Ambulatory Blood Pressure and Plasma Lipids in Older Persons," *Journal of Hypertension*, 18.4 (2000):411-415.

23 Gale, Catherine R., et al, "Vitamin C and Risk of Death from Stroke and Coronary Heart Disease in Cohort of Elderly People," *British Medical Journal*, 310 (1995):1563.

24 Cameron, Ewan, and Pauling, Linus Carl, *Cancer and vitamin C: a Discussion of the Nature, Causes, Prevention, and Treatment of Cancer with Special Reference to the Value of Vitamin C* (Menlo Park, CA: Linus Pauling Institute of Science and Medicine, 1979).

25 Timimi, Farris K., et al, "Vitamin C Improves Endothelium-Dependent Vasodilation in Patients With Insulin-Dependent Diabetes Mellitus," *Journal of the American College of Cardiology*, 31.3 (1998):552-557.

26 Davie, Sarah J., Gould, Barry J., and Yudkin, John S., "Effect of Vitamin C on Glycosylation of Proteins," *Diabetes*, 41.2 (1992):167-173.

27 Massip, Laurent, et al, "Vitamin C Restores Healthy Aging in a Mouse Model for Werner Syndrome," *The Journal of the Federation of American Societies for Experimental Biology*, 24.1 (2010):158-172.

28 Anderson, Richard A., "Chromium and Insulin Resistance," Nutrition Research Reviews, 16 (2003):267-275.

29 Hao, Cui, et al, "Insulin Sensitizing Effects of Oligomannuronate-Chromium (III) Complexes in C2C12 Skeletal Muscle Cells," *PLoS ONE*, 6.9 (2011): Accessed September 2012, http://www.plosone.org/article/info%3Adoi%2F10.1371%2Fjournal.pone.0024598.

30 Juturu, V., Komorowski, J.R., "Program Including Chromium Picolinate and Biotin to Reduce Blood Sugar Levels in Type 2 Diabetes," *Obesity Research*, 11 (2003): A106.

31 Komorowski, J.R., Juturu, V., "Chromium and Biotin Combination Improves Blood Sugar Control in People with Type 2 Diabetes Mellitus," Proc Intern Diab Fed Cong (18th) 2003.

32 Larrieta, E., et al, "Effects of Biotin Deficiency on Pancreatic Islet Morphology, Insulin Sensitivity and Glucose Homeostasis," *The Journal of Nutritional Biochemistry*, 23.4 (2012):392-399.

33 Yin, Jun, et al, "Efficacy of Berberine in Patients with Type 2 Diabetes," *Metabolism*, 57.5 (2008):712-717.

34 Prasad, K., "Tocotrienols and Cardiovascular Health," *Current Pharmaceutical Design*, 17.21 (2011):2147-2154.

35 Kuhad, A., and Chopra, K., "Attenuation of Diabetic Nephropathy by Tocotrienol: Involvement of NFkB Signaling Pathway," *Life Sciences*, 84.9 (2009):296-301.

CHAPTER 21: DRUGS AND DIABETES

1 Despres, Jean-Pierre, et al, "Hyperinsulinemia as an Independent Risk Factor for Ischemic Heart Disease," *The New England Journal of Medicine*, 334 (1996):952-958.

2 Mayo Clinic Staff, "Insulin and Weight Gain: Keep the Pounds Off," October 2011, Accessed September 2012, http://www.mayoclinic.com/health/insulin-and-weight-gain/DA00139.

3 Giovannucci, E., "The Role of Insulin Resistance and Hyperinsulinemia in Cancer Causation," *Current Medicinal Chemistry*, 5 (2005):53-60.

4 Research and Markets, "Analyzing the Global Diabetes Market," February 2012, Accessed September 2012, http://www.researchandmarkets.com/research/f5eb22/analyzing_the_glob.

5 The Diabetes Prevention Program Research Group, "Impact of Intensive Lifestyle and Metformin Therapy on Cardiovascular Disease Risk Factors in the Diabetes Prevention Program," *Diabetes Care*, 28.4 (2005):888-894.

6 The Diabetes Prevention Program Research Group, "10-year Follow-up of Diabetes Incidence and Weight Loss in the Diabetes Prevention Program Outcomes Study," *Lancet*, 374.9702 (2009):1677-1686.

CHAPTER 22: FIGHT HIDDEN CULPRITS

1 National Institutes of Health, *Progress in Autoimmune Diseases Research* (Washington, DC: U.S. Department of Health and Human Services, 2005).

2 Medline Plus, "Autoimmune Disorders," National Institutes of Health, Accessed September 2012, http://www.nlm.nih.gov/medlineplus/ency/article/000816.htm.

3 National Diabetes Information Clearinghouse, "Diabetes Overview," National institutes of Health, Accessed September 2012, http://diabetes.niddk.nih.gov/dm/pubs/overview/.

4 Landin-Olsson, M., "Latent Autoimmune Diabetes in Adults," *Annals of the New York Academy of Sciences*, 958 (2002):112-116.

5 Fourlanos, Spiros, et al, "A Clinical Screening Tool Identifies Autoimmune Diabetes in Adults," *Diabetes Care*, 29.5 (2006):970-975.

6 See Endnote 5.

7 Nakazawa, Donna Jackson, *The Autoimmune Epidemic* (New York, NY: Simon and Schuster, 2008).

8 Walsh, Bryan, "The Perils of Plastic," Time Specials, April 2010, Accessed September 2012, http://www.time.com/time/specials/packages/article/0,28804,1976909_1976908,00.html.

9 Center for Disease Control and Prevention, *Forth National Report on Human Exposure to Environmental Chemicals* (Washington, DC: Department of Health and Human Services, 2009).

10 Breast Cancer Fund, "Bisphenol A (BPA)," Accessed September 2012, http://www.breastcancerfund.org/clear-science/chemicals-glossary/bisphenol-a.html.

11 Centers For Disease Control and Prevention, "National Health and Nutrition Examination Survey," Accessed September 2012, http://www.cdc.gov/nchs/nhanes/nhanes2003-2004/nhanes03_04.htm.

12 Laks, Dan, "Dr. Dan Laks Discusses the Effect of Chronic Mercury Exposure IAOMT San Diego 2010," Youtube.com, April 2012, Accessed September 2012, http://www.youtube.com/watch?v=YHcfm83ncFA.

13 Laks, Dan R., "Assessment of chronic mercury exposure within the U.S. population, National Health and Nutrition Examination Survey, 1999–2006," *Biometals*, 2009, Accessed September 2012, http://xa.yimg.com/kq/groups/21183985/2110973354/name/laksBloodHglevelsinUSAwomen2009.pdf.

14 Laks, Dan, "Mercury levels in Americans rose from 2% in 1999 to 30% in 2006," Youtube.com, September 2010, Accessed September 2012, http://www.youtube.com/watch?v=aFc-sjNFgxY.

15 Guallar, Elisea, et al, "Mercury, Fish Oils, and the Risk of Myocardial Infarction," *The New England Journal of Medicine*, 347 (2002):1747-1754.

16 Silbergeld, E.K., Silva, I.A., and Nyland J.F., "Mercury and Autoimmunity: Implications for Occupational and Environmental Health," *Toxicology and Applied Pharmacology*, 207.2 (2005):282-292.

17 See Endnote 7.

18 Nakazawa, Donna Jackson, *The Autoimmune Epidemic* (New York, NY: Simon and Schuster, 2008) 227-228.

19 Nakazawa, Donna Jackson, *The Autoimmune Epidemic* (New York, NY: Simon and Schuster, 2008) 229-230.

20 American Academy of Periodontology, "Gum Disease Links to Heart Disease and Stroke," Perio.org, Accessed September 2012, http://www.perio.org/consumer/mbc.heart.htm.

21 Neri, M.C., et al, "Prevalence of Helicobacter Pylori Infection in Elderly Inpatients and in Institutionalized Old People: Correlation with Nutritional Status," *Age and Ageing*, 25.1 (1996):17-21.

22 Mitchell, H.M., "The epidemiology of Helicobacter pylori," *Current Topics in Microbiology and Immunology*, 241 (1999):11-30.

23 Amin, A.H., Subbaiah, T.V., and Abbasi, K.M., "Berberine Sulfate: Antimicrobial Activity, Bioassay, and Mode of Action," *Canadian Journal of Microbiology*, 15.9 (1969):1067-1076.

CHAPTER 23: REACH OUT FOR HELP

1 Potter, Beatrix, *The Tale of Peter Rabbit* (London, UK: Frederick Warne and Company, 1902).

2 Nerem, R.M., Levesque, M.J., and Cornhill, J.F., "Social Environment as a Factor in Diet-Induced Atherosclerosis," *Science*, 208.4451 (1980):1475-1476.

3 Gardner, Amanda, "Lonely? Your Health may Suffer," CNN Health, June 2012, Accessed September 2012, http://www.cnn.com/2012/06/18/health/mental-health/loneliness-isolation-health/index.html.

4 Nonogaki, Katsunori, et al, "Social Isolation Affects the Development of Obesity and Type 2 Diabetes in Mice," *Endocrinology*, 148.10 (2007):4658.

5 Tomaka, Joe, et al, "The Relation of Social Isolation, Loneliness, and Social Support to Disease Outcomes Among the Elderly," Journal of Aging and Health, 18.3 (2006): 359-384.

6 Ornish, Dean, *Dr. Dean Ornish's Program for Reversing Heart Disease* (Raleigh, NC: Ivy Books, 1995).

7 Ornish, Dean, *Love and Survival* (New York: Harper Collins Publishers, 1998).

8 Seeman, T.E., Syme, S.L., "Social Networks and Coronary Artery Disease: a Comparison of the Structure and Function of Social Relations as Predictors of Disease," *Psychosomatic Medicine*, 49.4 (1987): 341-354.

9 See Endnote 7, 24-25.

10 Madalie, J.H., et al, "The Importance of Biopsychosocial Factors in the Development of Duodenal Ulcer in a Cohort of Middle-Aged Men." *American Journal of Epidemiology*, 136.10 (1992):1280-1287.

11 See Endnote 7.

12 Viscott, David, *How to Live with Another Person* (New York, NY: Pocket Books, 1974).

13 Proverbs 18:24 (American King James Version).

14 Isaiah 58:8 (New International Version)

15 Ecclesiastes 4:10 (New International Version)

16 Williams, Redford, and Williams, Virginia, *Anger Kills: 17 Strategies for Controlling the Hostility that Can Harm Your Health* (New York, NY: Harper Collins, 1994).

17 Peck, M. Scott, *The Road Less Traveled* (New York, NY: Touchstone, 1978).

18 Tibbits, Dick, *Forgive to Live,* (Nashville: Thomas Nelson, 2008).

Index

C

D

E

U

V

W

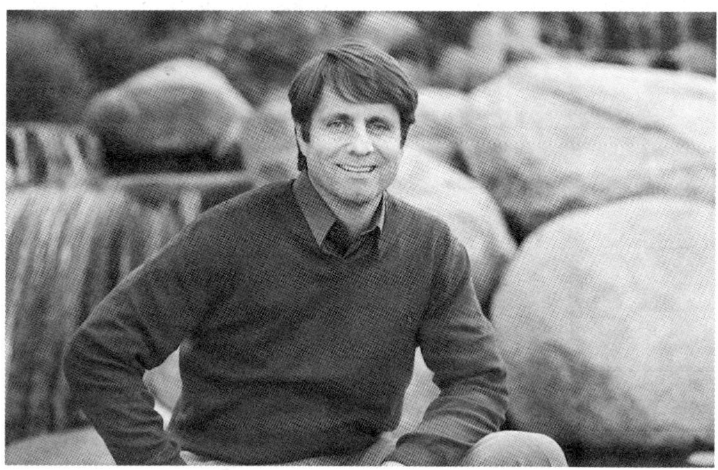

Wes Youngberg, DrPH, MPH, CNS, FACLM

Dr. Youngberg trained at Loma Linda University, where he earned a doctor of public health degree in clinical preventive care and a master of public health degree in nutrition. He is an assistant clinical professor for the Loma Linda University Schools of Medicine and Public Health. He is also a certified nutrition specialist and a founding director and fellow of the American College of Lifestyle Medicine.

Dr. Youngberg spent 14 years on the island of Guam, researching the diabetes epidemic on the Micronesian islands of the Western Pacific region and directing the Wellness Center at the Guam Seventh-day Adventist Clinic. He traveled throughout the islands, providing public health education, screenings, and professional training for diabetes prevention and care.

Dr. Youngberg was honored twice with the Heroes of the Pacific award by the Guam chapter of the American Diabetes Association. In 2007, he was awarded the Ancient Order of the Chamorri—the highest honor given by the governor of Guam for extraordinary contributions to the island community.

Dr. Youngberg has more than 20 years of clinical experience using integrative lifestyle therapies for diabetes control, depression recovery, cardiovascular disease reversal, and effective management of many chronic health conditions. He currently sees patients at the Youngberg Lifestyle Medicine Clinic in Temecula, California, where he lives with his wife Betsy and three children—Dakota, Madie, and Katie.

Notes: